MEDICAL MICROBIOLOGY

VOLUME 2

VIROLOGY, MYCOLOGY, PARASITOLOGY, AND INFECTION CONTROL

Ankur Mittal

ALLIED
HEALTH
PRESS

Medical Microbiology

Volume 2: Virology, Mycology, Parasitology, and Infection Control

Author: **Ankur Mittal**

Allied Health Press
4164 Lakeshore Road
Burlington ON L7L 1A4
Canada
www.alliedhealthpress.com
Email: orders@arclereducation.com

ISBN: 978-1-77956-781-9

ABOUT THE AUTHOR

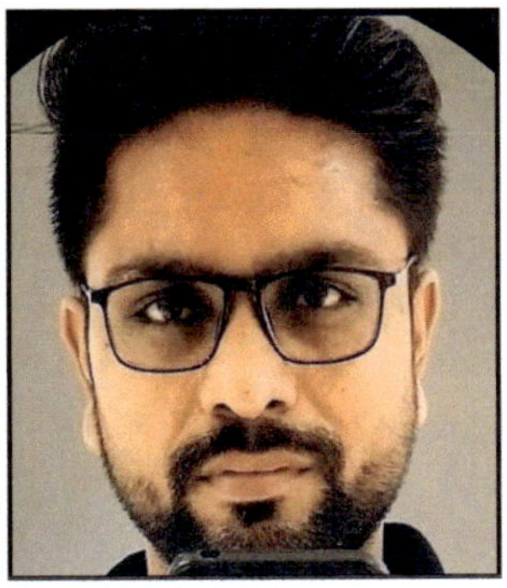

Ankur Mittal is a dedicated biomedical researcher specializing in molecular biology, microbiology, and clinical biochemistry, currently engaged in basic research on infectious and metabolic diseases. His work focuses on developing rapid molecular diagnostic platforms for Fungal Endophthalmitis and employing metagenomic sequencing for advanced microbial characterization. His research aims to integrate molecular diagnostics with clinical applications to enhance early disease detection and therapeutic outcomes.

He previously contributed to significant projects exploring Diabetic Retinopathy (DR) and Age-Related Macular Degeneration (AMD), particularly investigating the role and balance of VEGF165 and VEGF165b proteins in pathological angiogenesis. His work elucidated mechanisms underlying impaired protein expression in retinal disorders, contributing to a deeper understanding of molecular processes in ocular pathology.

Mr. Mittal completed his Master of Science (M.Sc.) in Biochemistry from the Postgraduate Institute of Medical Education and Research (PGIMER), Chandigarh (2014–2016), where he specialized in cell and molecular biology, immunogenetics, bioinformatics, and gene-based diagnostics. He earned his Bachelor of Science (B.Sc.) in Microbiology from Delhi University (2010–2013), graduating with a strong foundation in medical, industrial, and molecular microbiology.

His research contributions are documented through publications in reputed journals, including Kidney Diseases (2018), International Journal of Drug Development & Research (2016), and Pharmacology Research (2016). Additionally, he has presented his work at several national scientific conferences, such as ACBICON 2015 and the National Conference on Frontiers in Applied Biotechnology, and has participated in numerous workshops on flow cytometry, big data science, immunology, and biotechnology at leading institutions such as INSA, ILBS, and TERI University.

Brief Table of Contents

Getting Started with This Book

Chapter Openers

A list of Chapter Outline is presented providing a brief Introduction to what will be covered in the chapter.

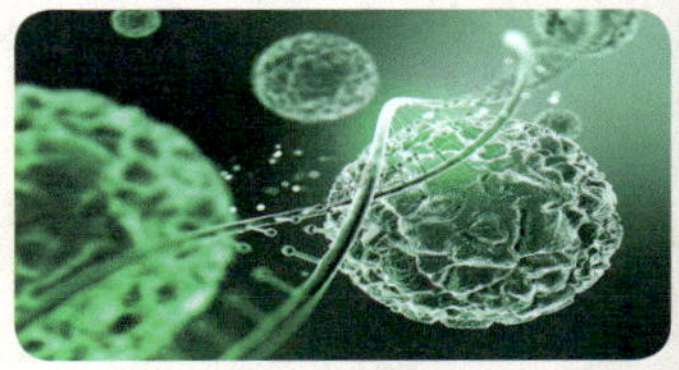

Introduction

Often referred to as the science of life, biology is a broad field of study aimed at comprehending the several kinds of life on Earth, from tiny creatures to sophisticated multicellular entities. Comprising several subfields, including molecular biology, ecology, and evolutionary biology, each of which advances our knowledge of living systems, this field clarifies the mechanisms controlling life events, including development, reproduction, and interaction with the surroundings, which is the central goal of biology. Moreover, biology fills in the void between the natural sciences and medicine by offering a necessary understanding of health, illness, and the interactions between organisms and their environments. Dealing with urgent global issues such as climate change, biodiversity loss, and new diseases depends on an awareness of these complex biological interactions, therefore highlighting the critical part biology plays in modern civilization. Fundamentally, biology explores and tests ideas about the living world using the scientific method. Through methodical observation and experimentation,

LEARNING OBJECTIVES

After studying this chapter, you will be able to:

1. Discuss the scientific method in biology;
2. Explain the cell theory;
3. Discuss the genetics and heredity;
4. Evolution and natural selection;
5. Focus on ecology and ecosystems;
6. Learn about human biology;
7. Evaluate the plant biology;
8. Explain the microbiology;
9. Focus on current trends in biology.

1.1. The Scientific Method in Biology

Learning Outcome

1. Describe the steps of the scientific method;
2. Focus on hypothesis formation;
3. Learn about experimental design.

Learning Outcomes

The beginning of each section of every chapter contains a set of Learning Outcomes that inform students of concepts they should understand. These outcomes help students understand what they should be able to do if they have mastered the material in that section.

Test Your Knowledge

Throughout each chapter, Test Your Knowledge cues you to note which topics have been covered and to self-test your understanding of the material presented.

Test Your Knowledge

1. Explain why correlation does not imply causation in scientific experiments.
2. How does the scientific method help reduce the influence of personal opinions in research?

Chapter Summary

The Summary Section appear at the end of each chapter and summarize main concepts covered throughout the chapter. These points provide key concepts in an engaging and meaningful way.

Summary

The investigation of biological principles highlights the importance of a comprehensive view of life by reflecting the intricate interactions that occur within living systems. The complexity of biology goes beyond individual species or systems, as this essay highlights; it also includes the interactions that mold ecosystems and affect biodiversity. Researchers can conduct in-depth analyses of metabolomic data using sophisticated technologies like MetaboAnalyst, which offer insights into the molecular mechanisms underlying these interactions. As demonstrated by the developments in MetaboAnalyst, for example, the integration of diverse omics data promotes a thorough understanding of metabolic pathways and helps identify important biological markers necessary for research on development and disease (Chong et al., 2018). Additionally, the phenomenon of ecological invasions is a key component of biological research and a vital field of study. The introduction of non-native species into unfamiliar habitats has significant ramifications and calls for multidisciplinary management strategies. Examining the origins and effects of these biological incursions, invasion science has become a crucial field that highlights the need to comprehend ecological dynamics and community interactions. As interest in biological invasions increases, new findings are emerging that put conventional ecological theories and practices to the test. The importance of incorporating various scientific viewpoints is shown by this developing discipline, which also highlights how invasive species shape ecosystems and advances our knowledge of ecological resilience (David et al., 2013). When taken as a whole, these discoveries from invasion science and metabolomics highlight the value of multidisciplinary biology research. Fostering cross-disciplinary collaboration and utilizing technological breakthroughs to improve our comprehension of intricate biological interactions are crucial as we look to the future of biological research. In addition to deepening our understanding of the complexities of life, this method lays the groundwork for tackling urgent environmental issues. Future studies can ensure the continued relevance of biology in a world that is constantly changing by acknowledging the interconnection of biological systems and opening the door to creative solutions that support sustainability and biodiversity conservation. We might imagine a thorough comprehension of life that serves both academia and society at large through ongoing investigation and integration of scientific knowledge.

Knowledge Assessment

The chapter includes material designed to review and reinforce each content. It includes Critical Thinking Questions to help test of your understanding of information presented in the chapter and Short answer Questions to review your understanding of the key concepts presented in the chapter.

Critical Thinking Questions

1. **Who is known as the "Father of Modern Biology"?**
   a. Aristotle
   b. Charles Darwin
   c. Gregor Mendel
   d. Louis Pasteur
2. **What is the basic unit of life?**
   a. Atom
   b. Molecule
   c. Cell
   d. Organism
3. **Which branch of biology studies the interaction of organisms with their environment?**
   a. Genetics
   b. Ecology
   c. Physiology
   d. Botany
4. **Which macromolecule is the main source of energy for living organisms?**
   a. Proteins
   b. Lipids
   c. Carbohydrates
   d. Nucleic acids
5. **DNA is primarily responsible for which function in living organisms?**
   a. Energy production
   b. Protein synthesis
   c. Storing genetic information
   d. Regulating body temperature

Short Answer Questions

1. What is biology, and why is it important to study biology?
2. What are the three main domains of life, and how are they different from one another?
3. Define homeostasis and give an example of how it works in living organisms.
4. What is the cell theory, and why is it fundamental to biology?
5. How do autotrophs and heterotrophs differ in the way they obtain energy?
6. What is the scientific method, and how is it applied in biological research?
7. Discuss how biology helps address global challenges such as climate change, disease, and food security.
8. Explain the levels of biological organization from the smallest unit to the largest. Provide examples at each level.
9. Describe the relationship between structure and function in biology, giving specific examples from cells or organs.
10. How has the discovery of genetics shaped our understanding of inheritance and variation among organisms?

Supplementary Materials

Key Terms: A list of key terms is given for quick reference

KEY TERMS FROM THIS CHAPTER

Annotation enrichment analysis	Biological structure	Cell
Cell theory	Cellular structure	Ecology
Ecosystems	Genetics	Human biology
Microbiology	Natural selection	Organism
Plant biology		

Further Resources: Recommendations for additional readings, websites, and multimedia resources.

References

1. Argelaguet, R., Velten, B., Arnol, D., Dietrich, S., Zenz, T., Marioni, J. C., Buettner, F., et al. (2018). Multi-omics factor analysis—A framework for unsupervised integration of multi-omics data sets. *Molecular Systems Biology, 14*. https://doi.org/10.15252/msb.20178124.
2. Bacher, S., Blackburn, T. M., Essl, F., & Genovesi, P. (2017). *Socio-Economic Impact Classification of Alien Taxa (SEICAT)*. https://core.ac.uk/download/286567949.pdf (accessed on 8th March 2025).
3. Barnett, R., Brace, S., Cucchi, T., & Dobney, K. (2013). *Divergent Evolutionary Processes Associated with Colonization of Offshore Islands*. https://core.ac.uk/download/20664364.pdf (accessed on 8th March 2025).

Detailed Table of Contents

CHAPTER 3

RNA Viruses 71

CHAPTER 4

Emerging and Re-emerging Viral Infections 109

CHAPTER 5

Medical Mycology 141

CHAPTER 6

General Parasitology 177

CHAPTER 7

Protozoan Infections 213

LIST OF FIGURES

PREFACE

The modern medicine has been significantly altered due to the progress in the knowledge of infectious agents during the last century. The microorganism research; viruses, fungi, parasites and bacteria, has revealed how the organisms cause the disease, their interaction with human host and their reaction to the treatment measures. With the transformation of scientific tools, the power to identify, describe, and manage infectious diseases has changed, resulting in better patient outcomes and population health approaches globally. The host-pathogen relationships are complex and indicate this growing body of knowledge and the relevance of microbiological principles in clinical practice.

In this dynamic field, infection detection and control have been important aspects of medical care. Infectious agents will always pose a problem with their varying biology, adaptability and new/drug resistant strains. Prevention of the spread of infections, particularly in health facilities, needs a combined effort that comprises microbiological diagnosis, monitoring, and control measures that are based on evidence. This knowledge on the biology of the pathogens coupled with the clinical manifestations is the basis of effective diagnosis, treatment and prevention measures.

This book, *Medical Microbiology: Volume 2*, is intended to serve as a reference text to give the reader an advanced but accessible summary of the important topics in medical microbiology. This book is dedicated to the viral, fungal and parasitic infections, practical issues of infection control in the hospital and microbiological diagnosis. It is a good reference book to students, clinicians, microbiologists, and health care personnel who need to advance their knowledge on infectious diseases and how they are handled. The book is rich in scientific information and at the same time clinically relevant, with clear explanations to connect the microbiological principles and patient care.

Chapter 1 is a comprehensive introduction to the study of virology, including basic principles of virology: structure, replication and classification of viruses. This background qualifies readers to comprehend the subsequent elaborate descriptions of individual groups of viruses.

Chapter 2 deals with DNA viruses and explains their biology, pathogenesis and clinical syndromes produced by these viruses.

Chapter 3 stays on the topic of RNA viruses and discusses their diversity, infection process, and diseases. Both chapters emphasize diagnostic methods and current therapeutic options.

Chapter 4 deals with emerging and re-emerging viral infections, and it focuses on those viruses that present special problems because of their evolving epidemiology, zoonotic causes, or pandemic capabilities. In this chapter, recent outbreaks and the response to them that are needed by the public health are discussed.

Chapter 5 moves on to medical mycology and describes the biology and classification of medically significant fungi, typical fungal infections, and the principles of antifungal therapy.

Chapter 6 begins with general parasitology, which is a review of parasite classification, life cycle, and interaction with the human host.

It is then followed by Chapter 7, which is devoted to the protozoan infections, in which the authors examine the diseases caused by single-celled parasites, their transmission, clinical presentation, and treatment.

Chapter 8 is about helminthic infections, which discusses the biology and clinical effects of the multicellular parasitic worms, diagnostic problems, and therapeutic approaches.

Chapter 9 concentrates on hospital-acquired infections (HAIs) and infection control measures. It covers the most frequent pathogens that cause HAIs, risk factors, monitoring methods, and precaution measures that are necessary to ensure patient safety in health care facilities.

Chapter 10 gives an in-depth discussion of the microbiological diagnostic techniques in the identification of infectious diseases. This encompasses specimen collection, laboratory methods, molecular diagnostics, and result interpretation which is important in making clinical decisions.

The book is meant to be used by medical students, microbiology trainees, clinicians and allied health professionals in need of a comprehensive, yet practical guide to medical microbiology. It facilitates learning because of its lucid arrangement and clinically applicable contents and can thus be used as both academic material and a clinical guide. Also, the chapters on diagnostics and hospital infection control will be useful to laboratory personnel and infection control practitioners.

The scope of this book, *Medical Microbiology: Volume 2,* is to provide the reader with the information necessary to appreciate infectious agents beyond their biological properties, with a heavy focus on their clinical significance, diagnostic problems and management. With the discipline still growing with new findings and technologies, this book has been a good starting point for the present practice and future study in the field of medical microbiology.

GENERAL VIROLOGY

1

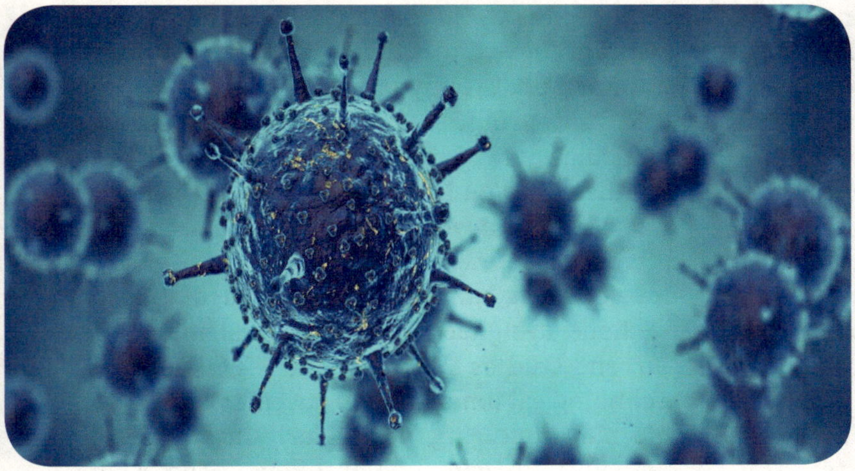

Introduction

The discipline of studying virology forms an essential area of medical microbiology and deals with the interaction, pathogenesis, and control of viruses. This discipline involves knowledge of virus structure, classification, and their mechanisms of replication. Viruses are peculiar organisms; consisting of nothing but genetic material wrapped in a protein shell, they defy conventional descriptions of living things. Notably, their need for host cell replication speaks to the complex interactions that viruses have with different biological systems. In medical microbiology, an understanding of these basic concepts is critical to designing diagnostic and therapeutic approaches to viral infections that critically influence human health and disease. As succinctly noted, practical training in medical education, such as "Practical Microbiology and Virology," demonstrates varying degrees of consensus among students as to their efficacy, implying a disconnect between theoretical knowledge and its application (Mazouchian et al., 2014). Advances in virology have been made possible through

LEARNING OBJECTIVES

After studying this chapter, you will be able to:

1. Know the structure and classification of viruses;
2. Discuss viral replication and life cycle;
3. Explain the pathogenesis of viral infections;
4. Describe diagnostic procedures in virology;
5. Handle treatment and prevention of viral infections;
6. Emphasize emerging viruses and worldwide health.

highly advanced technologies, especially the advent of molecular diagnostics, which have revolutionized the detection and monitoring of viral pathogens. Polymerase chain reaction (PCR) has proven to be a potent tool for the identification of viruses, particularly hard-to-culture viruses or those without appropriate animal models. For example, human caliciviruses (HuCVs) and small round-structured viruses (SRSVs) are such a challenge because they cannot be grown in laboratory settings (Butcher et al., 1997). The use of PCR-based techniques in diagnosing viral infections is an indication of the vital role genetic analyses play in virology. Such approaches not only deepen our knowledge of viral diversity but also allow us to identify certain viral strains, which is essential for epidemiological analysis and public health actions following outbreaks. In addition, the field of virology moves beyond the identification of pathogens and includes the examination of viral pathogenesis and host response. Understanding how viruses invade host cells, evade immune defenses, and cause disease is essential for developing effective vaccines and antiviral therapies. This dynamic interplay between host and virus often dictates the clinical outcomes observed in infected individuals. Moreover, the impact of viral diseases such as influenza, HIV/AIDS, and hepatitis on public health accentuates the need for extensive research and surveillance in virology. Accordingly, the combination of lab practical skills with theoretical knowledge is essential for future healthcare professionals. Being aware of the relevance of extensive training in virology, as demonstrated by surveys of student opinions towards lab practical courses, establishes the importance of focused education strategies in medical microbiology (Mazouchian et al., 2014).

Definition and Scope of Virology

Virology, as a subdiscipline of microbiology, is largely dedicated to the science of viruses, their composition, classification, and the process by which they infect host cells. It overlaps with disciplines like genetics, molecular biology, and immunology to gain a better insight into viral pathology and behavior. The word virus itself indicates not only the causal agent but also the intricacies associated with its life cycle, such as replication and mode of pathogenicity. The history of virology is instrumental because it developed as a separate branch of science in the early to mid-20th century, evolving from a specific study of observing viral pathogenicity to an expansive investigation covering virology methodology and theories. This evolution emphasizes the dynamic character of the field and provides a prelude to discussing particular viral interactions in human health and disease (Van Loon, 2002). The applications of virology go beyond basic research to medical microbiology practice. Examples include vaccine development, antiviral drugs, and diagnostic methods designed to prevent viral infections. Current studies highlight the significance of technological innovation in vaccine preparation and manufacturing, particularly in addressing new viral threats like influenza. The rising sophistication of viral strains requires novel measures, such as reverse genetics and recombinant technology, to ensure improved vaccine effectiveness (Cavicchi et al., 2012). In addition, virology also overlaps with public health in the sense that the knowledge of viral dynamics can guide reactions to epidemics and pandemics, demonstrating the real significance virologists have when it comes to protecting public health. As virology continues to grow, it is also confronted with the challenge of emerging viral challenges, demonstrating its continued importance in the medical microbiology field. Virology not only helps understand the intricacies of viral diseases but also the unraveling of the meaning of viral diseases for world health. The continuous research on virulence factors has become a priority in the field of virology due to the necessity of characterizing and controlling viral epidemics that reflect serious health threats. The overall interdisciplinary approach of virology makes it possible to study virus-host interactions from a multidimensional standpoint and derive therapeutic strategies to counter viral pathogenesis. With advancements in virology, its approaches have to be upgraded to cater to the new threats, leading to the need for ongoing research and development in this area. The relationship between virology and technology, particularly in vaccine development speed, underscores the importance of being vigilant in detecting and acting on viral outbreaks as an integral part of medical microbiology (Van Loon, 2002; Cavicchi et al., 2012) (Figure 1.1).

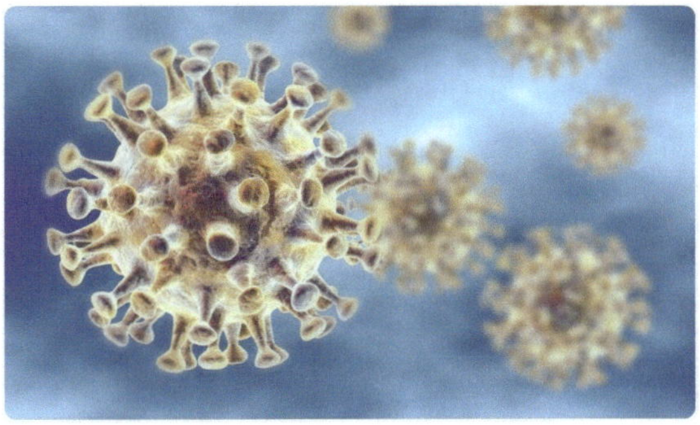

Figure 1.1. Illustration of the SARS-CoV-2 virus, responsible for COVID-19.

Source: https://www.news-medical.net/image-handler/ts/20210317042002/ri/673/picture/2021/3/shutterstock_1625661736.jpg.

Historical Context and Development of Virology

The evolution of virology has been characterized by milestones that have contributed to our understanding of viral pathogens and their intricate relationships with hosts. Initially, the concept of viruses emerged in the late 19th century with the realization that infectious agents could be smaller than bacteria and could pass through porcelain filters. This was exemplified by the discovery of the tobacco mosaic virus in 1892, which laid the groundwork for virology as a distinct scientific discipline. Later developments in the 20th century, such as electron microscopy and methods of molecular biology, allowed viruses to be visualized and controlled at the molecular level by researchers. These developments spurred the classification and description of many viral species, leading eventually to an organized framework for virus taxonomy. The establishment of the International Committee on Taxonomy of Viruses (ICTV) in 1966 was a turning point, offering a systematic approach to virus classification through structural and genetic properties (Adams et al., 2017). The development of virology has not only enriched our understanding of viral diversity but has also enabled key public health interventions.

Few of these are as significant as the advances in vaccine technology, which are a result of a better understanding of viral pathogenesis and immune response. As an example, the polio vaccine's successful creation in the mid-20th century constituted a remarkable victory for infectious disease control, which has seen the near eradication of a disease that used to paralyze thousands. In addition, the re-emergence and resurgence of arboviruses, as noted by recent research endeavors, illustrate the persistent difficulty experienced by the scientific community in controlling mosquito-borne diseases. Research has identified that the incidence of disease is highly variable across geographic areas and is influenced by ecological determinants such as climate and topography (Chrisafis, 2017). These discoveries highlight the value of historical context in virology, reinforcing the ways in which knowledge developed over the past has shaped disease prevention and control measures today. As virology evolves further, the connection between history and contemporary challenges becomes increasingly pronounced. Advances in global health consciousness, especially with regard to viral outbreaks such as HIV, Ebola, and SARS-CoV-2, have reiterated the need for sound virological studies and successful public health measures. The ICTV's effort to update and expand its resources indicates a larger trend in virology to connect with the changing environment of viral threats. Improved online information and community discussion spearheaded by the ICTV help to meet the urgent needs in virus classification and emergent viral diseases (Adams et al., 2017). With the advancement of virology as a field, it is still imperative that researchers and public health professionals leverage past knowledge while developing novel approaches to fighting viral diseases effectively and being prepared for future outbreaks and maintaining global health security (Figure 1.2).

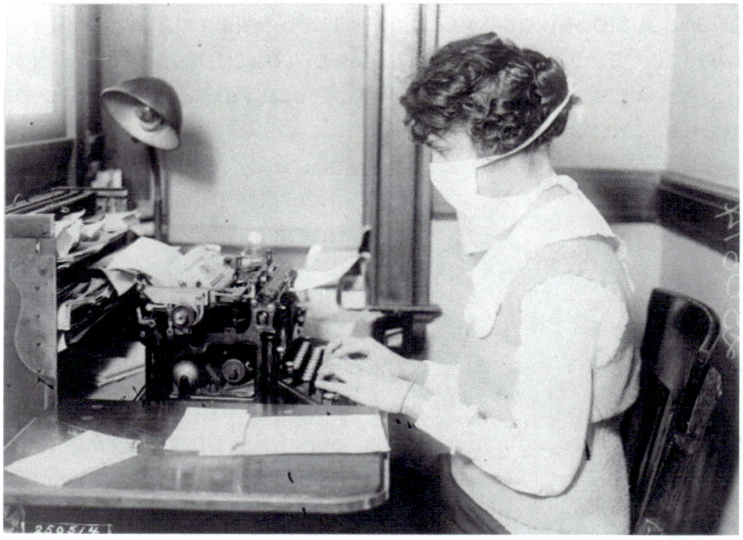

Figure 1.2. A woman working during the 1918–1919 influenza epidemic.

Source: https://upload.wikimedia.org/wikipedia/commons/9/9d/Influenza_Pandemic_Masked_Typist.jpg.

Importance of Virology in Medical Microbiology

Virology is important in the overall context of medical microbiology because it offers information about how viruses interact with their hosts and lead to disease. This information is essential in developing therapeutic as well as preventive modalities. Viruses have their own type of replication that interferes with cellular processes and creates a spectrum of pathophysiological consequences. As such, the science of virology underpins the knowledge of disease dynamics, particularly with reference to viral epidemics. The information acquired through virology research also helps determine possible viral pathogens in clinical specimens, ultimately enabling timely detection and treatment. Through explaining the lifecycle of a number of viruses, virology not only helps the healthcare field but also public health initiatives regarding the prevention of the spread of viral infections. The worldwide burden of viral infections in vulnerable populations is evidence that highlights the need for virology research. For example, respiratory syncytial virus (RSV) has a major impact on the health of children, with an estimated 33 million cases in children aged under five years, resulting in serious morbidity and significant healthcare expenditure (Jha et al., 2016). The recognition of the epidemiology and pathogenesis of viruses such as these allows health professionals to put in place efficient public health interventions and vaccination programs. In addition, virology progress is critical for discovering new antiviral agents and vaccines as new ways to treat presently untreatable viral infections. This is the aspect of virology that closes the gap between basic research and clinical medical science and highlights its importance in coming up with integrated strategies to counter viral attacks. Besides its direct application in the study of infectious diseases, virology is key in deciphering chronic health issues linked with viral infections. The association between serious infantile RSV bronchiolitis and future respiratory complications such as asthma is one illustration of this multifaceted interaction (Jha et al., 2016). Such long-term effect reflects the need for virology not just in the management of acute infection but also to deal with their possible long-term outcomes. In addition, the study of viral interactions in the immune system increases our knowledge of how viruses can take advantage of host defense, resulting in chronic disease or even cancer. As medical microbiology advances, incorporating virology into its fundamental principles guarantees total awareness of acute and chronic health issues, providing a foundation for novel diagnostic, therapeutic, and preventive methodologies.

1.1. Structure and Classification of Viruses

Learning Outcome

1. Appreciate fundamental virus components;
2. Describe the classification systems for viruses;
3. Make distinctions between DNA and RNA viruses.

Their composition as viruses is based on their uniquely simple but varied make-up that facilitates their efficient infection of a broad variety of hosts, including animals, plants, and bacteria. They have as their core a genome of DNA or RNA, which can be single or double-stranded, further dividing them according to the makeup of their genetic material. This genome is contained in a covering protein shell referred to as a capsid, which helps protect the viral nucleic acids during transfer. Furthermore, there are some viruses with an outer lipid envelope created from the host cell membrane, which helps facilitate the virus's capacity to infect new cells. The difference between enveloped and non-enveloped viruses is important; non-enveloped viruses are generally more resistant to environmental factors, while enveloped viruses can use their lipid membranes to aid entry into host cells and improve immune evasion (Cavicchi et al., 2012). Viruses are classified in an intricate process that embraces a number of criteria such as the nature of nucleic acid, whether they have an envelope or not, and their mechanism of replication. The International Committee on Taxonomy of Viruses (ICTV) classifies viruses into families, genera, and species based on these distinguishing characteristics. For example, DNA viruses, like the family Herpesviridae, are known to have double-stranded DNA, whereas RNA viruses can be classified into single-stranded and double-stranded types, represented by the families *Picornaviridae* and Reoviridae, respectively. The classification system is essential in medical microbiology, as it helps guide research agendas and therapeutic strategies. By recognizing the structure and classification of viruses, scientists are able to design effective vaccines and therapeutics to target particular viral families that have caused epidemics and pandemics, such as with influenza (Cavicchi et al., 2012). Viruses are not just genetically varied but also in the way they are transmitted, which impacts their influence on public health. The virion structure determines the way a virus infects, replicates, and spreads within populations. Enveloped viruses, such as the human immunodeficiency virus (HIV), often use the receptor-mediated endocytosis pathway to enter host cells, while non-enveloped viruses like norovirus may rely on direct cell lysis to release their progeny. Understanding these dynamics is crucial for developing effective public health measures and interventions, especially during outbreaks. The advancements in research on viral structure and classification have fueled the development of innovation in vaccine development, with research studies ongoing to advance the effectiveness of responses against new viral challenges. This sustained interest is critical, especially considering previous influenza pandemics that highlight the importance of being ready to deal with viral infections across the world (Orlova, 2012).

1.1.1. Basic Components of Viruses

Knowledge of the elementary parts of viruses is essential to an understanding of their place in medical microbiology. Viruses are essentially made up of genetic material, DNA or RNA, covered in a protective layer of protein called a capsid. The capsid protects the viral genome from destruction and helps the virus attach to host cells. Certain viruses, known as enveloped viruses, have an outer lipid bilayer from the host cell membrane that adds to their infectivity and immune evasion capabilities. Remarkably, family and genus classification of viruses is frequently based on these structural elements, showing the biological importance of their architecture in viral replication and pathogenesis within a host organism. In virology, the understanding of virulence and its objectification in science is of utmost importance. The evolutionary history of virology has shown that the knowledge of viruses as entities developed out of a complicated relationship between scientific practices and research methods. Viruses were hard to classify at first because of their peculiarities, i.e., being acellular and needing a host cell to replicate. Over time, the establishment of a distinct virology discipline allowed scientists to cultivate and study viruses systematically, paving the way for advancements in the identification and treatment of virus-related diseases. This discovery highlights the fact that understanding viruses as discrete biological particles was not merely an issue of observation but a systematic process demanding active scientific investigation and cross-disciplinary cooperation (Van Loon, 2002). Additionally, virology's application to public health and food safety is highlighted by its overlap with microbiological procedures. For example, the inactivation of foodborne pathogens by various means, like the use of ozone treatment, emphasizes the applicative relevance of our knowledge on viral components and their processes. Understanding the structural make-up and the life cycles of viruses enables scientists to investigate new biocidal approaches in order to prevent virus transmission in food products. This application of virological insights into everyday practice illustrates an important connection between laboratory science and everyday health issues. As pathogens such as *E. coli* and *Salmonella enteritidis* remain highly risky, effective microbial control systems should be based on a sound appreciation of the basic viral structures and functionalities to augment public health security (Willett & Hosie, 2013) (Figure 1.3).

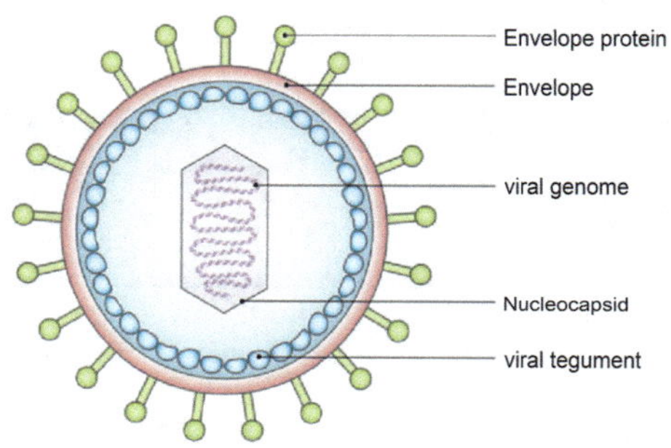

Figure 1.3. Basic structure of a virus.

Source: https://www.researchgate.net/profile/Olatunji-Kolawole-3/publication/340249925/figure/fig2/AS:874020920631297@1585394234735/Basic-structure-of-a-virus-Taylor-2019.png.

1.1.2. Classification Systems for Viruses

The virus classification systems are most important in the field of virology, particularly medical microbiology. These systems are critical in comprehending the diversity and complexity of viral pathogens. The International Committee on Taxonomy of Viruses (ICTV), which was put in place to systematize viral classification, has evolved greatly over the years to accommodate the increasing knowledge of virus diversity and the developments in characterization techniques. As noted, ICTV has opened a discussion with the virology community to solve the challenges in virus taxonomy and increase resources like the ICTV Virus Taxonomy Report, which provides up-to-date information regarding viral classifications and is an indispensable resource for researchers and medical practitioners (Adams et al., 2017). This careful system of classification not only facilitates communication among scientists but also informs the creation of specific medical treatments. Given the complexity of viruses, classifications tend to mirror numerous criteria, such as the type of nucleic acid, method of replication, and physical structure. Virus classification has transitioned from a strictly morphological view to one of genomic data, suggesting a more sophisticated appreciation for viral pathogens. This change highlights the complicity involved in objectifying viruses as independent entities within virology. The historical path of virology reveals that pathogen virulence has been studied with the use of stringent laboratory procedures and an extensive range of research tools. Consequently, the modern concept of viruses today includes inter-disciplinary methods that contribute to the simplification of the complex nature of viral categorizations, thereby making them more intelligible in medical microbiology (Van Loon, 2002). In the growing development of virology, there is a greater demand for dynamic classification systems that can embrace newly developed viruses and new strains. With advancements in molecular biology, new viral genomes are being identified at an unprecedented rate, necessitating continual updates and revisions to existing classification frameworks. The work of the ICTV remains vital in this context, providing a structured system that not only facilitates the organization of known viruses but also anticipates future developments in viral taxonomy. Such classification endeavors facilitate research and diagnostics simplification, thus translating into enhanced public health measures against viral epidemics. The incorporation of new methods and technological advancements into the then-existing classification schemes forms a pivotal step in advancing the field, once again emphasizing the significance of virus classification within the total medical microbiology spectrum (Adams et al., 2017) (Figure 1.4).

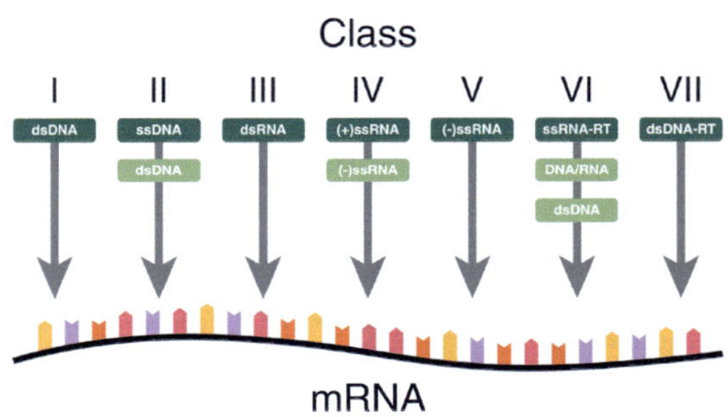

Figure 1.4. Viral classes.

Source: https://textimgs.s3.amazonaws.com/boundless-microbiology/rusbaltimoreclassification.svg#fixme.

1.1.3. Differences Between DNA and RNA Viruses

The differences between DNA and RNA viruses are central to appreciating their modes of replication, rates of mutation, and general pathogenicity. DNA viruses, including both double-stranded (dsDNA) and single-stranded (ssDNA) types, tend to be more genetically stable through their more precise processes of replication by DNA polymerases. That stability enables DNA viruses to preserve their genomes for longer intervals, thus having lower rates of mutation compared to RNA viruses. By contrast, RNA viruses, which are made up of single-stranded RNA (ssRNA) or double-stranded RNA (dsRNA), tend to mutate at a much higher rate due to the inherent error propensity of RNA-dependent RNA polymerases. Such variations in genetic material naturally influence how each virus would interact with host cells and the way the immune system would react, demonstrating the varied pressures of evolution that modulate viral behavior within the medical microbiological context. Aside from replication and mutation, DNA and RNA viruses also contrast with each other in overall strategies for hijacking host cellular machinery. DNA viruses generally invade the nucleus of the host cell and use the host's DNA replication and transcription apparatus to generate viral components.

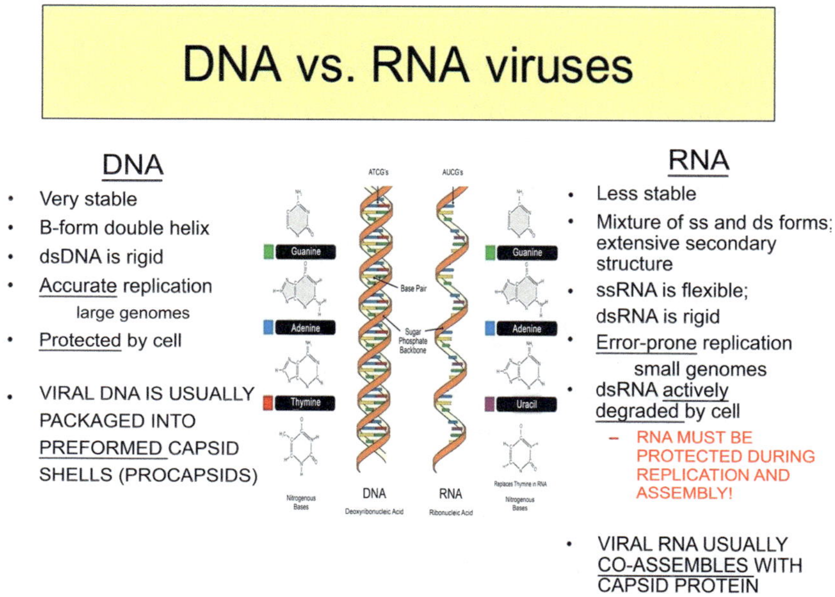

Figure 1.5. DNA vs. RNA viruses.

Source: https://slideplayer.com/slide/3864327/13/images/4/DNA+vs.+RNA+viruses+DNA+RNA+Very+stable+B-form+double+helix.jpg.

The process may involve viral DNA integration into the host genome and is followed by latency or oncogenic transformations. Conversely, RNA viruses prefer to replicate within the cytoplasm, hijack the host's ribosomes to synthesize viral proteins quickly, and frequently utilize sophisticated tactics to avoid immune detection. This difference underscores the versatility of both virus types in utilizing host cell mechanisms for replicating effectively. As discussed in current research, such differences have important implications on public health interventions and therapeutic regimes of certain categories of viral infections, such as respiratory viruses and foodborne viruses (Willett & Hosie, 2013). Further, the clinical relevance of such differences cannot be explained too much, especially in the context of virology and medical microbiology. RNA viruses' high rates of rapid mutations help make them quickly adaptable, rendering outbreaks difficult to control and treat. The development of new influenza and coronavirus strains, for example, shows how RNA viruses can swiftly change direction under environmental pressures, making it difficult to develop vaccines. Conversely, DNA viruses such as human papillomavirus have been determined to remain in existence for long periods of time, usually resulting in chronic infections and related malignancies, highlighting their long-term effects on human health. It is essential to comprehend the molecular foundations of these groups of viruses, as emphasized in the lengthy studies throughout the years, to realize effective preventive and therapeutic measures in clinical interventions (Van Loon, 2002) (Figure 1.5).

Test Your Knowledge

1. What are the fundamental structural elements of a virus?
2. What are the main distinctions between DNA and RNA viruses in structure and replication?

1.2. Viral Replication and Life Cycle

Learning Outcome

1. Appreciate the processes of viral entry into host cells;
2. Describe the phases of viral replication;
3. Outline the determinants of viral life cycles.

The viral life cycle and replication process are complex, with a sequence of well-established stages that end with the formation of new viral particles. First, viruses need to bind and enter their host cells, a stage dominated by the binding between viral surface antigens and particular cellular receptors. After they have entered the host, the viral genome is released into the cytoplasm, which hijacks the host's cell machinery for replication. This is a process of viral RNA transcription and protein synthesis, highlighting the virus's dependence on host cellular mechanisms to produce new viral material. Every successful replication leads to the formation of new viral particles that are then released and go on to infect new cells, continuing the viral life cycle and underlining the parasitic nature of these organisms as presented in the modern perception of viruses as molecular organisms (Bandea, 2009). The viral life cycle is more than merely biological significance, but rather has a great impact on medical microbiology. Viral pathogens tend to hijack host cell processes, thereby making it difficult to combat using conventional antimicrobial drugs. Consequently, new antiviral approaches aim to inhibit crucial phases of viral replication to hinder infection. For example, inhibiting the attachment phase using neutralizing antibodies prevents the virus from entering cells, while viral polymerases can be inhibited using antiviral drugs to stem replication. In addition, a thorough understanding of viral replication pathways dictates vaccine development, with an emphasis on how alterations in such pathways can enable scientists to pre-emptively resist viral outbreaks. Such comprehension is critical in the management of viral diseases, especially in scenarios where quick mutation results in novel viral strains that may frustrate current therapeutic approaches (Willett & Hosie, 2013). Rising studies continue to reveal the intricacies of viral evolution and its public health implications. The fusion hypothesis that suggests viruses could have evolved from parasitic cellular organisms reconstitutes our knowledge of viral biology. This view not only adds depth to the debate on viruses' central role in cellular evolution but also solidifies the call for further studies on their life cycles. Since certain parasites undergo conversion to viral forms, this evolutionary pathway emphasizes the dynamic interaction between viruses and hosts and offers information on the mechanisms of viral emergence and pathogenicity. As more and more evidence confirms this model, scientists are urged to study the phylogenetic connections of viruses to cellular life, eventually leading to new therapeutic strategies and further understanding of viral influence within the larger fabric of life (Bandea, 2009) (Figure 1.6).

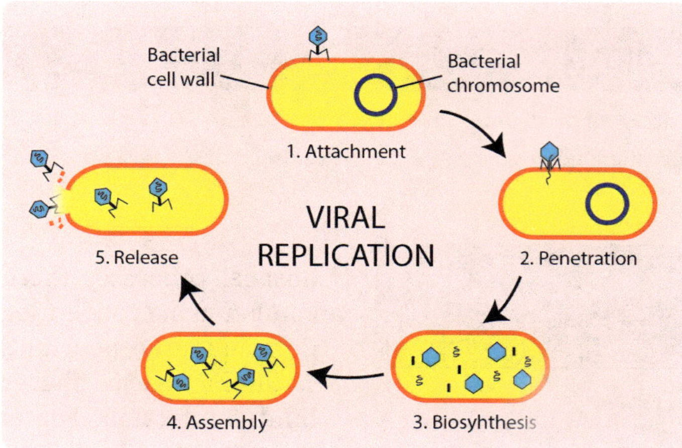

Figure 1.6. Diagram showing the viral replication cycle.

Source: https://teachmephysiology.com/wp-content/uploads/2023/07/Viral_replication.png.webp.

1.2.1. Mechanisms of Viral Entry Into Host Cells

Knowledge of the processes through which viruses infect host cells is important to the general area of virology and its applications in medical microbiology. Viruses typically have certain strategies that they use to take over host cell machinery, starting infection. The most well-known process involves an interaction between viral surface proteins and host cell receptors. This interaction can determine the specificity of a virus for its host. For example, proteins on the surface of the virus attach to host cell receptor proteins, resulting in either direct entry by endocytosis or fusion with the cell membrane. Various viruses use variations of these strategies, demonstrating the complex evolutionary dynamics that shape host-pathogen interactions. These approaches pose a delicate balance between viral infectivity and the host's immune defense systems, which lays the foundation for potential therapeutic interventions. Endocytosis is an important entry route for a majority of viruses that seek to invade host cells. It involves various types, such as macropinocytosis and clathrin-mediated endocytosis, that allow extracellular material to enter the cell. The virus first attaches to cell surface receptors, which signal the viral particle's internalization into an endosomal compartment. Upon entry into the cell, the acidic pH of the endosome may trigger conformational changes in viral proteins, facilitating the discharge of viral genetic material into the cytoplasm. The efficiency of this entry process is different between virus families, and some viruses, like influenza and HIV, have shown special aptitude for utilizing the endocytic pathway. Recognizing these entry strategies further guides the creation of antiviral drugs that can interfere with such essential early stages of infection. The study of viral entry mechanisms extends to the clinical therapeutic area, especially in the treatment of drug-resistant viruses. As illustrated with HIV, which has been a major challenge to treat effectively because it can resist immune attack and develop drug resistance, new strategies are essential (Dwivedi et al., 2011). Research is ongoing into methods like RNA interference (RNAi) to inhibit viral replication by degrading viral RNA or blocking viral proteins critical for entry selectively. Progress in nanotechnology also holds promising opportunities for the improvement of drug delivery systems with high specificity to target viral entry. With the improvements of these therapeutic interventions, public health issues arising from viral infections are better addressed, reducing their burden on health systems worldwide (Dwivedi et al., 2011). These collaborative efforts thus highlight the significance of knowledge on viral entry mechanisms in the development of innovative medical therapies (Figure 1.7).

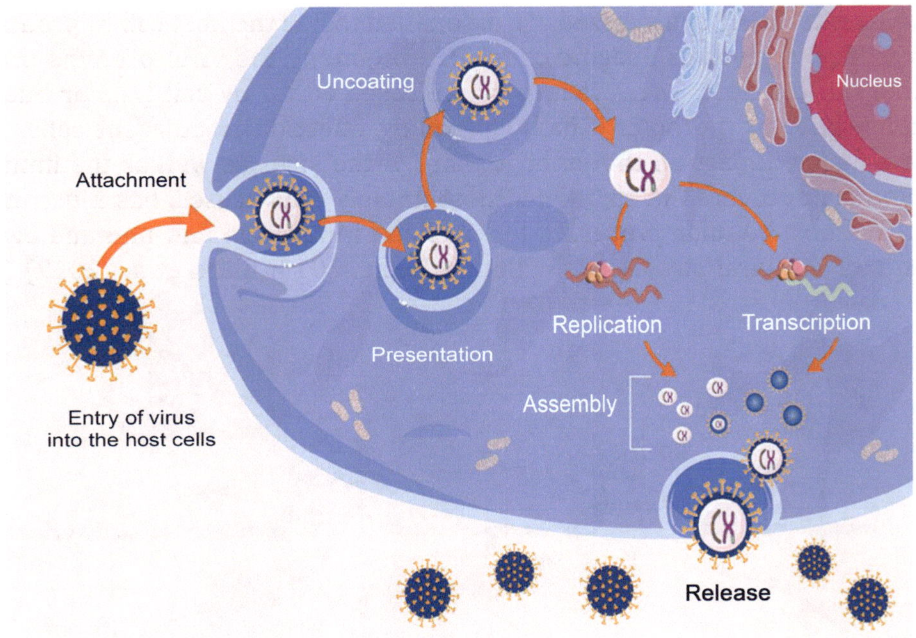

Figure 1.7. Mechanism of virus entry and replication in host cells.

Source: https://www.researchgate.net/publication/343804004/figure/fig1/AS:11431281212024262@1702524990492/Mechanism-of-virus-entry-and-replication-in-host-cells.tif.

1.2.2. Stages of Viral Replication

Viral replication is an intricate, multifaceted process of events central to the reproduction of viruses in host cells. Attachment and entry represent the start of this replication process. Viruses use specific surface receptors of the host cells to attach, then penetrate the cell membrane. This stage is of particular importance since the virus has to successfully evade host defenses in order to set up infection. After entering, the viral genome is uncoating, releasing genetic material into the cytoplasm of the host cell, a step that is critical for successful viral replication. These processes are critically important in medical microbiology, as they illuminate potential therapeutic targets for antiviral intervention. Future research can be based on these results to better understand mechanisms of viral entry and discover new ways to interfere with them, especially useful in managing major pathogens (Willett & Hosie, 2013). After the uncoating step, the process of viral replication continues on to the transcription and translation steps. At this time, the viral genome, either DNA or RNA, hijacks the host's cellular machinery to make viral proteins and copy its genetic material. The hijacking is essential because it enables the virus to make structural proteins required for assembling new virions. The complex interaction between viral and host elements during these functions provides opportunities for therapeutic gain by exposing vulnerabilities. Interestingly, most viruses have developed ways to circumvent host immunity during this phase, increasing their replication efficiency. Elucidation of the mechanisms employed in this phase can help researchers design vaccines and antiviral drugs targeting specific mechanisms, thus impeding the ability of the virus to replicate (Clark et al., 2017). The last phases of viral replication involve assembly and release, completing the cycle of replication by the formation of new virions that can infect new host cells. Viral components newly synthesized are assembled inside the host cell to produce intact viral particles. This assembly involves specific coordination among the viral proteins present and the cellular machinery of the host. Then, virions are released either by cell lysis or budding off from the cellular membranes of the hosts, finally spreading infection to adjacent cells. These release processes have a major impact on the pathogenicity of the virus as well as the immune response of the host. Significant research in this field, most notably flaviviruses, has illustrated the ability of viruses to hijack host cellular processes for maximal replication and immune evasion and has provided a basis for antiviral strategies (Willett & Hosie, 2013; Clark et al., 2017) (Figure 1.8).

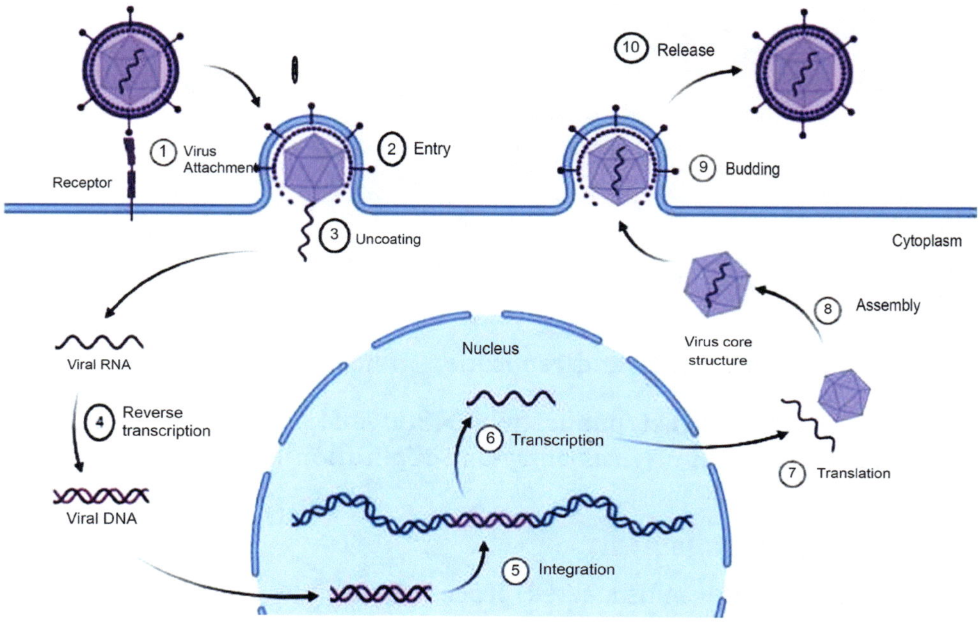

Figure 1.8. Diagram of viral replication process.

Source: https://www.researchgate.net/publication/348869255/figure/fig2/AS:986086943764480@1612112856637/Diagram-of-viral-replication-process-BioRendercom-Coronavirus-Replication-Cycle-2020a.jpg.

1.2.3. Factors Influencing Viral Life Cycles

The understanding of the determinants of viral life cycles is critical to understanding viral pathogenesis and transmission dynamics. A number of internal and external variables determine how viruses replicate, persist, and disseminate in host populations. Of these, the host availability and the population dynamics significantly impact viral prevalence. For example, investigations have shown that zoonotic viruses such as the Puumala virus (PUU) display spatio-temporal patterns highly correlated with host populations, i.e., bank voles (*Clethrionomys glareolus*), whose population size varies dramatically. In areas with high densities of nephropathia epidemica, high bank vole populations allow for the transmission of PUU to humans, especially in autumn when human exposure in infested areas increases. This interactive relationship indicates how ecological and environmental factors strongly influence viral life cycles, thus making them important factors in medical microbiology (Olsson, 2003). Environmental variables also strongly influence viral life cycles apart from host dynamics. The particular environments that harbor host populations can facilitate the transmission and persistence of viruses. For instance, research has shown that features like old-growth moist forests correlate with greater PUU-infected bank vole populations. Where there is dense vegetation and substrate available for cover, the availability of rodent habitats is likely to increase, thus facilitating favorable conditions for viral replication and transmission. In addition, environmental factors, such as temperature and humidity, have been found to affect both viral stability outside a host and host behavior. As such, appreciating the subtle interplay between environmental parameters and viral epidemiology is essential for epidemic prediction and designing successful control measures in public health policy (Willett & Hosie, 2013). In addition, the viral genome itself contains variations that affect a virus's adaptability and efficiency of the life cycle. Rates of mutation and the potential for genetic reassortment can give rise to new strains that can colonize alternative ecological niches or avoid host defenses. This element of viral evolution necessitates regular surveillance of viral populations, particularly in accordance with shifting environmental determinants or host dynamics likely to promote transmission. The intricate interplay between the viral genome and exogenous determinants best represents the dynamic, multifaceted nature of viral life cycles. Finally, understanding these dynamics is of immense value in the planning of strategies to prevent viral infections and the better understanding of virus-host interactions in medical microbiology (Olsson, 2003).

Test Your Knowledge

1. What are the primary mechanisms of entry of viruses into host cells?
2. What are the overall steps of the viral replication cycle within a host cell?

1.3. Pathogenesis of Viral Infections

Learning Outcome

1. Describe mechanisms of viral pathogenicity;
2. Comprehend host immune response to viral infections;
3. Provide examples of viral diseases.

The pathogenesis of viral infections is a multifaceted relationship between the virus and the immune response of the host. The infection process usually begins with the mucous membranes, with the viruses utilizing epithelial cells as a site of entry. After gaining entry, viruses take over the cellular machinery of the host to produce and form new virions. This process can give rise to cell death or dysfunction, usually leading to tissue damage and inflammation. For instance, respiratory viruses initiate extensive loss of epithelial cells, compromising airway epithelial integrity and facilitating secondary bacterial infections. It is important to know about these early events, as they determine the outcome of the disease and the hosts immune response, which can differ considerably among populations as a consequence of genetic and environmental variations. Mechanisms of immune evasion are the signature of viral pathogenesis. Numerous viruses have developed means to evade the host's immune system, thus ensuring continued infection and transmission. This comprises the inhibition of host antiviral responses, manipulation of major histocompatibility complex (MHC) expression, and modulation of apoptosis pathways. For example, some viruses can encode for proteins that suppress interferon signaling, which is important in the antiviral response. These evasion mechanisms not only enhance viral persistence but also magnify pathology through chronic inflammation, which may lead to disease progression. Immune pathway activation that is persistent, in turn, establishes an environment conducive to secondary infections and complications, illustrating the fine balance between viral replication and host defense mechanisms. The long-term effects of viral infections tend to go beyond acute illness, impacting chronic diseases. For instance, infections due to some viruses, like hepatitis B and C, correlate with the formation of chronic liver disease and hepatocellular carcinoma. They result from long-term results such as persistent viral replication, immune-mediated damage to the liver, and the formation of genetic mutations caused by the viral genome. In a general context, the interaction between viral pathogenesis and chronic disease outlines the significance of continued research to reveal viral pathogenesis mechanisms. This knowledge is crucial in establishing potent vaccines and treatment measures that could curtail the effects of viral infections on public health, as revealed by recent investigations on viral components and how these interact within host systems (Willett & Hosie, 2013; Frolova et al., 2016).

1.3.1. Mechanisms of Viral Pathogenicity

The study of viral mechanisms of pathogenicity is vital for the progress of medical microbiology, particularly in formulating effective treatments and prevention strategies. Viruses use different strategies to infect host cells, hijack cellular machinery, and avoid immune detection. For example, some viruses have the ability to modulate host cell signaling pathways, thus ensuring their reproduction while at the same time inhibiting host defense processes. This manipulation can result in cellular apoptosis, necrosis, or other pathophysiologic processes that aid in disease. Through analysis of these mechanisms, researchers are able to identify possible targets for antiviral drugs which reverse these viral mechanisms, further emphasizing the significance of viral pathogenicity in medical virology. The immune response's role in viral pathogenicity cannot be overemphasized, with viruses such as those in the genus Flavivirus displaying advanced ways to subvert host defense. Recent research has pointed out how flaviviruses, e.g., dengue and Zika, use mechanisms to inhibit type I interferon pathways—a major part of the host immune system. By these pathways, flaviviruses may reduce the antiviral function of interferons, permitting productive infection and virulence. This active process of interaction between the virus and the immune system of the host highlights the viral pathogenesis dilemma and the need for extensive studies to initiate new therapeutic strategies. Moving away from fundamental science, knowledge of these interactions can inform clinical practice and public health interventions focused on preventing viral disease and its attendant burden on healthcare systems (Clark et al., 2017).

Aside from immune evasion mechanisms, some viruses have evolved mechanisms directly affecting cell processes, increasing their capacity to survive and replicate within the host. For instance, viral protein interaction with host cellular mechanisms may result in dysregulation of cellular processes, creating a facilitative environment for viral replication. Of the foodborne pathogens, viruses such as those belonging to the enterovirus subgroup have been found to exploit such mechanisms, exemplified through investigations into the capacity of such viruses for survival under conditions involving various biocidal compounds used in food safety (Willett & Hosie, 2013). The complex character of viral pathogenicity makes it difficult for scientists to devise guidelines for infection control and treatment protocols. By examining these mechanisms, researchers can gain a greater understanding of the life cycle of viruses and create advanced strategies against the viral diseases that impact public health (Figure 1.9).

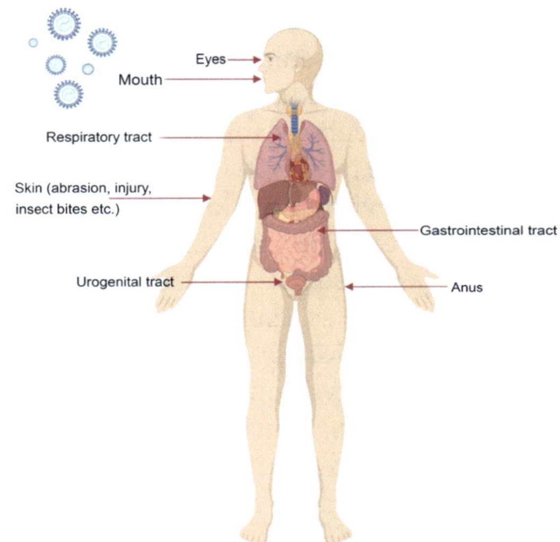

Figure 1.9. Typical sites of virus entry into the body: The first steps of viral infection is determined by the site at which the virus implants into the body. This would subsequently dictate the mechanisms of viral pathogenesis.

Source: https://upload.wikimedia.org/wikipedia/commons/thumb/2/29/Typical_sites_of_virus_entry_into_the_body.png/800px-Typical_sites_of_virus_entry_into_the_body.png.

1.3.2. Host Immune Response to Viral Infections

The host immune response to viral infections is a multifaceted coordination of innate and adaptive mechanisms aimed at recognizing and eliminating pathogens. On viral entry, the innate immune response is triggered, mainly by pattern recognition receptors (PRRs) that recognize viral components. This stimulates the release of type I interferons (IFNs) and other cytokines that create an antiviral state in neighboring cells. Moreover, triggering of natural killer (NK) cells and phagocytic cells contributes to the immediate response to viral insults. However, viruses have developed advanced methods to avoid these defenses, such as PRR signaling pathway downregulation and interference with interferon responses. Knowledge of these interactions is important for the effective design of therapeutic measures against viral infections, especially considering emerging and re-emerging viruses posing serious threats to human health, as reflected in the current research in the area of virology. Adaptive immunity also modulates the host response to viral infections by activating T and B lymphocytes. $CD8^+$ cytotoxic T-lymphocyte activation is an essential part of the cellular immune response, as they kill virus-infected cells directly. Additionally, $CD4^+$ helper T cells enable B cell activation and proliferation, which leads to the production of virus-specific antibodies. These antibodies inactivate viruses and block their binding and infection of host cells. Some viruses, like those in the Flavivirus genus, have, however, found ways to overcome these adaptive immune responses. For example, they can disrupt interferon-mediated signaling pathways in order to avoid immune detection and reduce the efficacy of the hosts antibody response. These adaptations highlight the need for continuous research into virus-host interactions, the knowledge of which can be used in the development of vaccines and therapeutic interventions to increase the host immune response (Clark et al., 2017). In spite of the adaptive and innate immune responses, most viral infections can cause extensive morbidity and mortality, highlighting gaps in host defenses. The difficulty is in the capability of certain viruses to evade the host immune system and cause persistent infections. As understood in current research, even in the context of foodborne pathogens, such as those discussed in microbial studies, environment and conditions can increase vulnerability to infection (Willett & Hosie, 2013). This highlights the complex interaction between the virulence determinants of the pathogen and the hosts immune environment. Tackling this complexity demands an interdisciplinary strategy that unifies immunology, microbiology, and virology, opening the doors for new therapeutic approaches. By demystifying these interactions, scientists are able to foretell viral behavior better and design improved treatment regimens that strengthen the host immune response, thus enhancing patient recovery in viral infections (Figure 1.10).

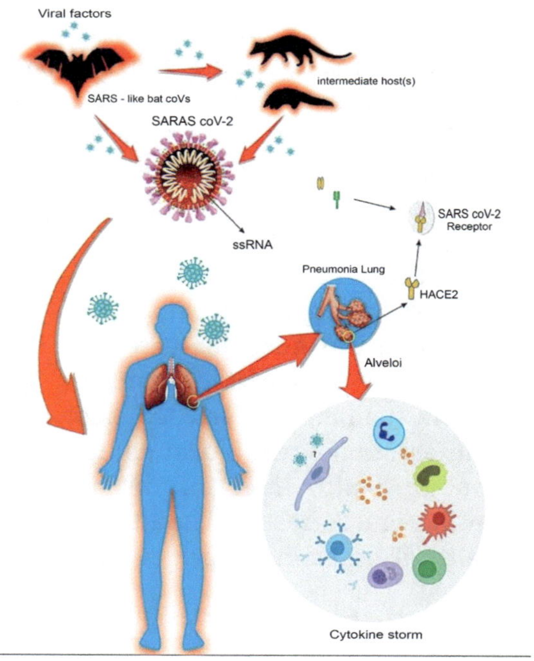

Figure 1.10. Proposed host immune response during SARS-Cov-2 infection.

Source: https://www.researchgate.net/profile/Adel-Elmaghrabi/publication/342889750/figure/fig1/AS:912806652174336@1594641473184/Proposed-host-immune-response-during-SARS-Cov-2-infection.jpg.

1.3.3. Examples of Diseases Caused by Viruses

The field of viral illness is vast and includes a range of infective agents causing severe morbidity and mortality globally. An example of this is the Human Immunodeficiency Virus (HIV), which results in acquired immunodeficiency syndrome (AIDS). This virus targets the immune system, weakening the body's capacity to fight infections and cancer. With progression of HIV, patients develop opportunistic infections that are essential markers of the diseases progression. In addition, Hepatitis B and Hepatitis C viruses are causative agents of liver diseases like cirrhosis and hepatocellular carcinoma, causing a huge healthcare burden worldwide. The viral pathogens express not only the complexity of viral interactions with human hosts but also the different implications they have on public health, which makes them the subject of extensive research in vaccine development and therapeutic interventions. Another viral infection of concern is the influenza virus, which is one of the primary causes of seasonal epidemics and the occasional pandemics. Influenza comes in many different forms, such as type A, B, and C, each with its own difficulties in the way of transmissibility as well as virulence. The seasonal flu that recurs each year can cause serious respiratory illness, with significant hospitalization as well as death, mainly among susceptible populations. The dynamic behavior of the influenza virus, in addition to being able to cause antigenic shift and drift, makes it challenging to develop an effective vaccine. This requires continuous monitoring to track circulating strains and tailor vaccination efforts accordingly. The circumstances of influenza highlight the significance of virology in deciphering transmission dynamics and instituting effective interventions for countering its effects on public health systems worldwide. Additionally, viruses like the norovirus and rotavirus illustrate the viral cause of gastroenteritis, producing acute gastrointestinal illnesses that afflict millions globally. Norovirus has a notorious reputation for spreading quickly, especially in close areas such as cruise ships and nursing homes, causing outbreaks that can paralyze entire populations. Rotavirus, however, has served as a leading causative agent of severe diarrhea among children. Immunization campaigns have dramatically curtailed the incidence of rotavirus disease, demonstrating the pivotal position of virology in preventive medicine. The difficulties presented by these viruses attest to the imperative for strong diagnostic processes and epidemiological surveillance to control outbreaks efficiently. Indeed, advancements in molecular techniques, as illustrated in the detection of human caliciviruses, are crucial for enhancing our response to these viral threats (Butcher et al., 1997; Willett & Hosie, 2013) (Figure 1.11).

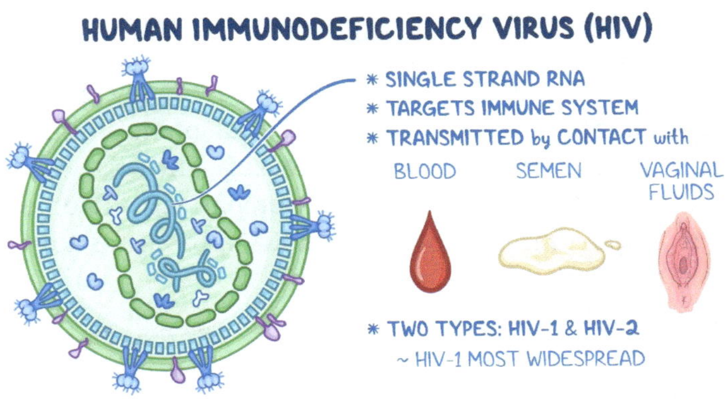

Figure 1.11. Human immunodeficiency virus (HIV).

Source: https://www.osmosis.org/_next/image?url=https%3A%2F%2Fd16qt3wv6xm098.cloudfront.net%2FZ4KjyynnSsSQvX1XlQ5Tc_NwRhSeEFMm%2F_.jpg&w=3840&q=75.

Test Your Knowledge

1. What are the main mechanisms by which viruses cause disease in the host?
2. How does the immune system respond to a viral infection?

1.4. Diagnostic Techniques in Virology

Learning Outcome

1. Describe traditional methods of virus detection;
2. Understand molecular techniques for viral diagnosis;
3. Discuss on serological assays and their applications.

Molecular diagnostics has transformed virology by providing a sensitivity and specificity in detecting viruses that was previously unknown. Techniques such as polymerase chain reaction (PCR) and reverse transcription PCR (RT-PCR) allow for the amplification of viral nucleic acids, making it possible to identify viruses even at low concentrations. This capability is especially crucial for monitoring infections like respiratory syncytial virus (RSV), which affects millions of children annually, resulting in significant morbidity and mortality (Jha et al., 2016). In addition, these molecular methods can also be used to give information about viral load and strain differences in addition to just presence of the virus, thus guiding treatment and epidemiology. With the development of the sphere, these technologies keep on improving our knowledge of the viral infections and it is important to note that accurate diagnostic method is the key to successful medical microbiology. Along with molecular techniques serological techniques are still important to diagnose viral infections by identifying the production of antibodies against a virus. Enzyme-linked immunosorbent assay (ELISA) and Western blot are examples of serological tests commonly employed in clinical settings. The methods are especially helpful in the diagnosis of infections where viral loads might be below the limit of detection by molecular assays or in the surveillance of immune response after vaccination. Serology tests may also be useful in detecting past infections, which is essential in the immunity of the population and epidemiology trends. The historical development of such diagnostic methods highlights the intertwined evolution of clinical virology and immunology, exemplified by the early studies on feline leukemia virus (FeLV) that paved the way for discovering new viral pathogens and the importance of antibody response in controlling viral diseases (Willett & Hosie, 2013). Emerging technologies such as next-generation sequencing (NGS) are setting a new paradigm for diagnostic virology. The NGS technology allows the complete study of viral genomes, which can give information on the genetic diversity and the evolutionary pattern of viruses in populations. This method has been invaluable in the tracing of the origin of outbreaks such as in viral epidemics whose high mutation rates pose a challenge to public health agencies. The possibility to rapidly sequence and analyze viral DNA or RNA in clinical samples provides diagnostic possibilities that cannot be compared to the traditional ones. Furthermore, NGS may help to detect co-infections and determine the effectiveness of treatment measures during the course of time. With increased use of these sophisticated diagnostic tools in everyday clinical practice, they hold the potential of improving our response to viral diseases and this will eventually translate to better patient outcomes and guide population health approaches to virology.

1.4.1. Traditional Methods of Virus Detection

Conventional virus detection techniques have traditionally been central to the diagnosis of viral infections especially in the days preceding the molecular techniques. Tissue culture assays are among the oldest and most basic detection methods, in which viruses are isolated in patients samples by inoculation of susceptible cell lines. In this method, cytopathic effects can be observed; here, the infected cells change their morphology. Although tissue culture is still considered a mainstay of viral diagnostics, it can be time-consuming and needs special facilities. Moreover, it does not apply to every virus, especially the ones that are hard to grow in vitro. The drawbacks of the conventional culture-based approaches have led to the constant search of faster and more sensitive detection methodologies, which further emphasizes the applicability of the combination of these classical methods with the newer molecular-based methods in order to increase the diagnostic possibilities. Another common conventional technique that has been used in detecting viruses is serology assays. The assays take advantage of this specificity of antibodies which can be utilized to detect virus-related antigens in patient samples. Techniques such as enzyme-linked immunosorbent assays (ELISAs) and hemagglutination inhibition tests have been successfully employed to detect antibodies produced in response to viral infections. For instance, serological testing has been critical in identifying diseases such as hepatitis and human immunodeficiency virus (HIV). Serology assays however have limitations because they depend on the host immune response which might not be apparent in the early stages of infection. This delay may result in false negative, especially among the immunocompromised hosts. Nevertheless, in spite of these difficulties serological techniques can still be useful epidemiological tools which can give information about population immunity and how infections have prevailed over time. There is growing importance of combining conventional procedures with modern technologies in clinical virology. For instance, the combination of conventional culture techniques with polymerase chain reaction (PCR) testing can enhance both the sensitivity and specificity of virus detection. Conventional approaches, which at times are viewed as outdated, still guide and confirm more recent molecular diagnostics. The complementarity of these methods also makes a significant contribution to the proper identification and surveillance of viral pathogens in the populations which contributes to the knowledge of viral epidemiology. With the changing landscape of medical microbiology it is important to maintain and streamline the already existing diagnostic modalities, especially in scenarios like the one involving emergent viral threats where speed of response is most important. Noteworthy, studies have shown the importance of maintaining a balanced diagnostic arsenal, maximizing the strengths of both traditional and modern techniques to address diverse clinical challenges, as evidenced in recent evaluations of various pathogens and their diagnostic requirements (Willett & Hosie, 2013; Jha et al., 2016) (Figure 1.12).

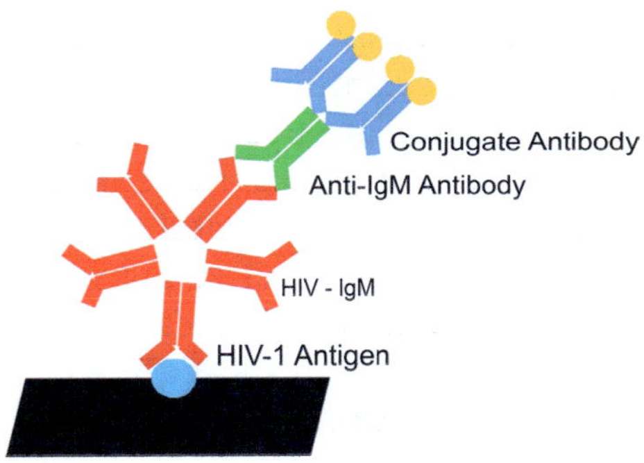

Figure 1.12. Enzyme-linked immunosorbent assay (ELISA) method for detecting anti-HIV1 IgM antibody captured by membrane-bound recombinant gp41.

Source: https://www.researchgate.net/publication/281340996/figure/fig7/AS:669650295734279@1536668480363/Enzyme-linked-immunosorbent-assay-ELISA-method-for-detecting-anti-HIV1-IgM-antibody.jpg.

1.4.2. Molecular Techniques for Viral Diagnosis

The diagnosis of viruses has undergone a molecular revolution, whereby the accuracy and speed of detection of the pathogen in a clinical environment has been greatly improved. Conventional diagnostic tools, including viral cultures and serological tests, are usually insensitive and can require days to provide an answer. In contrast, molecular techniques, including polymerase chain reaction (PCR) and next-generation sequencing (NGS), provide rapid identification of viral nucleic acids, enabling timely clinical decisions. This shift is particularly crucial in the context of infections such as respiratory syncytial virus (RSV), which has a substantial global incidence rate, particularly among young children and the elderly. The deployment of these molecular tools has transformed the landscape of viral diagnosis, allowing for prompt identification and management of viral diseases, thereby reducing the burden of morbidity and mortality associated with them (Jha et al., 2016). In addition to PCR and NGS, newer molecular techniques like reverse transcription PCR (RT-PCR) and in situ hybridization are becoming increasingly integral to viral diagnostics. Not only can viral RNA be detected by these methods but they also enable the study of viral distribution in tissues to be studied. Advanced techniques such as quantitative PCR (qPCR) enable quantification of viral load, which is essential for monitoring the progression of infections and the effectiveness of antiviral therapies. The implementation of these molecular methods in medical practice is supported by the fact that they can deliver essential data regarding the severity of diseases and possible epidemics. As molecular diagnostics continue to evolve, they hold promise for enhanced surveillance and outbreak management, further solidifying their role in addressing public health challenges related to viral infections (Van Loon, 2002). The theoretical development of molecular methods in virology is also associated with a deeper comprehension of the pathogen virulence and its role in medical microbiology. The historical development of virology as a science has highlighted the importance of using an interdisciplinary approach to understand the behavior of viruses and their interactions with host systems in all respects. The process represents a wider tendency in scientific study, as the objectification of viruses in the laboratory has given way to new approaches to viral classification and diagnostics. With the help of a combination of various technological and methodological innovations, scientists will be able to gain more knowledge about the pathogenesis of viruses and increase the level of diagnostics. Consequently, the ongoing evolution of molecular techniques will not only advance the field of virology but will also facilitate the development of targeted therapeutics and vaccines, ultimately aiming to mitigate the impact of viral diseases globally (Jha et al., 2016) (Figure 1.13).

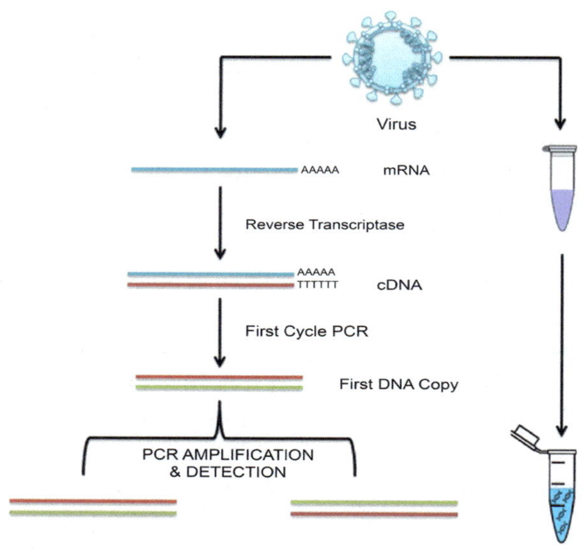

Figure 1.13. Graphical illustration of RT-PCR.

Source: https://www.researchgate.net/profile/Fakhar-Khan-6/publication/343407421/figure/fig2/AS:921968421392386@1596825809346/Graphical-illustration-of-RT-PCR.png.

1.4.3. Serological Assays and Their Applications

The value of serological tests in clinical diagnosis is a prerequisite of medical microbiology, especially when discussing viral diseases. The assays are meant to identify the presence of particular antibodies in the serum of a patient and, therefore, can indicate previous infections as well as continuing immune responses. For instance, the development of enzyme immunoassays (EIA) has greatly enhanced the ability to diagnose infections like RSV and influenza by determining the presence of virus-specific antibodies. Traditional methods often focus on single analyte formats, however, the move towards multiplex microarray immunoassays (MAIA) enhances the capability to assess multiple viral infections simultaneously, offering a more comprehensive assessment of a patient's immune status. This shift not only streamlines diagnosis but also supports large-scale serosurveillance efforts in populations, thereby improving public health monitoring and response strategies, particularly in young children who are at high risk for severe viral infections (Kazakova et al., 2019). Besides enhancing the effectiveness of diagnosis, serological assays are critical in measuring vaccine effectiveness. The study of the antibodies produced after vaccination presents the essential information about the immunity of the population to certain viral infections. Serological assays like the multiplex microarray immunoassay have been demonstrated to be correlating well with traditional techniques thereby making its use valid in both clinical and research applications. As an illustration, investigations with the usage of MAIA allowed identifying IgG and IgM antibodies against several types of influenza, which proved its efficiency in immunity monitoring in children and adult groups. This enhanced capability is paramount in conducting epidemiological studies, tracking the spread of viruses, and tailoring vaccination campaigns to effectively address emerging public health threats (Kazakova et al., 2019). Moreover, other sampling techniques are also advancing with serology-based technologies to enhance access and subject adherence to immunization activities. As an example, oral fluid as a source of antibodies detection is a non-invasive method that has a potential to enhance the recruitment of subjects in longitudinal studies. The development of assays like the IgG antibody capture enzyme-linked immunosorbent assay (GACELISA) for mumps-specific antibodies illustrates this trend. Such methods have demonstrated sensitivity and specificity of 100% compared to traditional serum samples, which underline the potential of non-invasive samples to broaden the boundaries of serological monitoring. Nevertheless, there are still challenges including the dilution of antibodies in oral fluids, which requires developments in the sensitivity of the assays. Exploring the incorporation of recombinant antigens and innovative technologies like immuno-polymerase chain reaction (I-PCR) might enable future enhancements in the effectiveness of serological assays in both clinical and research applications .

Test Your Knowledge

1. What are the traditional methods used for virus detection in clinical samples?
2. What is the role of serological assays in viral diagnostics?

1.5. Treatment and Prevention of Viral Infections

Learning Outcome

1. Describe antiviral therapies and their mechanisms
2. Focus on vaccination strategies against viral diseases
3. Understand public health measures for virus control

Viral infections and their treatment and prevention are the significant aspects of public health and clinical practice in the field of medical microbiology. The new knowledge on the pathogenesis of viruses has resulted in new methods of controlling viral diseases. For many viral infections, particularly respiratory syncytial virus (RSV) and human immunodeficiency virus (HIV), prevention strategies are paramount. Healthcare providers use supportive treatment methodologies in the case of RSV because there are no highly effective antiviral agents. Palivizumab has emerged as a licensed preventive measure for select high-risk infants, showcasing the necessity of targeted prophylaxis in vulnerable populations, particularly given the significant morbidity associated with RSV in children and the elderly (Jha et al., 2016). The dynamic nature of antiviral therapeutics is evidenced by the continuous development of vaccines and antiviral drugs, to lessen the burden of disease and death. HIV is a more complicated problem in the field of treatment and prevention because it remains at a high prevalence level especially in such areas as southern Africa. The efficacy of antiretroviral therapy (ART) as a method of prevention, commonly referred to as treatment as prevention (TasP), exemplifies a strategy that can mitigate viral transmission. A large community-randomized trial in Botswana provides an example of the complex strategy that needs to be used to fight HIV. The trial is combining ART with other preventive strategies and therefore the need to stress the value of HIV testing, male circumcision, and clinical linkage to achieve comprehensive care. By utilizing viral phylogenetics, researchers can elucidate the dynamics of transmission and gauge the effectiveness of various interventions, thereby committing to a data-driven approach in public health initiatives (Essex, 2014). Such combination of prevention methods plays a crucial role in managing the current epidemic. Within the framework of viral diseases, the situation in the field of therapy and prevention is still changing in connection with the appearance of new antiviral agents and complex immunization programs. Indicatively, the genomic innovations have resulted in the formulation of vaccines that are likely to induce strong immune responses and reduce the chances of disease enhancement. The main issue is still to work out efficient and safe therapeutic guidelines against different viral diseases, and even those ones which do not have therapeutic alternatives yet. Education, accessibility and availability of preventive options and advances in molecular diagnostic tools will be important as the public health structures readjust to cope with these challenges. This comprehensive strategy will not only address the short-term health issues but also aims at achieving resilience towards any future viral pandemics, thus improving the overall health outcomes in all countries.

1.5.1. Antiviral Therapies and Their Mechanisms

The invention of antiviral agents is thus far one of the major achievements in the discipline of medical microbiology, especially in countering the viral diseases that are a real threat to health. Antivirals act by inhibiting a certain phase of the viral life cycle, viral replication, and reducing the severity of the disease. As an illustration, nucleoside analogs are made to target the replication of viral genome by resembling natural nucleotides, which may cause the stalling of viral DNA or RNA production. This process is especially clear in the treatment of chronic viral diseases like hepatitis B where development of drug resistance may complicate the treatment plan. Knowing how these antivirals work, medical practitioners can design therapeutic courses in a way that would maximally benefit patients and minimize the impact of viral diseases on the overall population worldwide. In the case of respiratory syncytial virus (RSV), which is associated with significant morbidity among vulnerable populations, antiviral options are limited, necessitating a focus on research for novel treatments. The management currently used is mainly supportive with the passive immunity of high-risk infants being offered by the monoclonal antibody palivizumab. Irrespective of these constraints, there are current research efforts into novel antiviral agents that propose the possibility of new therapeutic agents which target specifically RSV entry or replication. The pathophysiological knowledge of the RSV-caused bronchiolitis, which is marked by a considerable airway inflammation, is used to develop specific immunomodulatory treatments that could be applied to the currently used treatment patterns. As our understanding of viral mechanisms expands, the prospect of developing effective antiviral agents for RSV and similar viral infections becomes increasingly feasible, highlighting the need for continued research in this field (Jha et al., 2016). Viral infections and especially chronic infections such as hepatitis B are complex enough to highlight the importance of close attention paid to antiviral resistance. With the evolution of strains and their attainment of mutations, as in the case of hepatitis B virus reverse transcriptase, the effectiveness of treatment may be highly reduced and an initial characterization of the virus is important in determining the course of treatment. Research has also demonstrated that naturally occurring resistant mutations can persist even in treatment-naive individuals thus making the treatment situation more complex. This is because the information on these mutations before the antiviral therapy is initiated will enable the clinicians to tailor the treatment in a way that will reduce the chances of selecting the resistant strains. This nuanced approach exemplifies the critical intersection of virology and clinical microbiology, advocating for tailored treatment strategies that acknowledge the adaptive capabilities of viruses and the necessity for continuous evaluation of antiviral effectiveness (Bedfordi et al., 2013) (Figure 1.14).

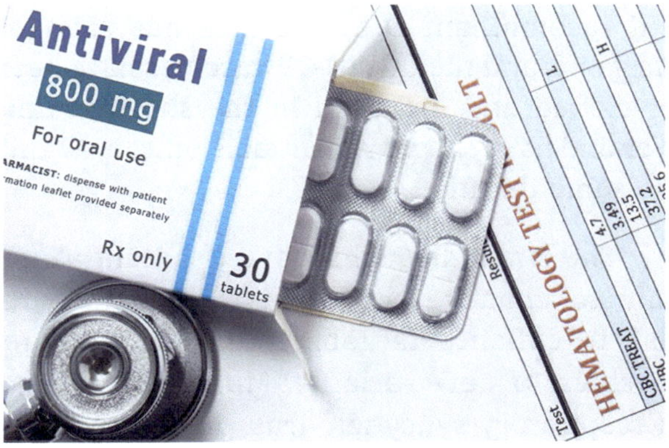

Figure 1.14. Antiviral medication.

Source: https://www.eehealth.org/-/media/images/modules/blog/posts/2021/06/hd-life-covid-antiviral-medication.jpg?h=499&w=750&hash=77E351993CAEB6CDA4FEF99E14A3D9B9.

1.5.2. Vaccination Strategies Against Viral Diseases

The growing threat of viral diseases all over the world has created the necessity of paying immediate attention to efficient vaccination practices. Vaccination is an important tool of conferring immunity against certain pathogens and thereby checking the spread of the viruses and protecting the populations especially the children and the aged who are the most susceptible. There are several types of these vaccines, live-attenuated, inactivated, subunit vaccines, with different immunological profiles and benefits. As an illustration, live-attenuated vaccines usually prime strong immune response and durable immunity, whereas inactivated vaccines offer a safer version, particularly in high-risk populations. As viral pathogens continue to evolve, refining these vaccination strategies remains paramount to address public health challenges effectively (Willett & Hosie, 2013). The recent success in the use of new vaccine technology underscores the importance of focusing on viral diseases that are well known to have high morbidity and mortality rates. The entry of mRNA-based technology and recombinant DNA vaccines has changed the game, and the COVID-19 vaccines have been developed and deployed in the shortest time ever and have shown remarkable efficacy within the same duration.

The breakthroughs have a potential not only to enhance the immune response but also to enhance the ability to quickly adapt vaccines to new variants. Moreover, as seen in respiratory syncytial virus (RSV) infections, which account for millions of cases among young children, the pursuit of novel vaccines is of paramount importance (Jha et al., 2016). As the strategies are still under development, they can be applied in the reduction of the severe complications of the viral infections, which ensures enhanced health outcomes. The problem of vaccine hesitancy, unequal access, and varying public health policies also weighs down on vaccination strategies. These elements explain the significance of extensive educational programs to sensitize the population regarding the effectiveness and safety of vaccinations. It is also important to educate the populations on the preventative powers of the vaccines so that herd immunity can be achieved which is very important in curtailing the spread of viral diseases. Governments, healthcare delivery organizations, and communities ought to collaborate to overcome the barriers to vaccination and attain equal distribution, particularly in settings that are resource-limited. The success of vaccination programs hinges not only on the scientific advancements in vaccine development but also on the societal commitment to fostering a culture of health and prevention (Willett & Hosie, 2013) (Figure 1.15).

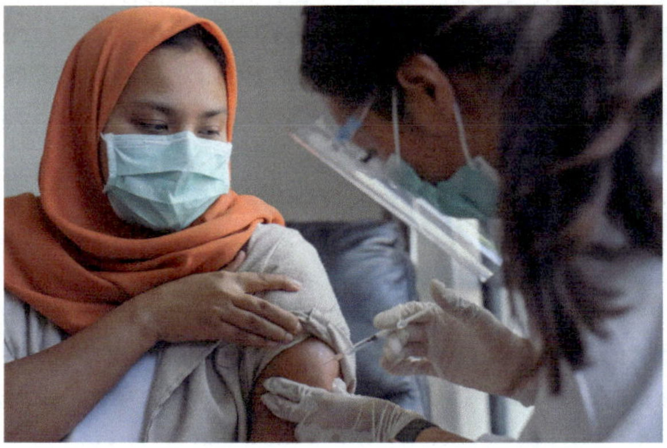

Figure 1.15. Vaccination against viral diseases.

Source: https://www.bread.org/wp-content/uploads/2024/03/iStock-1320262755-scaled.jpg.

1.5.3. Public Health Measures for Virus Control

In the control of viral infections, public health measures are very crucial especially the use of vaccination programs. Vaccination not just helps in protecting the person but also helps in herd immunity, where the occurrence of infectious diseases in a community is lowered. As an illustration, influenza immunizations considerably reduce the transmission of the virus, alleviating the morbidity and fatality rates related to it. The persisting problem, though, is that the viruses capability to perform antigenic drift requires the annual change of the formulations of the vaccines. Research has revealed that A/H3N2 evolves at a faster rate than other influenza lineages, driving yearly variations in immunity needed for effective vaccine deployment (Bedford et al., 2013). Therefore, it is important that public health agencies constantly survey the strains of the virus in circulation so as to maximize the benefit of vaccination, thus the connection between virology and population health efforts in controlling infectious disease. Diagnostic testing is another pillar of virus control in the population in addition to vaccination. A fast and correct diagnosis of viral infections will enable timely measures, lowering the rate of transmission. The advent of molecular-based diagnostic tools has revolutionized our ability to diagnose complex viral infections such as respiratory syncytial virus (RSV), which poses significant risks to children and vulnerable populations. With an estimated 33 million cases annually among children under five, effective diagnostics enable healthcare providers to deliver appropriate management options and support resources where they are needed most (Jha et al., 2016). This is because early detection not only assists in protecting the vulnerable populations, but it can also be used to guide wider population health interventions geared towards managing outbreaks, a fact that highlights the importance of ensuring that laboratory capacities are aligned with epidemiological activities. Moreover, non-pharmaceutical interventions, which include hygiene and social distancing, have been effective in reducing the spread of the virus, especially in the case of a pandemic. The strategies will minimize the susceptible hosts and hence the infection will spread slowly. Societies that implement such measures as mask-wearing, regular hand-washing, and avoidance of social gatherings have shown low levels of spread of the virus in case of an outbreak. They complement vaccination efforts synergistically, which explains the need to adopt a multidimensional perspective on population health. The contradiction between the evolution of viruses and the actions of public health services requires an active reaction. Based on this, public health officials should be more attentive, and they should adjust their approaches to the constantly evolving situation with viral pathogens, thus making sure that the containment of outbreaks will be scientifically literate and methodologically reasonable.

Test Your Knowledge

1. How do antiviral drugs work to inhibit viral infections?
2. What is the distinction between live attenuated and inactivated vaccine?
3. Which prevention measures of public health can aid in preventing the transmission of viral infections?

1.6. Emerging Viruses and Global Health

Learning Outcome

1. Explain causes of new virus emergence;
2. Highlight recent viral outbreaks case studies;
3. Describe the contribution of worldwide surveillance in virology.

The occurrence of new viruses poses a serious challenge to world health, most notably because they cross with shifting environmental and social factors. Of particular concern are zoonotic viruses that have their origins in wildlife reservoirs because they have the ability to quickly adapt to human hosts. An example is the epidemiology of nephropathia epidemica (NE), which presents the complex interaction between ecological processes and viral transmission. In northern Sweden, studies have shown that Puumala virus (PUU), the cause of NE, is closely related to the population dynamics of its key host, the bank vole. Since these rodents live in specific environmental conditions, e.g., old-growth moist forests, human exposure risk is enhanced during the peak vole populations, particularly in autumn (Olsson, 2003). Knowledge of such interactions is important for the design of effective preventive strategies against emerging viral infections. The effect of environmental determinants on the cyclic emergence of viruses highlights the importance of interdisciplinary research in virology and environmental science. In addition to epidemiological trends, demographic influences also add significantly to the comprehension of emerging disease spread. Information from Sweden-based studies illustrates that middle-aged men are disproportionately impacted by NE, which implies that certain lifestyle choices, like engaging in outdoor activities in close proximity to rodent habitats, could place these men at increased risk of infection. These types of discoveries highlight the necessity of integrating demographic information into evaluation calculations for predictions of risk from emerging viruses. Public health education for high-risk groups would be critical in preventing the consequences of these infections and is key to a robust global health response. In facing the threat of emerging viruses, global collaboration and interconnected health systems are imperative. Interconnectedness in the world today means that viral epidemics do not stay localized; they can mount to international pandemics. For this reason, surveillance systems need to be modified to incorporate not just conventional virology indicators but also ecological and demographic information feeding into risk assessment models. Efforts aimed at increasing community preparedness and awareness of local outbreaks are most crucial. For example, combining veterinary and environmental health surveillance could provide early warning systems for viral emergence among wildlife populations to enable early and proactive intervention for human health risk management. In this constantly dynamic context of emerging viral risks, common approaches are necessary to ensure public health and narrative resilience (Olsson, 2003).

1.6.1. Factors Contributing to the Emergence of New Viruses

New virus emergence is more and more determined by several ecological and anthropogenic drivers of viral transmission and evolution. A main driver is the process of zoonotic spillover, as a result of viruses transferring from animal reservoirs to humans. Such transfer frequently follows the expansion of human activities into wildlife habitats, promoting contact between species. For instance, the transmission dynamics of CPV provide evidence of how interspecies associations can lead to the adaptation of viruses to novel hosts. The evolutionary patterns of CPV, which has experienced extensive genetic diversification in

Europe and South America, show how local adaptation and migrations lead to the emergence of new viral strains. As viruses evolve and change through these interactions, they can develop new abilities that endanger public health within different populations, thereby highlighting the linkage between ecological disturbance and viral emergence. Another factor that aids the emergence of new viruses is antigenic evolution, as demonstrated by the ongoing changes seen with influenza viruses. These viruses use tactics such as antigenic drift, whereby they are able to counteract host immunity derived from previous strains. The rapid evolution of influenza lineages, especially A/H3N2, points to the viruses capability to generate mutant strains less identifiable to the immune system. This antigenic drift is important in defining the efficacy of current vaccines since the introduced genetic diversity through mutation can cause large disparities between circulating strains and vaccine antigens. Through the simulation of such antigenic and genetic patterns, scientists have come to understand how viral strains evolve with time, a crucial point for comprehending the viral infection rates' dynamics and transmission within populations and developing successful public health measures, including vaccination, as emphasized in Bedford et al., (2013). In addition, climate change induced by global warming, urbanization, and globalizations enable geographic virus spread. Climate change shifts the habitats and migration patterns of vectors as well as hosts and can create new interactions capable of triggering viral emergence. For example, increased temperature can spread the range of certain zoonoses, such as those that involve ticks and mosquitoes, a development that poses the risk of introducing previously isolated viruses to new human populations. The constant movement of viral strains, as exemplified in studies on canine parvovirus populations, shows how waves of viral genetic material are able to sweep across continents, mixing local strains with those from other regions, as discussed in Aldaz et al., (2018). This interconnectedness underscores the need for global surveillance and collective public health action in monitoring and addressing potential viral threats in development, which is subject to intricate environmental and social determinants (Figure 1.16).

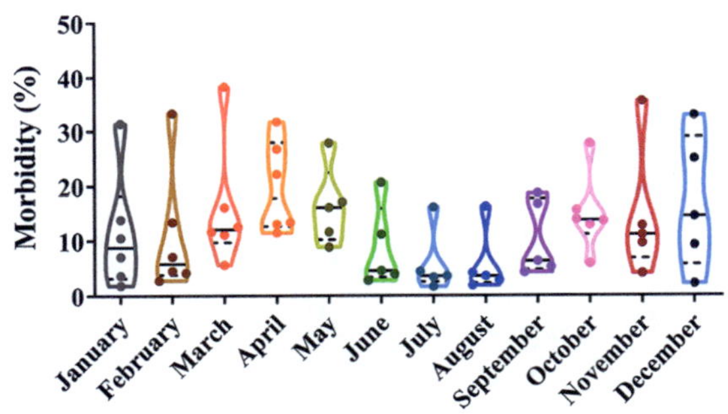

Figure 1.16. Monthly correlation analysis of canine parvovirus (CPV) infections in China.

Source: https://www.researchgate.net/publication/339383394/figure/fig3/AS:1143128124165591 6@1715185322446/Monthly-correlation-analysis-of-canine-parvovirus-CPV-infections-in-China.tif.

1.6.2. Case Studies of Recent Viral Outbreaks

The development of viral outbreaks like hand, foot, and mouth disease (HFMD) has become a major public health concern, especially in highly populated areas of the Asia Pacific. This disease, which is mostly caused by human enteroviruses, is frequently self-limiting but may develop severe neurological and cardiopulmonary morbidities in susceptible individuals. It has been shown that

HFMD is mainly transmitted through the faeco-oral route in developing regions but is altered towards respiratory droplets in industrialized countries, making it harder to control. The geographic distribution of severe outbreaks within the Asia Pacific could be the result of environmental hygiene and host population genetic predisposition. This epidemiologic model emphasizes the importance of ongoing surveillance, since the quick evolution and genetic recombination of the virus can bring unpredictable outbreaks, which require an integrative approach to disease management and surveillance (Willett & Hosie, 2013). The recent case studies have shed light on the shocking potential of viral pathogens to evolve and survive across various environments with major public health significance. As an example, research into viral inactivation processes has shown ozone to be an effective biocidal agent against well-known foodborne pathogens like *Campylobacter jejuni* and *Salmonella enteritidis*. Studies show that treatment conditions such as population and temperature variations can significantly determine the efficacy of ozone in eliminating these risks. This application extends beyond food safety; viral outbreak control, particularly in disease-intensive facilities, is essential in preventing large-scale epidemics. Comprehension of the dynamics of these pathogens in their own environment is essential to shaping effective interventions to counter the risks identified in these case studies (Willett & Hosie, 2013). In addition, the dynamic between environmental influences and viral persistence identifies the complexities involved in containing viral outbreaks in the globalized world. Enterovirus outbreaks are especially severe in places with poor sanitation and health infrastructure, permitting extended survival and transmission of the pathogens. The development of new viral variants makes vaccine creation more challenging because of their rapid genetic evolution and because the diseases they produce are mild, leading to possible underreporting and inadequate public health responses. As seen from the HFMD case, the identification of genetic recombination's and surveillance of outbreaks are critical to preparing effective public health strategies. A boost in research is necessary to evaluate the treatment alternatives, e.g., the use of intravenous immunoglobulin for severe complications, which may result in more effective and targeted interventions in the viral infection outbreak (Lau et al., 2010) (Figure 1.17).

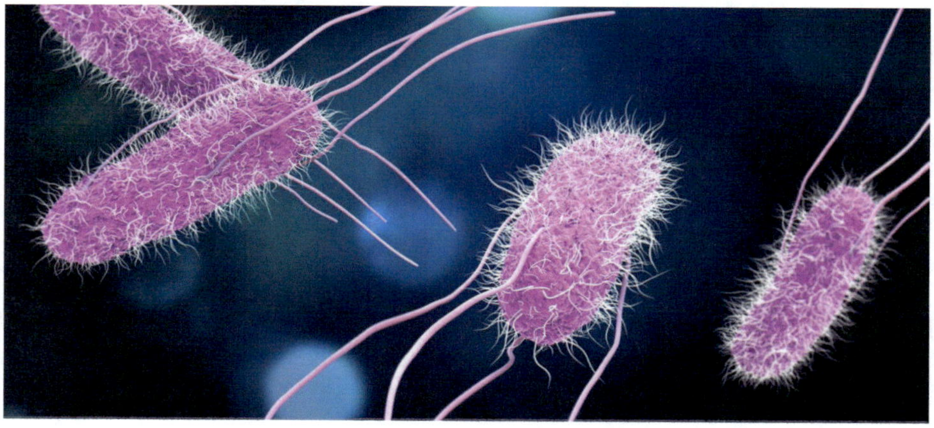

Figure 1.17. *Salmonella enteritidis.*

Source: https://cdn-dblhd.nitrocdn.com/baaZZsBRyWsSkxvRjeuJnYOHtwzeoEKd/assets/images/optimized/rev-95552f6/microbe-investigations.com/wp-content/uploads/elementor/thumbs/Salmonella-Enterica-qyn0kjeycjhbzea47298yx8ixprvfqh4cgryknd5ew.jpg.

1.6.3. The Role of Global Surveillance in Virology

Global surveillance is a central function in virology, especially in observing and studying viral outbreaks globally. Through routine collection and analysis of information on viral infections, organizations responsible for health can determine patterns of infection and emerging viral hotspots. This kind of surveillance is very important in the management of infectious diseases and guiding early public health interventions. The incorporation of genomic data into surveillance systems allows scientists to monitor mutations and viral evolution, gaining valuable insights into how viruses spread and adapt. Such surveillance empowers health authorities to make effective vaccination policies and resource allocation, saving lives and cost in healthcare. Global surveillance is even more important when dealing with respiratory viruses, specifically the influenza virus. Influenza viruses have antigenic drift, which results in seasonal epidemics and the infrequent pandemics. The monitoring strategies are aimed at following the antigenic changes in order to anticipate future epidemics and advise vaccine formulation procedures. Through methods like the hemagglutination inhibition (HI) assay, scientists can prepare antigenic maps that define the current evolution of influenza strains. Current research emphasizes the dynamic trends of antigenic drift in viral lineages, which reveal that ongoing surveillance can significantly increase knowledge of viral activity and related epidemiological trends (Bedford et al., 2013). Such data is critical in carrying out preemptive strategies to reduce influenzas impact on a worldwide scale. Global surveillance goes beyond influenza; it includes a variety of viral pathogens, particularly those with high disease burdens in areas like those mentioned. For instance, global surveillance of HPV and HIV infections in sub-Saharan Africa shows high correlations with rising cervical cancer incidence. The interaction between viral infections and cervicovaginal microbiota is an expanding field of research, where dysbiosis increases the risk of cancer in vulnerable populations (Angeletti et al., 2020). Through such relations by virtue of thorough surveillance, public health programs can design interventions to address viral persistence and resultant diseases. Essentially, global surveillance serves as a pillar of virology in medical microbiology, providing us with information needed to make informed, productive public health actions.

Test Your Knowledge

1. What are the principal determinants of the emergence and re-emergence of viral disease?
2. How does global surveillance contribute to the control of viral outbreaks?

Summary

In summarizing an investigation of general virology in medical microbiology, there is a need to acknowledge the revolutionized progression that virology has experienced from its beginning as a scientific field. The development of virology into a recognized scientific field was characterized by major leaps in pathogen virulence understanding, resulting in objective virus characterization. This path necessitated more than the mere aggregation of facts; it involved the complex process of objectification, where virulence concepts were actively produced and constructed through a number of different scientific practices. As outlined within the discussion of the objectification of the virus, the science of virology was developed from decades of dispersed research, readjusting methodologies and technologies in order to form a coherent picture of viral agents (Van Loon, 2002). This groundwork impacts current strategies in virology and its place within medical microbiology. Additionally, the continuous evolution of virology emphasizes the dynamic interplay between scientific breakthrough and technological innovation. The International Committee on Taxonomy of Viruses (ICTV) has been instrumental in curating and categorizing viral diversity, which acts as a foundation for future investigation and clinical utility. Looking back on the last half-century of the ICTV's history, it is evident that there has been a dedication to keeping in line with technological progress and facilitating communication among members of the virology community. The recent projects funded by grants, designed to advance online resources and facilitate dialogue, indicate an active response to challenges in virus taxonomy and characterization (Adams et al., 2017). Such collaborative work is essential in addressing the intricacies of viral diseases, highlighting a multidisciplinary model that remains essential in medical microbiology. In conclusion, the summary of this discussion underscores that general virology is a vital aspect of medical microbiology, intimately interconnected with scientific progress and public health. As our knowledge of viruses grows and develops, its implications for medical science grow ever more profound. The intricate interplay between scientific research, technological advancement, and practical utility makes ongoing research and interdisciplinary collaboration ever more essential. An awareness of historical context and current developments in virology enables us to grasp the essential contribution it is making towards solving global health issues. Finally, the history of virology is not just one of scientific success but also one of public responsibility in safeguarding public health from viral infection.

The history of virology, as it is portrayed in the context of medical microbiology, highlights the evolutionary process through which viruses evolved in scientific knowledge. At first, the research on viruses was characterized by experimental work devoid of an integrated approach, and there were difficulties in comprehending pathogen virulence. With time, technological and methodological advancements have enabled the objectification of viruses, making it easier to study them in a more complete manner. The development was not a straight line but a series of interactions between different branches of science that helped develop virology as a separate science. The creation of a purported "virology-assemblage" in the early 1950s was decisive, for it enabled the collaborative development of knowledge and techniques, which ultimately provided researchers with the ability to investigate viruses with some coherency not before attained (Van Loon, 2002).

The emergence of human cytomegalovirus (HCMV) further demonstrates the vital convergence of virology and medical microbiology. HCMV illustrates the intricacies of viral pathology since it can be latent in the host for life and reactivates with potentially devastating consequences, especially in vulnerable groups such as congenitally infected infants or immunocompromised patients. Among the primary challenges of HCMV infection control is the development of antiviral resistance, coupled with the unavailability of effective vaccines. This complexity is increased by the ability of HCMVs to evolve fast, using immune evasion tactics that make therapies challenging. The research on HCMV's genetic makeup and evolutionary patterns continues to demonstrate how recombination processes contribute to high genetic diversity, making treatment more challenging and highlighting the importance of new methodologies in developing vaccines (Atkinson et al., 2016). Finally, the analysis of viral dynamics in the context of medical microbiology presents the complex interactions between host immune responses and viral evolution. The potential of viruses like HCMV to quickly evolve and diversify by homologous recombination has important consequences for clinical management and the development of antiviral therapies. As emphasized, the hyper-variable zones within the viral genome that code for proteins important in immune evasion not only indicate a survival strategy but also shed light on the continuous arms race between host defenses and viruses. Through ongoing research into these evolutionary trends, medical microbiology can lead to greater knowledge of virus-host interactions and ultimately drive the efforts toward fruitful treatments and vaccines specifically designed to address the constantly evolving threats of viral pathogens (Atkinson et al., 2016).

KEY TERMS FROM THIS CHAPTER

- Antimicrobial drugs
- Chronic infections
- DNA integration
- Double-stranded (dsDNA)
- Health threats
- Histocompatibility complex (MHC)
- Host-pathogen interactions
- Human immunodeficiency virus
- Immune system
- Antiviral drugs
- Diagnostics simplification
- DNA viruses
- Hand, foot, and mouth disease (HFMD)
- Healthcare professionals
- Host defense
- Human health
- Human papillomavirus
- Influenza pandemics

Critical Thinking Questions

1. **Which of the following best describes a feature of viruses?**
   a. They have both DNA and RNA within the same viral particle
   b. They can replicate independently without a host cell
   c. Their genetic material can be single or Double-stranded
   d. They have ribosomes for protein synthesis
2. **During the viral replication cycle, which step involves the synthesis of viral nucleic acid and proteins?**
   a. Attachment
   b. Penetration
   c. Release
   d. Biosynthesis
3. **Which of the following best explains how viruses cause disease in the host?**
   a. By directly damaging or killing host cells during replication
   b. By replicating independently in host tissues
   c. By inducing uncontrolled cell division in all cases
   d. By synthesizing toxins like bacteria
4. **What is the most commonly used method to detect viral nucleic acids in patient samples?**
   a. ELISA
   b. PCR (Polymerase Chain Reaction)
   c. Western blot
   d. Viral culture
5. **Which of the following is an effective preventive measure against many viral infections?**
   a. Broad-spectrum antibiotics
   b. Vaccination
   c. Corticosteroids
   d. Antifungal medications

Short Answer Questions

1. Outline the key structural elements of an average virus and describe how the viral structures lend themselves to viral classification.
2. Distinguish between DNA and RNA viruses based on genome structure, replication strategy, and examples of clinically important viruses.
3. Describe the overall steps in the viral replication cycle and the role of host cell machinery in each process.
4. Contrast the replication strategies of lytic and lysogenic viruses, providing an example of a virus that uses each strategy.
5. Describe the most important mechanisms involved in the pathogenicity of viruses in humans, such as direct cytopathic effects and immune-mediated injury.

Answer to Critical Thinking Questions

1. (c); 2. (d); 3. (a); 4. (b); 5. (b)

References

1. Bedford, T., Suchard, M. A., Lemey, P., Dudas, G., Gregory, V., Hay, A. J., McCauley, J. W., Russell, C. A., Smith, D. J., & Rambaut, A. (2014). Integrating influenza antigenic dynamics with molecular evolution. *eLife, 3*, e01914. https://doi.org/10.7554/eLife.01914 (accessed on 13th June 2025).
2. Abedi, F., Alavian, S. M., Ataei, B., Azad, R., et al. (2013). *Drug-Related Mutational Patterns in Hepatitis B virus (HBV) Reverse Transcriptase Proteins from Iranian Treatment-Naïve Chronic HBV Patients.* https://core.ac.uk/download/52204674.pdf (accessed on 13th June 2025).
3. Adams, M. J., Davison, A. J., Gorbalenya, A. E., Harrach, R., et al. (2017). *50 Years of The International Committee on Taxonomy of Viruses: Progress and Prospects.* https://core.ac.uk/download/78908153.pdf (accessed on 13th June 2025).
4. Aldaz, J., Alfieri, A., Alfieri, A., Calleros, L., et al. (2018). *Inter- and Intracontinental Migrations and Local Differentiation Have Shaped the Contemporary Epidemiological Landscape of Canine Parvovirus in South America.* https://core.ac.uk/download/287884512.pdf (accessed on 13th June 2025).
5. Willett, B. J., & Hosie, M. J. (2013). Feline leukaemia virus: half a century since its discovery. *Veterinary journal (London, England : 1997), 195*(1), 16–23. https://doi.org/10.1016/j.tvjl.2012.07.004 (accessed on 13th June 2025).
6. Anderson, J. G., Goudie, A. C., MacGregor, S. J., Olateju, B., et al. (2003). *Inactivation of Pathogens on Food and Contact Surfaces Using Ozone as A Biocidal Agent.* https://core.ac.uk/download/9020578.pdf (accessed on 13th June 2025).
7. Angeletti, P. C., Kahesa, C., Klein, C., Mwalselage, J., et al. (2020). *How the Cervical Microbiota Contributes to Cervical Cancer Risk in Sub-Saharan Africa.* https://core.ac.uk/download/287614750.pdf (accessed on 13th June 2025).
8. Atkinson, C., Balloux, F., Breuer, J., Brown, R., et al. (2016). *Islands of Linkage in An Ocean of Pervasive Recombination Reveals Two-Speed Evolution of Human Cytomegalovirus Genomes.* https://core.ac.uk/download/96882557.pdf (accessed on 13th June 2025).
9. Bandea, C. I. (2009). *The Origin and Evolution of Viruses as Molecular Organisms.* https://core.ac.uk/download/pdf/288872.pdf (accessed on 13th June 2025).
10. Jon R. Cavicchi, Stanley P. Kowalski, et al, "Patent Landscape of Influenza A Virus Prophylactic Vaccines and Related Technologies" (2012). (accessed on 13th June 2025).
11. Butcher, S. A., & Gould, E. A. (1997). *Production of Positive Controls for Calicivirus-Specific PCR Using Recombinant Baculovirus Technology.* https://core.ac.uk/download/11020756.pdf (accessed on 13th June 2025).
12. Chrisafis, G. C. (2017). *Historical Patterns of Arboviral Seroprevalence Across Africa and Asia.* https://core.ac.uk/download/84397690.pdf (accessed on 13th June 2025).
13. Clark, J. J., Cumberworth, S., Donald, C. L., Kohl, A., et al. (2017). *Inhibition of Type I Interferon Induction and Signaling by Mosquito-Borne Flaviviruses.* https://core.ac.uk/download/80697084.pdf (accessed on 13th June 2025).
14. Dwivedi, L., & Shrivastava, M. (2011). *Anti-HIV Therapy: Pipeline Approaches and Future Directions.* https://core.ac.uk/download/pdf/289772.pdf (accessed on 13th June 2025).

15. Essex, M. (2014). *140 Reversing the Epidemic of HIV-1C in Southern Africa with Treatment as Prevention.* https://core.ac.uk/download/28951260.pdf (accessed on 13th June 2025).

16. Jha, A., Jarvis, H., Fraser, C., & Openshaw, P. J. M. (2016). Respiratory Syncytial Virus. In D. S. Hui (Eds.) et. al., *SARS, MERS and other Viral Lung Infections.* European Respiratory Society. (accessed on 13th June 2025).

17. Frolova, A. V., & Generalov, I. I. (2016). *Instructions for Laboratory Training in Special Microbiology and Virology for Students of Faculty of Dentistry.* https://core.ac.uk/download/53875198.pdf (accessed on 13th June 2025).

18. Kazakova, A. (2019). *Multiplex Diagnostics: Development of Serological Dual-Mode Multiplex Microarray Immunoassay and Analysis of Influenza and Respiratory Syncytial Virus Disease Burden in Early Childhood.* https://core.ac.uk/download/275894270.pdf (accessed on 13th June 2025).

19. Kinney, A. L. (2007). *National Scientific Facilities and Their Science Impact on Non-Biomedical Research.* http://arxiv.org/abs/0705.1797 (accessed on 13th June 2025).

20. Lau, S. K. P., Wong, S. S. Y., Yip, C. C. Y., Yuen, K. Y., et al. (2010). *Human Enterovirus 71 and Hand, Foot and Mouth Disease.* https://core.ac.uk/download/37950461.pdf (accessed on 13th June 2025).

21. McKie, A. (2003). *Immunity Surveillance of Mumps and Rubella: Improved Methods for The Detection of Virus-Specific Antibody.* https://core.ac.uk/download/9657304.pdf (accessed on 13th June 2025).

22. Nguyen, T. G. (2018). *Risk Assessment of Norovirus Infection Considering Indirect Impacts of Seasonal Flood in Southeast Asia.* https://core.ac.uk/download/636363275.pdf (accessed on 13th June 2025).

23. Olsson, G. E. (2003). *Nephropathia epidemica and Puumala Virus Occurrence in Relation to Bank Vole (Clethrionomys glareolus) Dynamics and Environmental Factors in Northern Sweden.* https://core.ac.uk/download/11694648.pdf (accessed on 13th June 2025).

24. Orlova, E. (2012). *Bacteriophages and Their Structural Organization.* https://core.ac.uk/download/19509491.pdf (accessed on 13th June 2025).

25. Hossein Mazouchian, Leila Roshangar*, Fariba Salek Ranjbarzadeh, Reza Piri, Mahdi Karimi Shoar, Leila Rasi Marzabadi. (2014). *Medical Students' View About the Effects of Practical Courses on Learning the General Theoretical Concepts of Basic Medical Sciences. Res Dev Med Educ.* 2014;3(1): https://core.ac.uk/download/pdf/27043736.pdf (accessed on 13th June 2025).

26. van Loon, J. (2002). A Contagious Living Fluid. *Theory, Culture & Society, 19*(5-6), 107-124. https://doi.org/10.1177/026327602761899174 (Original work published 2002)

DNA VIRUSES

2

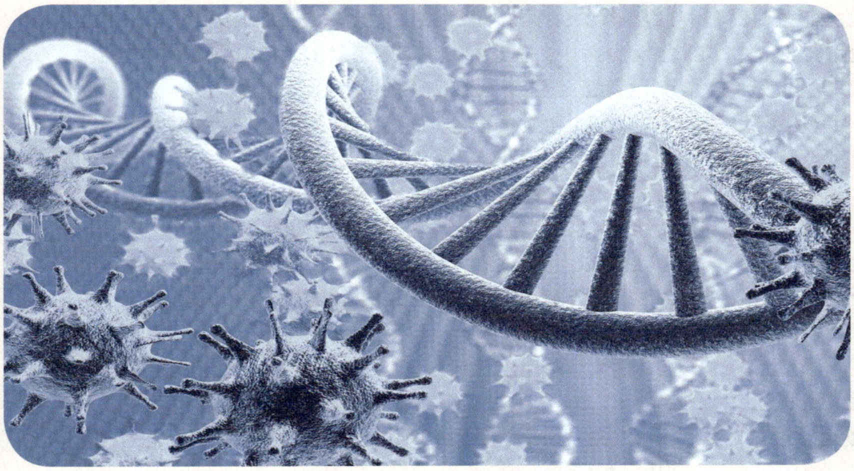

LEARNING OBJECTIVES

After studying this chapter, you will be able to:

1. Identify the category of DNA viruses;
2. Explain the DNA virus structure;
3. Describe the DNA virus replication cycle;
4. Discuss the pathogenesis of DNA viruses;
5. Coordinate DNA virus infection diagnosis;
6. Highlight the prevention and treatment of DNA virus infection.

Introduction

DNA virus research has become a more and more applicable field of study in the field of virology, especially when taking variability and complexity into consideration. These pathogens, with deoxyribonucleic acid as their genetic material, have a myriad of forms and patterns of infection. Unlike RNA viruses, DNA viruses are more stable in terms of their genome, which can be a key component in replication and pathogenicity. The necessity of these organisms' study cannot be overstated, as they are the etiologic agents of a wide variety of diseases in humans and animals, from benign to malignant. Understanding the mechanisms of DNA virus replication and pathogenesis has the potential to lead to new therapeutic agents, especially for viral infections that have been recalcitrant to conventional therapy. Advances in molecular techniques and sequence technology over the past few years have fueled the investigation of DNA viruses, allowing for more accurate analysis of their genomic structure and function. Techniques such as next-generation sequencing provide high-resolution descriptions of viral diversity and can be employed to detect less common viral strains responsible for disease. These tools allow researchers to detect a range of viral genomes from a variety of sources, expanding our knowledge of their epidemiology and evolutionary processes. For example, much has been learned about the role of certain DNA viruses, such as human papillomavirus (HPV), in carcinogenesis, with data indicating its prevalence in cervical cancers (Mensaert et al., 2015). These advances provide not only a basic understanding but also critical data to be employed to inform public health policy for viral disease prevention. Secondly, the importance of DNA viruses is not merely clinical in nature; they are also components of the broader ecological landscape. They interact with host cellular machinery and other microbes in complicated relationships that regulate health and disease states. These dynamics are worth grasping, as DNA viruses can modulate host cellular processes, impacting everything from cell cycle control to immune response modulation. Chronic infection by certain DNA viruses, for example, creates latent reservoirs, excluding therapy against viruses such as HIV-1 (Cole et al., 2020). Thus, knowledge of DNA viruses in the ecological landscape enhances our ability to develop integrated models of viral behavior and intervention strategies, further highlighting the need for specialized research in this field to address current global health challenges.

Definition of DNA Viruses

DNA viruses are a specialized group of viruses characterized by their genetic material consisting of deoxyribonucleic acid (DNA). The characteristic features differentiate them from RNA viruses, whose genetic material consists of ribonucleic acid. DNA viruses are classified into two broad groups based on their DNA structure: double-stranded DNA (dsDNA) viruses and single-stranded DNA (ssDNA) viruses. The structural features of the viruses play a major role in determining their replication processes and pathogenicity profiles. The classification of these viruses is significant not just to identify and study their biological impacts but to find effective antiviral drugs and vaccines. As sequencing technologies improve, a comprehensive database of genomic sequences aids to describe these viruses evolutionary relationships, further emphasizing the need to classify DNA viruses as a specialized group of viruses in virology (Fiscon et al., 2016). The replication processes of DNA viruses are relatively more stable compared to those of RNA viruses due to the semi-conservative mode of DNA replication. The characteristic leads to reduced mutation in DNA viruses, which potentially determines the degree of their evolutionary processes and interactions with host immune systems. In host-parasite co-evolution studies, the genetic stability of DNA viruses will frequently be consistent with an aligned rate of mutation that maximizes survival across a large host species range. Surprisingly, mutation rates in semi-conservative DNA viruses differ from conservative viruses, demonstrating how their genetic construction affects adaptability and virulence. This relationship is pivotal to virological research, as it reflects the interaction between genetic flexibility and stability, which in turn directs the formation of potential treatment and protective measures against DNA virus infection (Voet et al., 2004). From basic classification and replication of DNA viruses to the exploration of their pathological process within disease is crucial. For instance, certain DNA viruses are involved in oncogenic processes, where viral DNA inserts into the host genome and potentially leads to the formation of cancer. DNA virus mechanisms of inducing cellular transformation are complex and involve interaction within host cell pathways regulating growth and apoptosis. Furthermore, research into DNA virus diversification expands knowledge of their ecological roles and host interactions. With genomic sequencing continuing to identify new DNA viruses that were uncharacterized, the science of virology expands, requiring ongoing re-evaluation of current classifications and potential implications for public health (Voet et al., 2004; Fiscon et al., 2016).

Importance of Studying DNA Viruses

Understanding the significance of DNA virus research is not only crucial to medical science but also to the understanding of evolutionary biology and biotechnology applications. DNA viruses, like the human papillomavirus, are major disease contributors, of which cancers are included. HPV, for example, has been reported to have the potential to cause squamous cell carcinomas, hence its significance to oncological research. Over the past decades, scientists have put more effort into understanding the transcription machinery and viral protein interactions like the E2 protein of HPV5. This research will seek to understand how such viruses hijack cellular host mechanisms, potentially informing therapeutic interventions and an appreciation of virology's contribution to human health. By understanding specific viral interaction with cellular components, researchers can come up with effective prevention and treatment strategies against diseases caused by DNA viruses, a demonstration of the significance of ongoing research in the topic (Sankovski et al., 2018). In addition, DNA virus research extends beyond the appreciation of pathogenesis; it also aids in the understanding of viral evolution and mechanisms of gene transfer. Most DNA viruses have intricate life cycles that explain how viral genomes are inserted into the host DNA, influencing environmental adaptations as well as the evolution of the host organisms. Interestingly, during the process of cell division, some DNA viruses can utilize the mitotic process to partition their genomes into daughter cells, a process seen in major viruses like retroviruses and latent DNA viruses. This process not only provides insight into the virus-host interaction but also poses interesting questions about the evolutionary strategy utilized by such viruses to maintain their presence in the host population (Braeckmans et al., 2012). Understanding these mechanisms allows researchers to make more precise predictions about viral action and create new and innovative methods of gene delivery and therapeutic intervention. Aside from their biomedical importance, DNA viruses are also powerful tools in genetic engineering and biotechnology. What has been discovered from these viruses has facilitated great advances in gene therapy, vaccine technology, and delivery systems for genetic material. For instance, certain DNA viruses are genetically modified to produce viral vectors that introduce therapeutic genes into target cells with high efficiency. The capacity of viruses to target-specifically infect and integrate genetic material into host cells speaks to their usability. These applications not only demonstrate the usability of DNA viruses in human health but are also a testament to their utility in developing novel biotechnological solutions. Thus, studies on DNA viruses offer an integrated understanding that includes public health, evolutionary biology, and innovative approaches to therapy and are thus essential to future research (Sankovski et al., 2018).

2.1. Classification of DNA Viruses

Learning Outcome

1. Explain the types of DNA viruses;
2. Describe major families of DNA viruses.

The classification of DNA viruses is mainly determined by their structure and their replication mechanism. Scientists divide them based on their genome organization, for instance, whether they are single- or double-stranded DNA. Double-stranded DNA viruses, like herpesviruses and adenoviruses, are structurally more complex and may repurpose host cell machinery to replicate. Single-stranded DNA viruses, like parvoviruses, have less complex life cycles. The classification is important not just in the comprehension of the viruses' biological characteristics but also in the design of targeted therapy and vaccination. As research goes on, it has become clear that constantly evolving sequence information from next-generation sequencing platforms demands more sophisticated classification tools, highlighting the value of tools like phylogenetic trees and statistical models in illuminating evolutionary relationships in the vast DNA virus universe (Fiscon et al., 2016). Additionally, the DNA virus lifestyle dictates their classification, with cytopathic viruses that cause cell damage in contrast to non-cytopathic viruses.

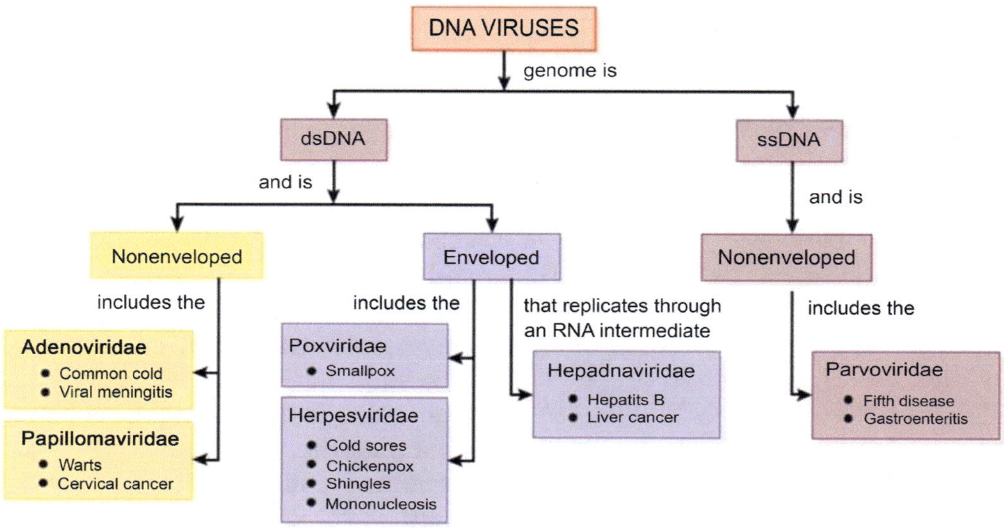

Figure 2.1. DNA virus classification.

Source: https://media.licdn.com/dms/image/v2/D4D22AQGgGyvDW46s9g/feedshare-shrink_800/feedshare-shrink_800/0/1695383159817?e=2147483647&v=beta&t=2ybGcKDQxZlpY2hfmZjlVfk0Gu5YQGnfud3XxGfwM_4.

For instance, some herpesviruses have latent infections that reactivate under specific conditions, positioning them in a different class compared to more virulent viruses. The comprehension of such lifestyle factors not only aids grouping but also influences public health activities, particularly in vaccine design and antiviral measures. The classification system has to be dynamic, embracing advances in genomic comprehension while highlighting viral behavior that guides epidemiological patterns. Thus, comprehensive databases and networks to facilitate tracking of such viruses are essential, affirming that multi-faceted objectives in virology aim towards an in-depth understanding of virus-host interactions (Cavicchi et al., 2012). The intricate taxonomy of DNA viruses eventually reflects the synergy between genetic diversity and pathogenic potential. Taxonomic systems emphasize the importance of central genetic features that establish such viruses, permitting systematic classification and identification. Secondly, with an increasing volume of research on DNA viruses, comprehension of their evolutionary trajectories becomes increasingly vital. New technologies, including comparative genomics and bioinformatics, permit researchers to categorize vast volumes of genomic data into meaningful classifications, shedding light on results previously masked. A stable taxonomy not only benefits scientific inquiry but also public health efforts by facilitating rapid responses to outbreaks through effective vaccine development and antiviral therapy. An ever-present revelation of DNA virus taxonomy is thus still of paramount significance in virology, as it guides research, clinical practices, and global health readiness (Fiscon et al., 2016) (Figure 2.1).

2.1.1. Types of DNA Viruses (Single-Stranded vs. Double-stranded)

Classification of DNA viruses into single-stranded (ssDNA) and double-stranded (dsDNA) viruses is key to their biology and pathogenicity. Single-stranded DNA viruses are usually smaller and less complex than dsDNA viruses. This category includes well-studied viruses such as Parvoviruses with limited genetic content and reliance on host cell systems for replication. Their simplicity can, however, make them effective adversaries for the host immune system, and they are successful in some niches. Since ssDNA viruses are most commonly associated with animal and human disease, their interaction with host systems advances our understanding of viral pathogenesis and treatment. The host immune system, on the other hand, may be more successful at combating dsDNA viruses, and studies have examined their specific mechanisms of evasion, an area of interest in the field of virology. Double-stranded DNA viruses provide a more complex model for investigation due to large genome size and heterogeneity in structure. This category includes large pathogens such as Herpesviruses and Adenoviruses, which include complex mechanisms of host defense evasion. For instance, Herpesviruses have evolved the capacity to integrate into the host genome to allow persistent infection and reactivation upon immune suppression. Their capacity to form stable reservoirs within the host makes treatment difficult, as conventional antiviral treatments may only affect active replication cycles. Additionally, dsDNA viruses have a tendency to give rise to a multifaceted immune response through multiple pathways, influencing the potential to induce autoimmunity under certain conditions. Information gained by the investigation of these viruses can shed light on general biological processes, as well as form the basis for therapeutic strategies to contain infection or autoimmunity caused by these pathogens, such as those involving Toll-like receptors (Anders et al., 2005). In addition, structural characteristics of ssDNA and dsDNA viruses are responsible for their functionality and interaction with host cells. Virus capsids with genetic materials possess distinctive charge distributions and geometry.

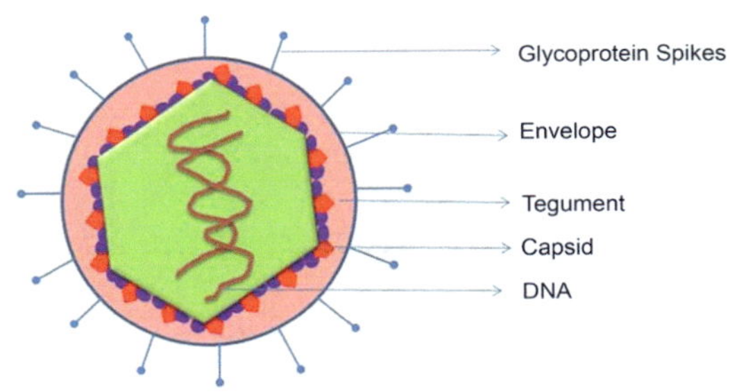

Figure 2.2. Double-stranded DNA viruses.

Source: https://www.researchgate.net/profile/Amit-Gaba/publication/235634464/figure/fig3/AS:578783715524608@1515004199804/Herpesviruses-are-enveloped-double-stranded-DNA-viruses-They-have-an-icosahedral-capsid.png.

Charge properties and geometry of viral capsids are able to provide profound insight into infectivity and entry processes of viruses into host cells. Surface charge, for instance, may influence binding affinity to cell receptors and consequently host range and tissue tropism. Charge distribution analysis based on integrative models is still unveiling our knowledge of viral behavior, as demonstrated in a prospective study (Božič et al., 2012). Implications of the results appear in vaccine design and antiviral strategy, indicating the significance of further study of the structural dynamics of ssDNA and dsDNA viruses (Figure 2.2).

2.1.2. Major Families of DNA Viruses (e.g., Adenoviridae, Herpesviridae)

The Adenoviridae family is vital in the study of DNA viruses because they possess a wide range of hosts, including mammals, birds, and reptiles.

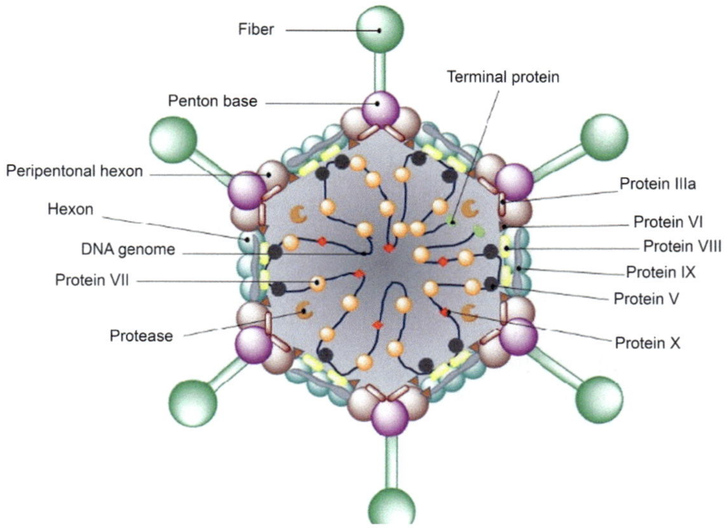

Figure 2.3. General structure of the Adenoviridae family.

Source: https://www.researchgate.net/profile/Jesus-Lujan-Montelongo/publication/357470377/figure/fig5/AS:1121095864332289@1644301491065/General-structure-of-Adenoviridae-family.png.

Adenoviruses have also been used in gene therapy and in vaccine production because they can induce immunity without the integration of the virus into the host genome. The viruses are also unique because they possess non-enveloped icosahedral capsids and double-stranded DNA, features that make them stable in the environment and effective as vectors. The adenoviruses have also contributed to the discovery of numerous types, including those from avian hosts, such as the fowl adenovirus (Hanson et al., 2006). The genomic diversity in the family makes the viruses promising as tools in the development of vaccines and in therapeutic strategies, thus making them vital in virology and public health. Herpesviridae is also a vital DNA virus family, and they are known to possess a complicated life cycle and the capability of causing lifelong infection in the host. The family includes well-studied pathogens such as Herpes Simplex Virus (HSV) and Varicella-Zoster Virus (VZV), both of which contribute significantly to morbidity in humans. The distinguishing feature of herpesviruses is their large double-stranded enveloped DNA genomes that can encode for over 100 proteins, thus making the possibility of complicated mechanisms of pathogenesis and immune evasion feasible (Figure 2.3).

Notably, research on various stratifications of herpesviruses in animals, e.g., those of bats, provides hints at their zoonotic transmission and emergence of novel viral strains (Allander et al., 2013). Understanding the clinical implications of herpesvirus infection enables specific therapeutic intervention and informs public health intervention in outbreak prevention. In addition to adenoviruses and herpesviruses, several other DNA virus families, such as *Papillomaviridae* and *Poxviridae*, contribute to the diversity of DNA viruses across different taxa. *Papillomaviridae*, in particular, are well known for their role in human papillomavirus (HPV) infections, which can result in cervical cancer and other cancers, making the importance of vaccination programs such as those for Gardasil all the more pertinent. In contrast, *Poxviridae*, which includes *variola virus* causing smallpox, presents a classic case of the potential threat of DNA viruses. The success of smallpox eradication demonstrates the efficacy of vaccines, while renewed interest in poxviruses as bioweapons underscores the importance of ongoing surveillance and research. All these families, thus, mirror the complexities of DNA viruses and their importance to human health, agriculture, and new paradigms for emerging infectious diseases (Figure 2.4).

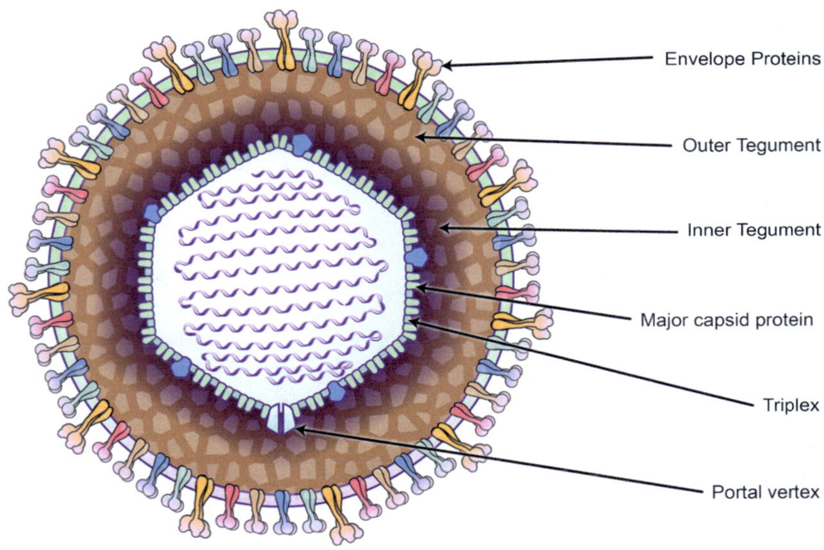

Figure 2.4. Herpesviridae.

Source: https://lsbio-7d62.kxcdn.com/Content/Images/Virology/Herpesviridae/Herpesviridae-Labeled.jpg.

Test Your Knowledge

1. What are the two main types of DNA viruses based on their genome structure?
2. Name at least three major families of DNA viruses and one disease associated with each.

2.2. Structure of DNA Viruses

Learning Outcome

1. Describe the capsid structure of viruses;
2. Know the composition of genetic material;
3. Focus on the existence of an envelope in DNA viruses.

DNA viruses possess intricate structural designs that allow for their survival and replication. Enveloping the viruses at their core is the genetic material, typically a single or double strand of DNA. This genetic code is contained in a protective envelope in the shape of a protein outer casing referred to as the capsid, which not only shields the viral DNA but also propels the virus's attachment and invasion of host cells. The capsid can take a broad range of shapes, from icosahedral to helical forms, depending on the adaptation to its specific biological niche. Some DNA viruses also possess an outer lipid envelope that comes from the host cell membrane and enhances their infectivity. These structures combined confer DNA viruses with the resilience they require to withstand environmental stress while effectively transmitting and infecting host organisms and facilitating a broad range of genetic and serological characteristics among various strains of DNA viruses (Orlova, 2012). The intricacy of DNA virus structures also manifests in the evolution of their capsid proteins, which demonstrate high heterogeneity among viral families. This heterogeneity is more than mere form; it has functional significance that enhances viral fitness and virulence. Some DNA viruses have also evolved sophisticated forms of packaging and delivering their genetic information, a process that is closely intertwined with their capsid design. For instance, some viruses employ specialized proteins to compact their DNA into the confined space of the capsid, while others can possess host-derived proteins that aid in immune evasion. Second, the interaction of the virus structure with the host cellular machinery is important because some DNA viruses hijack these pathways for assembly and replication. The data on these structural features give the key to the evolution and persistence of DNA viruses in ecological niches (Bandea, 2009).

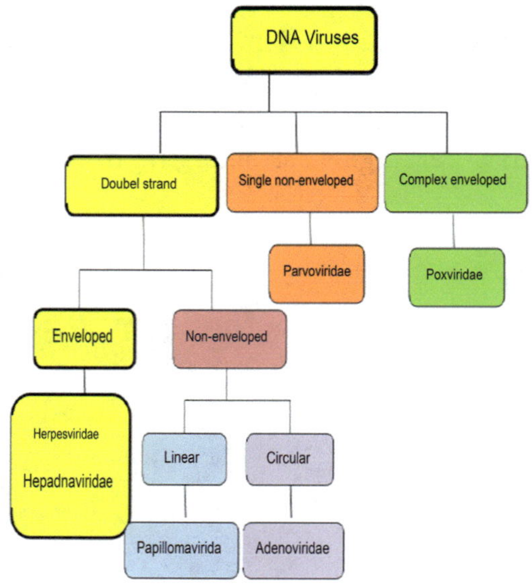

Figure 2.5. General DNA virus structure.

Source: https://www.researchgate.net/profile/Ahmed-Alzohairy/publication/260186052/figure/fig2/AS:297185636831234@1447865985926/General-DNA-Virus-structure.png.

Beyond fundamental biology, structural features have implications for the fields of therapeutics and vaccine development. Data gained from the investigation of DNA viral structures has resulted in novel approaches in the treatment of viral infections, such as the development of antiviral drugs that target viral targets. For instance, it is the knowledge of the capsid interaction with the cellular receptors that has resulted in the design of drugs that inhibit viral entry. In addition, the distinctive properties of DNA viruses are blueprints for synthetic biology applications, where aspects of their architecture can be utilized to design new vectors for gene therapy. As a result, research aimed at DNA viral structure not only improves our understanding of viral biology but also reveals opportunities for advanced medical procedures, rendering their importance in the overall context of infectious disease control (Orlova, 2012) (Figure 2.5).

2.2.1. Composition of Viral Capsids

Capsid structure is central to the understanding of viral form and function, particularly in DNA viruses. Capsids, composed of protein subunits assembling protective casings, are crucial to protecting the viral genome from damage by the outside environment while allowing for efficient infection of host cells. The architecture of the capsid protein subunit can be diverse; however, most DNA viruses exhibit icosahedral symmetry, which provides an extremely efficient and stable structure. Geometric organization minimizes the extent of encoded genetic information and provides space for additional function, such as receptor recognition sites that increase the infectivity of the virus. Structural complexity of such capsids is in line with principles outlined in the Caspar and Klug model, where regularity in protein shell organization creates stability and hardiness needed in viral transmission (Caspar et al., 2006). Beyond structural hardiness, the viral capsid structure also relies on the nature of encapsulated genomic material. In most DNA viruses, the virion encloses long stretches of genomic nucleic acids that must be efficiently packaged to avoid degradation and deliver to host cells. Evidence indicates that viral genomes will evolve to compact forms optimized for encapsulation; compactness is not merely beneficial for physical containment of the genome but also maximizes stability in transmission. Of particular importance, the complex folding and branching of viral RNAs allow them to be packed into minimal volumes without loss of structural integrity required for replication. As emphasized in earlier research, such characteristics reflect the evolutionary constraints placed on viral genomes to maximize fitness for successful infection and progeny production (Ben-Shaul et al., 2014). Heterogeneity of protein composition and structure present in viral capsids reflects DNA virus plasticity to accept changing environmental conditions and host interactions. Flexibility of capsid size, shape, and surface features can have a significant influence on the survival and virulence of a virus. In the context, the viral capsid composition study not only illuminates basic viral biology considerations but also informs regarding how such entities interact with host organisms. Knowledge of these processes is critical for the design of targeted antiviral therapies and vaccines. As researchers continue to investigate the complex relationship between capsid structure and viral virulence, detailed studies will progressively elucidate the subtleties of viral evolution and their influence on public health countermeasures to emerging viral threats (Figure 2.6).

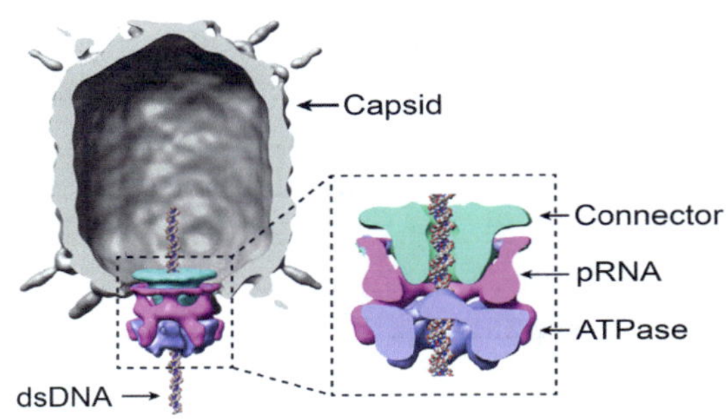

Figure 2.6. Cryoelectron microscopy reconstruction of the Phi 29 capsid (gray), connector (cyan), pRNA (magenta), and ATPase ring (blue).

Source: https://scx2.b-cdn.net/gfx/news/hires/2014/1-allintherota.jpg.

2.2.2. Genetic Material and Its Organization

Genetic organization is a fundamental characteristic of cellular and viral life that dictates their functionality and evolutionary dynamics. Genetic organization and structure in DNA viruses dictate how such pathogens interact with their hosts. DNA viruses, double-stranded DNA viruses, or single-stranded DNA viruses have evolved means of hijacking host cellular machinery for replication and transcription. Such complex interaction is facilitated by the particular organization of their genomic sequences, which may consist of functional genes, regulatory elements, and host interaction elements. This structural feature enables DNA viruses to optimize their reproductive strategies and respond to varied environmental signals, suggesting the importance of genetic organization in viral biology and evolution. Interestingly, virus-bacterial host interaction can have profound effects on genetic material and organization. Some bacterial strains have specialized capacities in communication and coordination, facilitated in part by their interaction with viruses, which may induce horizontal gene transfer and vertical colonization in ecological niches. This interaction not only contributes to the genetic diversity of the bacterial community but also illustrates how viruses, once thought to be simple infectious agents, influence the genetic makeup of their hosts. As Witzany (2008) surmises, the role of viruses extends beyond pathogenesis; they drive dynamic reorganization of genetic material in the bacterial world, exposing a rich interrelation that enhances evolutionary resilience in microbial communities. Moreover, the evolutionary history of viruses renders it impossible to view them as simple parasites; rather, they can be an independent and central lineage that drives the evolution of cells. The thesis that viruses originated from parasitic cellular organisms opposes the traditional perceptions and suggests that their genomic organization is the result of a sophisticated evolutionary process. As Bandea (2009) posits, this thesis provokes a reevaluation of viral taxonomy and its functional placement within the Tree of Life. The suggestion that viruses are molecular organisms exposes their potential to be actors in genomic reorganization and innovation, with serious implications for our comprehension of the organization of genetic material across all lines of life. This continued exploration of the texture of viral genomes points to the need for an interrelated methodology in the study of genetic material, filling the cellular and viral biology gap.

2.2.3. Envelope Presence and Its Significance

The presence of an envelope in DNA viruses plays a critical role in determining their pathogenicity and modes of transmission. Enveloped viruses are characterized by the presence of a lipid membrane derived from the plasma membrane of the infected cells, which covers their viral capsid and genetic material. The envelope, in addition to providing a protective sheath against environmental elements, also facilitates the fusion of the viral membrane with the host cell membrane. Through this, it facilitates the entry of the viral genome into the host cell, which is a central event in the viral life cycle. The envelope also carries glycoproteins of significance in the recognition and attachment to host cell receptors, hence enhancing the virus's infectivity as well as host adaptability to various hosts in various ecological niches. Additionally, the envelope role extends beyond the question of entry into host cells; it is implicated in evading the host immune system. For instance, enveloped DNA viruses can distort or shed their envelope proteins, which can be misleading to the host's immune system, and hence, vaccine design and therapeutic intervention become complicated. The hepatitis B virus (HBV), a DNA virus with a described envelope, has an impressive genetic variability, rendering it difficult to eliminate (Cuestas et al., 2015). The presence of surface gene variants, which occur under selective pressure from vaccination and antiviral therapies, implies the role of the viral envelope not only as an infectivity determinant but also as a critical determinant of the capacity to evade immune detection and persist in the host. Unlike enveloped DNA viruses, non-enveloped ones depend on other strategies of immune avoidance and invasion of cells. Non-enveloped DNA viruses, like adenoviruses, are more compact in shape and use alternate pathways for entry into host cells. They use capsids made of proteins that are resistant to harsh conditions and are therefore highly stable. But the absence of an envelope also constrains them from being as capable of modulating immune responses as enveloped viruses. Non-enveloped viruses possess certain surface features that can make them more detectable by host immune cells, both as a plus point for making vaccines and as a weakness to be avoided for long-term immunity. Therefore, it is essential to understand the differences between enveloped and non-enveloped DNA viruses to design effective vaccines and treatments against these numerous viral pathogens (Cannon et al., 2002).

Test Your Knowledge

1. What is the major function of the viral capsid in DNA viruses?
2. What is the overall makeup of the genetic material of the DNA virus within the capsid?

2.3. Replication Cycle of DNA Viruses

Learning Outcome

1. Explain the entry of DNA viruses into host cells;
2. Comprehend DNA virus replication and transcription mechanisms;
3. Describe how assembly and release of newly synthesized virions are crucial phases in the life cycle of DNA viruses.

The DNA virus replication cycle constitutes a sophisticated interaction of viral and host cell machinery that results in effective viral offspring transmission. To initiate the replication, DNA viruses initially bind to host cell receptors that enable entry into the cytoplasm or directly into the nucleus, where they can utilize host nucleotides and host enzymes. Upon entry into the nucleus, the viral DNA is typically brought into chromatin, utilizing the host's transcription machinery for replication. This is significant since the interaction between the viral genome and the host's cellular transcription factors has the potential to radically change the overall cellular environment, enabling the virus to exploit the host's cell cycle machinery. Unlike RNA viruses, DNA viruses significantly rely on host DNA replication machinery, and thus, it is critical to comprehend these mechanisms to formulate therapeutic responses against viral infections (Needham et al., 2023). As DNA viruses progress through their replication cycles, they induce crucial changes in the host cell's physiological states by coordinating changes in the cell cycle. For instance, most DNA viruses effectively arrest the cell cycle at specific checkpoints to enable the availability of cellular resources required for effective viral replication. This manipulation is typically accomplished through the expression of viral proteins that influence significant regulatory proteins of the host cells. Of significant note, the large T antigen of BK polyomavirus induces entry into the S phase while triggering the DNA damage response (DDR), though paradoxically, the DDR is meant to arrest over-replication (Needham et al., 2023). This hijacking of host processes not only facilitates viral replication but also constitutes a precarious balance between viral persistence and host cell integrity. It has been determined in studies that such dynamic interaction may lead to chronic infection if the viruses successfully evade host immune responses. In addition, the

DNA damage response is pivotal to the DNA virus replication cycle and impacts the life processes of the host and virus. Viruses such as human papillomavirus (HPV) utilize DDR pathways so as to create favorable conditions for their replication. Through interaction with the ATM and ATR signaling pathways, HPV suppresses the host's immune response and avoids mechanisms that would be counterproductive to viral infection. Such manipulation of cellular stress responses reflects the evolutionary mechanisms employed by DNA viruses to gain persistence in hosts while ensuring widespread transmission. Complete comprehension of such mechanisms, therefore, not only provides insights into viral pathogenesis but also determines potential targets for antiviral therapies that could disrupt such interactions. Finally, the DNA virus replication cycle constitutes the dynamic interaction between pathogen exploitation and host cellular regulation, a crucial area of study for the elimination of viral diseases (Figure 2.7).

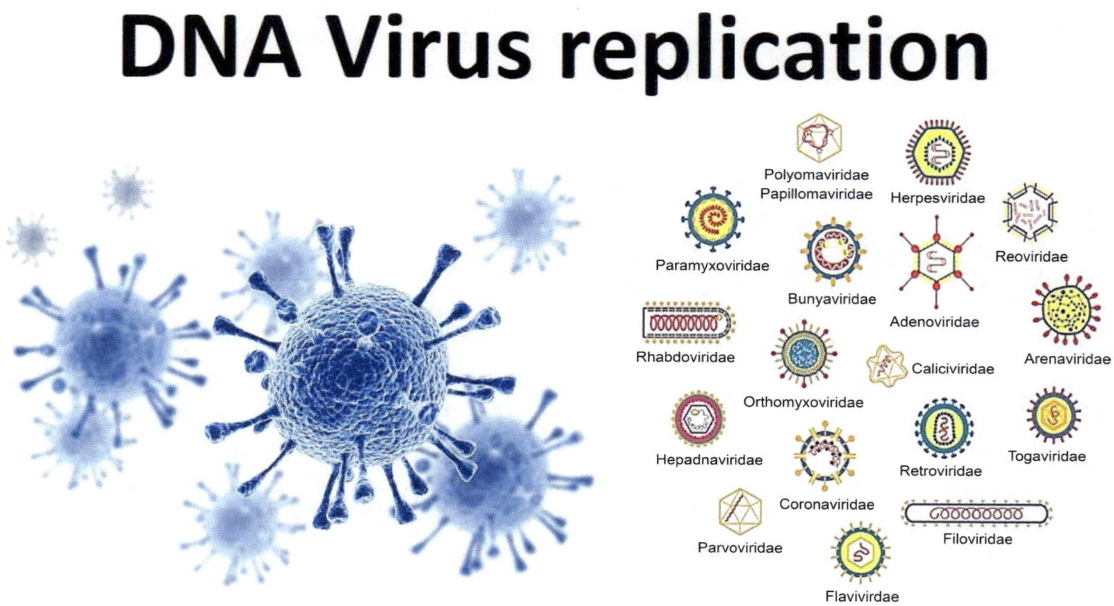

Figure 2.7. DNA virus replication.

Source: https://i.ytimg.com/vi/nR9e7eXm7gk/maxresdefault.jpg.

2.3.1. Entry Into Host Cells

The entry of a DNA virus into the host cell is complex and well-regulated and is pivotal in the initiation of viral replication. Primarily, this entry is facilitated through specific virus surface protein-receptor host interactions, which facilitate attachment and subsequent fusion. Following attachment, other pathways such as receptor-mediated endocytosis are employed for the delivery of the virus to the host cytoplasm. Through this mechanism, the virus can circumvent the host defense system, thereby ensuring the potential for successful infection. Interestingly, viral entry is not just virus nature but also host immune response and cellular environment status dependent, suggesting a dynamic interaction that modulates the virus's capacity to infect and transmit within the host (Blanc et al., 2012). Following entry and attachment, the transfer of the viral genome into the host cell nucleus is pivotal to the infection process. DNA viruses must ensure that their genomes are successfully imported into the nucleus, a process typically mediated by viral proteins that mimic cellular host processes. Interestingly, this entry serves to set the stage for viral gene transcription and viral DNA replication, ultimately leading to the assembly of new virions. The efficiency of this nuclear entry can play a critical role in viral pathogenesis, as interference at this juncture can lead to reduced viral loads or even immunological clearance of the host (Blanc et al., 2012). An in-depth understanding of the molecular mechanisms through which DNA viruses enter host cells is thus of absolute importance to the design of therapeutic interventions against these processes. Additionally, the evolving landscape of genome editing technologies, such as CRISPR-Cas9, presents promising options in the battle against viral infection through direct viral DNA targeting. The technologies can potentially make feasible the precise editing of the host genome to inhibit DNA virus replication by interfering with critical viral genes. Besides showing the versatility of modern antiviral methods, this approach also highlights the need for efficient delivery mechanisms to make possible the effective use of these technologies in the clinic. However, it is crucial to address the problems that accompany it, such as the risk of off-target effects and the development of viral escape mutants that would render such therapies useless. Thus, promising as it is, the application of genome editing to treat DNA viruses requires continued studies and careful consideration of the various factors involved in viral entry and pathogenesis (Figure 2.8).

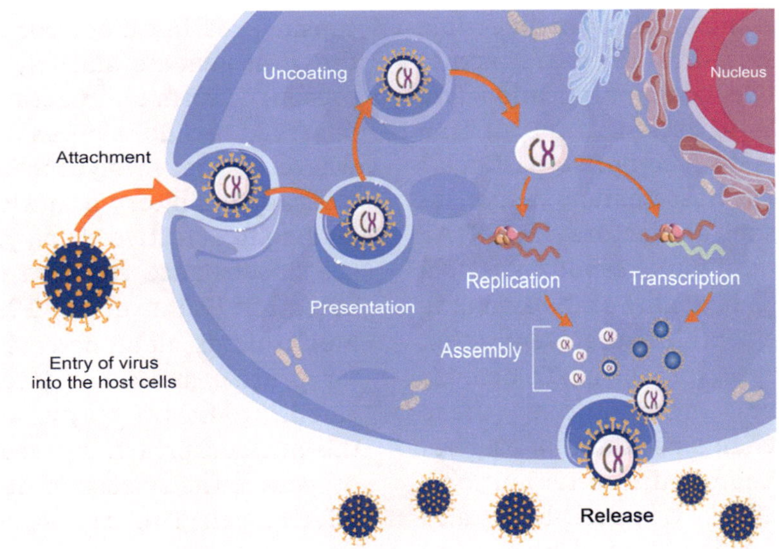

Figure 2.8. Mechanism of virus entry and replication in host cells.

Source: https://www.researchgate.net/publication/343804004/figure/fig1/AS:11431281212024262@1702524990492/Mechanism-of-virus-entry-and-replication-in-host-cells.tif.

2.3.2. Mechanisms of Replication and Transcription

The DNA virus replication and transcription mechanisms are extremely intricate, allowing them to hijack the host cell machinery to replicate. Unlike RNA viruses that utilize RNA-dependent RNA polymerases for replication, DNA viruses tend to utilize host DNA-dependent DNA polymerases. Upon infection of the host cell, the viral genome is brought into the nucleus, where it may integrate into the host's genomic DNA or replicate autonomously. While doing so, the virus might hijack the regulation of the host's cell cycle, making a welcoming environment for replication. For instance, some viruses, like the human papillomavirus (HPV), utilize the cellular DNA damage response (DDR) pathways to facilitate viral genome replication while concurrently suppressing the hosts innate immunity, hence evading detection and enabling persistent infection. This viral-host machinery interaction is a testament to the strategic complexities DNA viruses employ in their life cycles (Bordignon et al., 2017). Gene transcription of DNA viruses tends to involve the utilization of the host's transcriptional machinery. Upon infection of a cell by a DNA virus, it must utilize mechanisms to ensure its genome is effectively transcribed into mRNA for it to synthesize needed viral proteins. The viral DNA comprises early genes that are expressed immediately upon infection, which can proceed to control the expression of subsequent genes needed for replication and assembly. Most DNA viruses, like the African swine fever virus (ASFV), comprise particular proteins that suppress host immune responses or bind to transcription factors like STAT proteins, crucial for antiviral responses (Costa et al., 2011). Through hijacking of the signaling pathways, viruses can optimize their replication while efficiently suppressing the host's defense systems. Therefore, understanding these transcriptional mechanisms illuminates viral pathogenesis and therapeutic interventions. Mechanisms of viral transcription and replication not only facilitate viral replication but also provide therapeutic opportunities. Understanding how DNA viruses hijack host cell machinery will inform the development of antiviral interventions to interfere with these mechanisms. Interfering with the hijacking of viral proteins of DDR pathways or modulating the host's transcriptional responses, for example, will enhance treatment efficacy. In addition, understanding the nuances of these interactions enables the design of vaccines that can efficiently elicit robust immune responses against viral infection. With new evolving viral strains and the identification of new DNA viruses, the study of these mechanistic features remains essential in the ongoing efforts to counteract viral disease effects in agricultural and human contexts (Bordignon et al., 2017).

2.3.3. Assembly and Release of New Virions

The assembly and release of new virions are central processes in the DNA virus life cycle and dictate the efficiency of viral replication. Following replication of the viral genome, assembly initiation commences with encapsidation of the nucleic acid into the protein shell, or capsid. This is governed by intricate interactions between viral proteins and the host cell environment. In particular, viral capsid proteins must correctly interact with the viral genome and any structural proteins present to form an intact nucleocapsid. This is observed in Sindbis virus mutant experiments, where defects in glycoprotein interaction are critically inhibitory to nucleocapsid formation, leading to defective virion yield, demonstrating the fine balance required for successful viral assembly (Hahn et al., 1989). Such complex mechanisms demonstrate the requirement for precise molecular interactions to confer viability to the progeny virions assembled. With the nucleocapsid fully assembled, the second process is the release of new virions from the infected cell. This can occur through a variety of routes, such as cell lysis or budding. For enveloped DNA viruses, budding is the most prevalent route, which involves incorporation of viral glycoproteins into the host cell membrane. These proteins are responsible for the addition of a lipid bilayer, creating an envelope around the newly formed viral particle. Development of envelopes is not merely a structural modification; it also facilitates protection of virions from the host immune system and facilitates subsequent infection of new host cells (Orlova, 2012). Glycoprotein expression failure or glycoprotein-nucleocapsid interaction abnormalities may lead to non-infectious particles, suggesting coordination of molecular components during this important step in the viral life cycle. Assembly efficiency and release of virions significantly impact the virus's virulence and transmissibility. Control over the assembly processes can lead to a range of outcomes, from the production of fully infectious virus to defective virions that are unable to transmit the infection. Investigation of mutant strains, including glycoprotein mutant strains, demonstrates how single genetic changes can disrupt the intricate assembly process, leading to a lower yield of viable virions (Hahn et al., 1989). This advanced understanding of viral assembly and release processes guides the design of therapeutic agents that target these processes. By inhibiting individual interactions or channels of virion assembly, antiviral agents can effectively reduce viral titers and reduce the impact of DNA virus infection on host organisms. The exploration of assembly and release thus not only contributes to our knowledge of virology but also guides potential interventions in infectious disease (Figure 2.9).

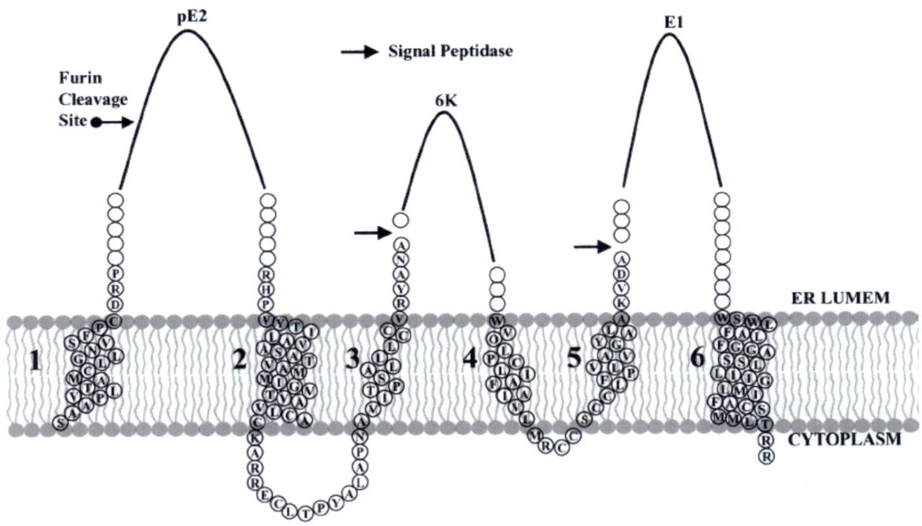

Figure 2.9. A schematic representation of the organization of the Sindbis virus structural proteins in the membrane of the ER. The integrated polyprotein has six transmembrane domains labeled 1 to 6.

Source: https://www.researchgate.net/profile/Raquel-Hernandez-14/publication/9015712/figure/fig1/AS:280168108183561@1443808690552/A-schematic-representation-of-the-organization-of-the-Sindbis-virus-structural-proteins.png.

Test Your Knowledge

1. Through what mechanism do DNA viruses generally enter host cells?
2. Where in the host cell does DNA virus replication and transcription usually occur?

2.4. Pathogenesis of DNA Viruses

Learning Outcome

1. Identify the mechanisms of viral infection and disease;
2. Give the examples of DNA virus-induced disease;
3. Host immunity to DNA virus infections emphasis.

The process of DNA virus pathogenesis is a complex interaction between viral replication mechanisms and host immunity. Upon entry of DNA viruses into the host cell, they hijack the cellular machinery for viral genome replication, transcription, and translation. For instance, herpesviruses, favorite member of DNA viruses, are known to cause lifelong latent infections through integration into the host genome, evading immune detection. This latency is crucial because it leads to periodic reactivation, which appears in the form of clinical manifestations ranging from asymptomatic to severe manifestations. This duality, where a virus remains dormant but disrupts cellular functions upon reactivation, illustrates the challenge in the creation of effective vaccines and therapeutic agents. Hence, understanding viral-host interactions, particularly in asymptomatic infections, is essential to understand the way such viruses toggle between latency and active disease progression (Gentile et al., 2016). Another key aspect of DNA virus pathogenesis is the way that these viruses manipulate host immune responses to facilitate infection and persistence. Most DNA viruses have evolved different mechanisms to evade the innate and adaptive immune mechanisms. For instance, some viruses can inhibit MHC molecule expression, precluding the presentation of viral antigens and disrupting T-cell responses. This mechanism not only inhibits the immune system's detection of the virus but also allows for the virus to be present in the host persistently. In addition, viral non-structural protein interactions with host cellular processes are able to remodel the immune landscape, promoting a viral survival niche (Kohl et al., 2013). By deciphering the complexity of these immune evasion strategies, researchers are able to better understand the pathogenesis of DNA viruses and achieve more targeted therapeutic interventions. In addition, the pathogenesis of DNA viruses is further complicated by the co-infection phenomenon, which has a significant impact on disease outcome. When a host is co-infected with multiple viruses, including DNA viruses and other viral genera, the interaction can modulate the expression of clinical symptoms and the immune response. This is especially true in herpesviruses, in which co-infections are able to complicate the severity of the causative diseases, turning otherwise harmless or asymptomatic infections into debilitating health states. The implication of such interactions highlights the importance of considering a broader viral ecosystem in the context of studying pathogenesis. The integration of understanding of asymptomatic chronic infection with current research in host-virus dynamics is essential to an overall understanding of DNA virus pathogenesis and the corresponding public health implications (Gentile et al., 2016).

2.4.1. Mechanisms of Viral Infection and Disease

The innate immune system plays a crucial role in the defense against viral infections, particularly those caused by DNA viruses. Upon detection of viral invaders, host cells use receptors known as pattern recognition receptors (PRRs) to recognize pathogen-associated molecular patterns (PAMPs), such as viral DNA. These PRRs trigger a sophisticated cascade of signals that lead to the production of interferons (IFNs), which are central cytokines of the antiviral defense system. IFNs can trigger the expression of over 300 interferon-stimulated genes (ISGs) for a range of antiviral functions, boosting the host's ability to combat the viral threat. DNA viruses have, however, developed sophisticated mechanisms to evade this immune system, thus making the host-pathogen interaction sophisticated and the knowledge of such mechanisms essential for therapeutic interventions to be rendered effective (Costa et al., 2011). The African Swine Fever Virus (ASFV) is a classic representation of the sophisticated interaction between viral pathogenesis and host immune responses.

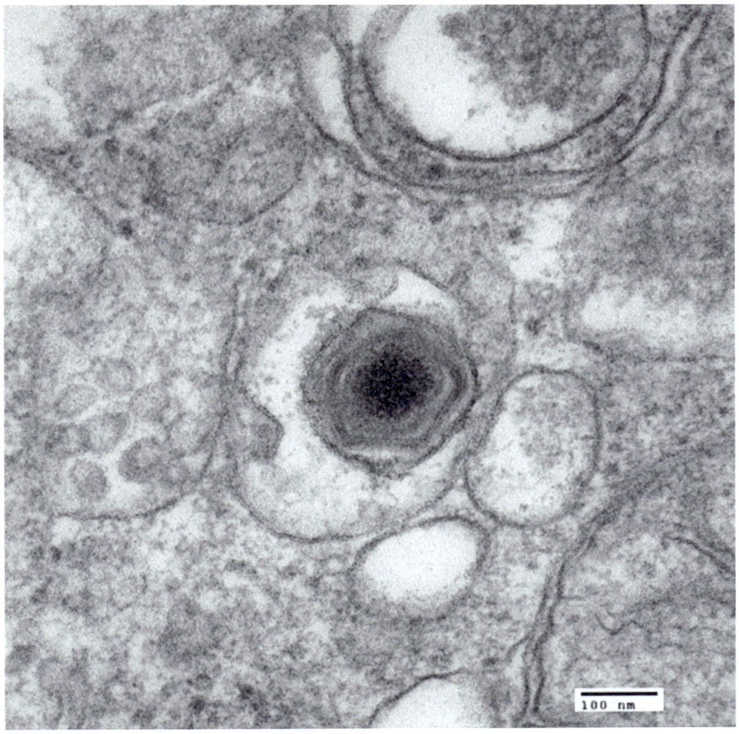

Figure 2.10. A photograph of an African Swine Fever virus.

Source: https://upload.wikimedia.org/wikipedia/commons/5/55/African_swine_fever_piadc.png.

Being a large DNA virus, ASFV infects monocytes and macrophages, exploiting the host cellular processes for survival and replication. Interestingly, ASFV has been found to encode genes for inhibiting apoptotic signaling and modulating immune responses, but curiously, no ASFV proteins to date have been known to inhibit the IFN response. This questions how ASFV survives and causes persistent infections in the presence of host defenses. Elucidating this viral evasion is essential as it may contribute to the development of targeted antiviral therapy and understanding the long-term impact on infected groups, thus enhancing the control of outbreaks in endemic and non-endemic regions (Gentile et al., 2016). Additionally, the interaction of chronic viral infections with host immune responses is key to disease outcome. Asymptomatic infection with some DNA viruses can have varied clinical presentations ranging from benign to severe disease. The impact of co-infections complicates the above, as they serve to modulate the immune response to the etiologic viral infection, determining its severity. The dynamic interaction calls for a keen understanding of host-viral interactions and the potential of resulting unforeseen complications of what might seemingly manifest as mild infection. As investigators re-engineer the traditional causality criteria by Koch's postulates to such modern complexities, they are headed towards a more sophisticated understanding of the way DNA viruses work in host systems, allowing for public health interventions and therapeutic interventions in curtailing their impact effectively (Gentile et al., 2016) (Figure 2.10).

2.4.2. Examples of Diseases Caused by DNA Viruses (e.g., Herpes, HPV)

DNA virus domain is a heterogeneous group of pathogens that infect and produce a large range of diseases in humans, including herpes simplex virus (HSV) and human papillomavirus (HPV). HSV is most well-known to produce painful oral and genital ulcers, but its impact is more extensive than the local ulcers. The virus may cause severe sequelae such as viral encephalitis, resulting in extensive neurological damage. HPV is also well-known to cause cervical cancer, one of the most prevalent cancers among women worldwide. The correlation between persistent HPV infection and oncogenesis is the virus's capability not only to cause benign warts but also to cause malignant transformation of epithelial cells, showing the range of diseases produced by DNA viruses (Thaker et al., 2019). The pathogenic action of such viruses is exacerbated by their capability to counteract the host immune system, enabling them to establish persistent infections. For example, HSV causes latency in neuronal cells, enabling it to remain dormant for a duration of years before reactivation, usually in stress or immunocompromised states. Such latency is especially difficult to prevent and treat. Likewise, some high-risk HPV types can integrate into the host genome, disrupting crucial oncogenes or tumor suppressor genes. The mechanisms by which such viruses counteract host cellular processes tend to be a complex interplay of viral and cellular mechanisms, which will need to be further studied to uncover their metabolic effect on host cells and potential therapy (Barzon et al., 2017) (Figure 2.11).

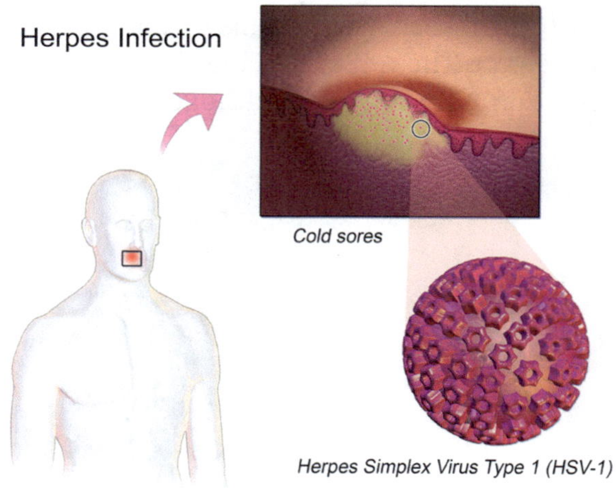

Figure 2.11. Herpes infection.

Source: https://upload.wikimedia.org/wikipedia/commons/thumb/7/71/Herpes_Infection.png/800px-Herpes_Infection.png.

With the growing disease burden due to DNA viruses, new therapeutic strategies are being developed. The emergence of genome editing tools such as CRISPR-Cas9 offers a promising solution for the targeting and inactivation of viral genomes, which will disrupt viral replication and subsequent disease progression. This approach would be directed against individual viral genes required for viral replication, and their expression suppression would be utilized to disrupt the life cycle of the virus. Off-targeting and resistant virus strains present challenges. These challenges would be significant to overcome for the successful translation of genome editing technologies from the lab to the clinic that could address the wide range of conditions caused by DNA viruses, including those involving HSV and HPV infections (Barzon et al., 2017; Thaker et al., 2019) (Figure 2.12).

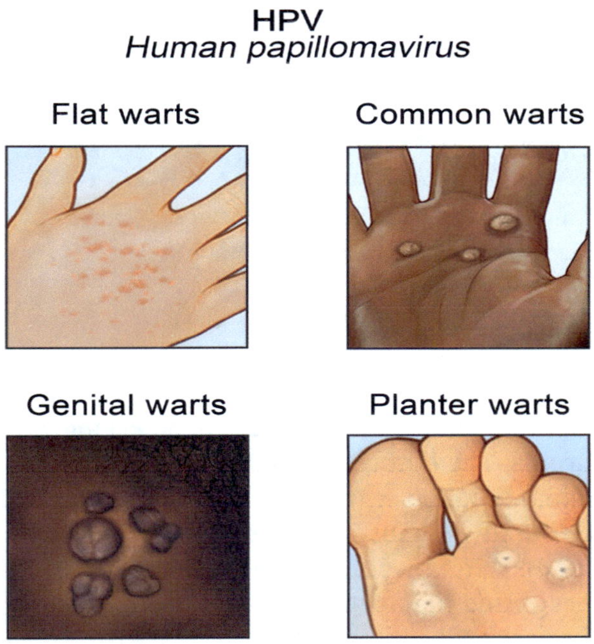

Figure 2.12. Human papillomavirus (HPV).

Source: https://my.clevelandclinic.org/-/scassets/images/org/health/articles/11901-hpv-human-papilloma-virus.

2.4.3. Host Immune Response to DNA Virus Infections

Host immune response to DNA virus infection is a multifaceted process, involving innate and adaptive processes that act together in harmony to clear the viral infection. When viruses infect the host, pattern recognition receptors such as toll-like receptors (TLRs) identify viral components, triggering activation of innate immune pathways. Activation triggers the production of pro-inflammatory cytokines and interferons that mediate the recruitment and activation of immune cells such as macrophages and natural killer (NK) cells. These innate responses form the basis of adaptive immunity, where T cells and B cells are activated to identify and kill infected cells specifically. Chronic infections, however, can result in immune evasion mechanisms developed by the virus, rendering it difficult to develop an effective immune response and causing chronic infection. Understanding these multifaceted dynamics is essential in developing effective therapeutic strategies against DNA viruses. Immune response in chronic DNA virus infections, such as those caused by hepatitis B virus (HBV) and human papillomavirus (HPV), is typically hijacked, with a good environment for viral persistence. Cellular components, such as Top2α, have been shown to play an important role in immunomodulation. In particular, various studies have shown that low expression and decreased activity of Top2α in T cells of chronically infected individuals lead to T cell dysfunction, inhibiting the body from mounting an effective immune response. Inhibition of Top2α has been shown to silence important pathways associated with DNA repair processes and cell proliferation, further complicating immune dynamics during chronic infections. This exchange underscores the need to investigate mechanisms of reversing such cellular functions to strengthen immune responses against chronic viral diseases, with host-pathogen interactions being of paramount importance. In addition, the DNA damage response (DDR) pathways also feature prominently in how DNA viruses can hijack host defense, ultimately causing chronic infection. For instance, human papillomavirus has been found to utilize the ATM and ATR DDR pathways, which are responsible for maintaining genomic integrity and cell cycle regulation. Through hijacking these pathways, HPV can extend the host immune response, allowing successful viral replication and immune evasion. This manipulation not only allows the virus to survive in the host but also allows the periodic release of infectious particles into the environment. As DNA viruses continue to evolve to improve survival and dissemination, comprehension of the mechanisms that govern their interaction with the host immune system is still pertinent. Investigation of the DDR and its association with viral life cycles may reveal opportunities for innovative therapeutic strategies to strengthen host defenses against DNA virus nfections.

Test Your Knowledge

1. What are the common mechanisms by which DNA viruses infect and produce disease in the host?
2. Name three diseases caused by DNA viruses and their respective causative viruses.
3. How do herpesviruses and other DNA viruses become latent in the host?

2.5. Diagnosis of DNA Virus Infections

Learning Outcome

1. Appreciate laboratory techniques for DNA virus detection in clinical practice;
2. Offer definitions of clinical symptoms of DNA virus infections;
3. Explain the importance of proper diagnosis in the management of DNA viruses.

Diagnosis of DNA virus infections is a critical component of virology that can play a significant role in the patient's prognosis and therapeutic management. Diagnostic strategies have advanced significantly with the advancement of technology, now facilitating rapid and precise identification of viral pathogens. Traditional methods such as viral culture and serology are increasingly being supplemented or replaced with molecular techniques, such as PCR and next-generation sequencing. These advanced technologies enhance the sensitivity and specificity of virus detection and thus hasten intervention. With the increasing diagnostic virology services, healthcare providers are increasingly involved in performing procedures involving these advanced methods, ultimately with the objective of minimizing the burden of viral outbreaks on public health. Furthermore, guidelines for interpreting results based on different tests need to be developed to allow clinicians to make informed decisions based on laboratory results (Drew et al., 1987). A clear case for the need for rapid diagnostic capacity is illustrated in the management of emerging viral threats. The outbreak of 2019-nCoV in Wuhan, China, resulted in the realization of the need for rapid diagnostic interventions (Du et al., 2020). Within weeks of the outbreak, the WHO recognized the need for early detection to stop the outbreak and prevent further transmission. The experience illustrates the dynamics of viral infections and the need for responsive diagnostic tools. By giving top priority to rapid diagnosis for new DNA viruses, scientists can not only deploy resources efficiently but also enhance surveillance systems to respond quickly to a similar health emergency. Ultra-rapid molecular assays to identify viral nucleic acid in clinical specimens within hours are a breakthrough in the ongoing struggle against infectious diseases, particularly against the background of global health interests around new viral strains. To bring diagnostic advances to the clinic has transformed the face of DNA virus infection management, enhancing patient care outcomes and justifying antiviral regimens. Integrated diagnostic approaches are applied not only to identify a pathogen but also to quantify viral load and antiviral drug resistance. Integrated diagnostic protocols allow healthcare professionals to tailor interventions based on patient-specific profiles rather than employing a blanket strategy. As increasingly targeted antiviral therapies are developed, the importance of proper diagnosis will escalate. Research into diagnostic innovation must, therefore, remain a priority of healthcare systems everywhere. This emphasis will not only enhance patient management but also enhance public health responses to rising and emergent DNA virus threats (Drew et al., 1987).

2.5.1. Laboratory Techniques for Detection (e.g., PCR, Serology)

The advent of molecular techniques has transformed the clinical detection of DNA viruses, and polymerase chain reaction (PCR) is a keystone technique. PCR enables amplification of target DNA sequences, which allows for sensitive and rapid detection of viral genomes even in low-abundance samples. This is significant in emergent infectious diseases since it offers early diagnosis and enables the use of public health interventions to prevent viral spread. The family of PCR-based assays, including quantitative PCR (qPCR) and nested PCR, can be designed for use with particular viruses and optimized for specificity and sensitivity for diagnostic tests. Such advances underscore the utility of molecular detection techniques for the realization of the rapid diagnostic promise, which is critical in the outbreak management of DNA viruses, particularly when the initiation of intervention is necessary to control transmission and improve patient outcomes.

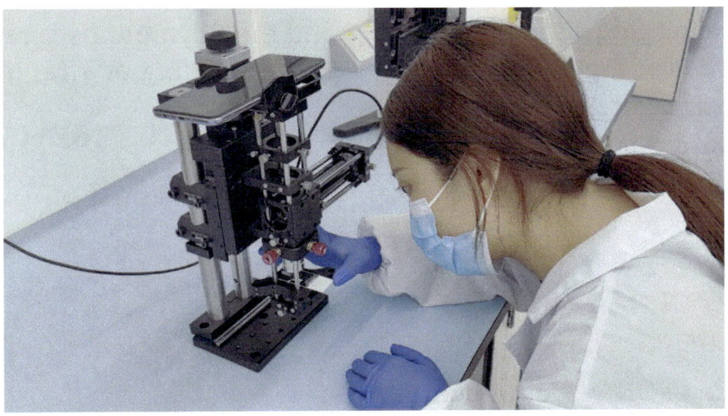

Figure 2.13. DNA virus detection system.

Source: https://cloudfront.jove.com/CDNSource/teasers/64833.jpg.

Serological tests supplement molecular techniques by the detection of antibodies induced by viral infection, which can be employed to gain information on the immune response of the host. The tests are particularly informative where direct detection of viruses by PCR is not feasible, e.g., in viral latency or chronic infection. They can identify infections of the past and apply them to identify epidemiological patterns useful in the design of public health interventions. Techniques, including enzyme-linked immunosorbent assays (ELISA) and Western blotting, can be employed to identify specific antibodies, which offer qualitative and quantitative information useful in informing vaccination policy and population immunity studies. Serological tests are also informative in the assessment of the efficacy of vaccines against DNA viruses through the measurement of the degree of antibodies post-immunization. Thus, the synergy between serological methods and molecular detection gives a panoramic view, enabling enhanced insights into viral dynamics and informing effective public health interventions. With advancing technologies, laboratory techniques for viral detection are increasingly sophisticated, with next-generation sequencing (NGS) being a new player in the field. NGS allows comprehensive genomic characterization of viral pathogens, including the detection of new strains and variants that potentially pose public health threats. The technique surpasses traditional approaches through the ability to sequence complete viral genomes from patient specimens, thus making it possible to correct epidemiologic tracking and investigation of outbreaks. However, the intricacies of NGS data become a challenge to researchers and clinicians as it demands cutting-edge bioinformatics capabilities in deciphering the huge volumes of generated data. However, the capacity of NGS to detect new DNA viruses quickly and accurately plays a key role in infectious disease management. As illustrated in recent reports, such as the ones addressing such emerging threats as the 2019-nCoV outbreak, the synergy of advanced detection methods continues to play a central role in facilitating global preparedness against future viral threats (Chiu et al., 2013; Du et al., 2020) (Figure 2.13).

2.5.2. Clinical Symptoms Associated with DNA Virus Infections

The clinical presentation of DNA virus infection is very variable depending on the virus and host determinants. For instance, herpesvirus infection, such as herpes simplex virus (HSV) and cytomegalovirus (CMV), typically presents with mild to severe symptoms ranging from lesions, fever, and fatigue. For instance, recrudescence can occur in HSV infection, leading to pain and discomfort in infected tissues. Similarly, CMV infection can lead to severe morbidity in immunocompromised hosts, leading to symptoms of hepatitis, pneumonitis, and retinitis. The variation in symptoms thus mirrors the variation in DNA viruses and the complexity of virus-host immune system interaction, which demands a multifaceted approach to diagnosis and treatment. In addition, the high prevalence of clinical symptoms of DNA virus infection demands effective treatment interventions. Herpesviruses, for instance, have a bifacial infection phase: an acute symptomatic infection phase and a latent phase. Current antiviral treatments can reduce the severity of clinical symptoms and suppress the frequency of recrudescence, but are not able to clear the virus effectively from the host system. Recently, the application of CRISPR/Cas9 technology has been explored to target and inactivate the genomes of latent herpesviruses, such as HSV and Epstein-Barr virus. The strategy has the potential to revolutionize antiviral therapy by providing a system to clear the virus completely from infected cells, potentially enhancing patient outcomes and alleviating the burden of recurrent symptoms of these infections (Chen et al., 2018). In addition, identification of new DNA viruses and their symptoms is required to enhance our understanding of viral pathogenesis.

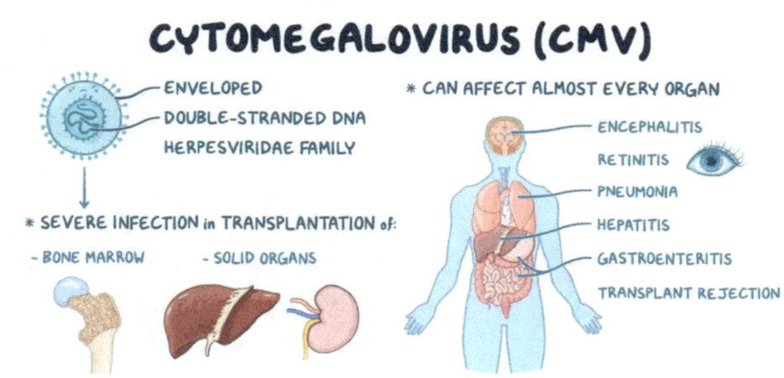

Figure 2.14. Cytomegalovirus (CMV).

Source: https://gccbiotech.in/wp-content/uploads/2024/03/CMV.png.

Human rhinovirus (HRV) strains have been the focus of recent studies, which have shown their extensive influence on respiratory well-being. Specifically, the emergence of HRV-C has been linked to a rise in rates of upper and lower respiratory tract infections among young children. Research has shown that HRV-C infection is frequently co-infecting with other respiratory viruses, allowing for the complex interplay to increase symptom severity. This requires the need for extensive diagnostic testing to determine co-infections that may further exacerbate clinical presentations. As researchers make further discoveries regarding mechanisms of these infections, it is crucial to implement more advanced diagnostic methods and treatment interventions to cover the wide range of clinical symptoms in DNA virus infections (Heim et al., 2009) (Figure 2.14).

2.5.3. Importance of Accurate Diagnosis for Treatment

Precise diagnosis is a predictor of successful treatment, particularly in the case of DNA viruses, where the clinical implications are severe. Early recognition of the viral agent provides specific therapeutic interventions that can optimize patient outcomes and avoid complications. For instance, the application of ultra-modern technologies such as clinical metagenomic next-generation sequencing (mNGS) enables clinicians to diagnose viral infection with precision. The method not only identifies the viral agent rapidly but also provides hints towards potential co-infection or co-microbial resistance, hence informing more effective treatment regimens. The integration of precise diagnostic methods is thus crucial since misdiagnosis can result in inappropriate therapies, further complicating the patient's condition, and increasing the public health burden (Chiu et al., 2019). The necessity for precise diagnosis is most evident in cases of outbreaks of new viral agents, such as the coronavirus known as 2019-nCoV. The speed of the virus's spread underscores the importance of rapid diagnostic methods to facilitate early intervention and control. In cases where misdiagnosis may potentially delay therapy, the implications can be disastrous, resulting in increased morbidity and mortality. Research into rapid diagnostic methods is thus crucial, not only to inform treatment regimens but also to inform public health interventions. Effective tracking and management of outbreaks largely rely on the ability to detect the causative agent accurately since this enables health authorities to institute prophylactic interventions in time (Du et al., 2020). Accurate diagnosis is thus not only beneficial to individual patient care but also to public health models. Moreover, the implications of accurate diagnosis extend beyond short-term treatment to long-term health models. Identification of the exact DNA virus causing an infection may affect vaccine development and the creation of specific therapies. For instance, identification of the genetic makeup of a viral strain enables the creation of vaccines and therapeutic tools to prevent subsequent epidemics. The healthcare system, therefore, needs to provide diagnostic credibility to inform research and development activities to effectively fight DNA viruses. Furthermore, integration of new diagnostic technologies into routine clinical settings will enhance our preparedness to fight emerging viral challenges, ultimately ensuring individual and community health. Continued development of diagnostic attributes emphasizes the significance of accurate diagnosis in optimizing treatment efficacy and minimizing the burden of infectious diseases (Chiu et al., 2019).

Test Your Knowledge

1. What are the most common laboratory tests employed to diagnose DNA virus infections?
2. Why is early and proper diagnosis of DNA virus infections critical in treating the patient?

2.6. Treatment and Prevention of DNA Virus Infections

Learning Outcome

1. List antiviral medications used against DNA viruses;
2. Describe vaccination procedures for DNA viral infections;
3. Emphasize public health strategies to manage DNA virus outbreaks.

Preventive and therapeutic strategies for DNA virus infections have much to catch up with, especially with the advent of vaccination approaches. Vaccines have remained the mainstay of prophylaxis against most viral diseases by eliciting an effective immune response upon exposure to the pathogen. The possibility of vaccine production, however, largely depends on the virus, and many of the most important DNA viruses remain far out of the reach of effective vaccines. New advances have seen new approaches being introduced, including passive transfer of monoclonal antibodies, as in the case of Synagis, to prevent and treat respiratory syncytial virus (RSV) infection. That trend more towards biochemical prevention highlights the need for developing alternative modes of immunological intervention that can supplement classic vaccination approaches, ultimately leading to our augmented arsenal against DNA virus infections (Fang et al., 2004). As researchers push for more effective means to bridge the gap of conventional therapy, breakthrough technologies such as the CRISPR/Cas9 system have emerged as powerful therapeutic agents. This genome editing system has the potential to target and eradicate the latency of herpesviruses, such as those causing herpes simplex virus and Epstein-Barr virus. The integration and efficiency of CRISPR/Cas9 enable viral genomes to be manipulated in ways previously not feasible, allowing us to analyze viral mechanisms and identify potential targets for therapy. With the current antiviral therapies against the latency of these infections having been shown to be of limited efficacy, the CRISPR/Cas9 system is being repurposed as a potential agent of viral eradication and long-term control of these DNA viruses (Chen et al., 2018). Successful management of DNA virus infections requires a multi-pronged strategy involving vaccination, monoclonal antibodies, and novel technologies such as CRISPR/Cas9. The heterogeneity of the DNA viruses requires specialized strategies involving prevention, treatment, and public health. Public health education campaigns directed at vaccination and herd immunity are paramount in reducing transmission rates. In addition, continued research into novel strategies for treatment, including the development of antiviral agents capable of synergizing with genome-editing technologies, will increase our ability to counter these infections. The combined strategy not only seeks to cure patients infected with DNA viruses but also to establish a sustainable reservoir for the reduction of the overall burden of DNA virus infections in communities globally.

2.6.1. Antiviral Therapies Available for DNA Viruses

The therapeutic landscape of DNA viruses has been revolutionized over the last few decades, in tandem with advances in molecular biology and pharmacology. Among antiviral therapies available, nucleos(t)ide analogs have emerged as a first-line treatment for many DNA virus infections, most notably those involving the hepatitis B virus (HBV). Lamivudine, entecavir, and tenofovir disoproxil fumarate are some examples of these agents, which inhibit viral polymerases and thereby viral replication. Their use has been vital in reducing HBV-related complications, including hepatocellular carcinoma (HCC). Nonetheless, it is important to note that although these agents can make serum HBV DNA undetectable, they do not remove covalently closed circular DNA (cccDNA) from hepatocytes, a reservoir that makes it difficult to treat (Coben et al., 2019). Hence, although effective treatment is possible for HBV, eradication is a gigantic unmet need. Another possible route of antiviral therapy for DNA viruses is the use of new biologic agents, most notably in the case of human papillomavirus (HPV) and associated malignancies. Immunotherapy, including therapeutic vaccines and immune checkpoint inhibitors, seeks to engage the patient's immune system against HPV-infected cells. These have been promising in clinical trials and may deliver a functional cure for HPV-related diseases by generating robust virus-specific T-cell responses. Lastly, the identification of genetically engineered technologies, including CRISPR-Cas9, has the promise of targeting and eliminating viral DNA in the host's genome specifically. This revolutionary approach has quenched interest in the development of therapeutic agents that can successfully target HPV by removing integrated viral sequences, arresting tumorigenesis. Collectively, these new strategies can result in effective antiviral treatments for DNA virus-related diseases, a paradigm shift in therapeutic models. The interplay of antiviral treatment and the application of induced pluripotent stem cells (iPSCs) has been a revolutionary new frontier in the prevention of DNA viruses. iPSCs provide a new platform upon which to construct patient-specific models to research the pathogenesis of viruses and host-pathogen interactions. These models enable researchers to provide greater insight into viral entry, replication, and persistence in human tissues, particularly in permissive cell types such as liver and neural cells. Furthermore, advances in genetic engineering techniques with iPSCs provide the potential to modify these cells to render them antiviral resistant, paving the way for new therapeutic strategies that target viral infection at its source (Barzon et al., 2015). As additional studies explore the enormous potential of iPSC technology, hope exists to find new antiviral therapies that not only improve patient outcomes but also resolve the long-standing conundrum of effective curative therapies for DNA viruses (Figure 2.15).

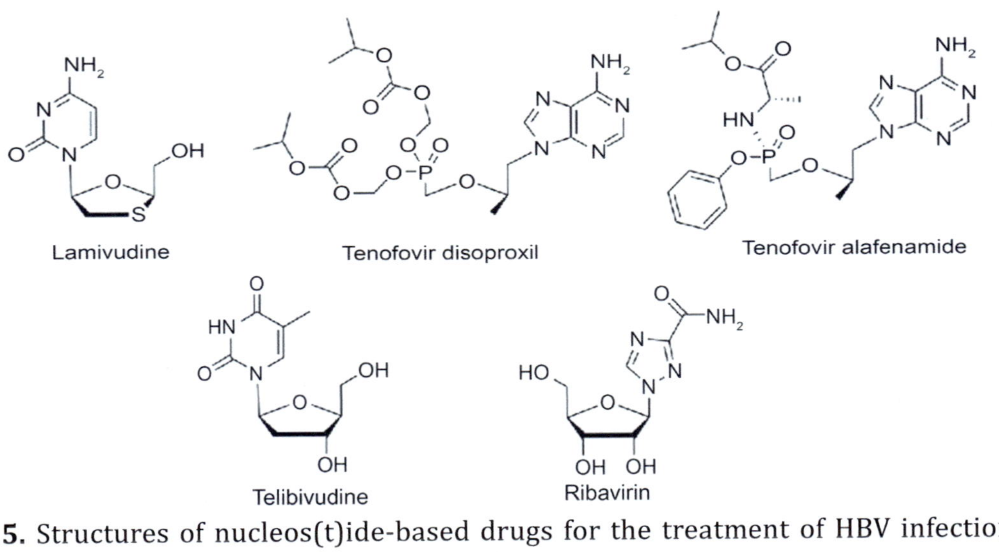

Figure 2.15. Structures of nucleos(t)ide-based drugs for the treatment of HBV infections.

Source: https://www.researchgate.net/publication/336660067/figure/fig1/AS:867977662582786@1583953409971/Structures-of-nucleostide-based-drugs-for-the-treatment-of-HBV-infections.png.

2.6.2. Vaccination Strategies (e.g., HPV Vaccine)

The development of vaccine approaches against DNA viruses has revolutionized public health, particularly in cancer prevention against viral diseases. Human papillomavirus (HPV), a major etiology of cervical and other anogenital cancers, has led to the development of vaccines for the prevention of its incidence. The vaccine application of Gardasil and Cervarix is a case in point of a preventive measure against HPV-induced diseases. The vaccines function by eliciting a robust immune response against the oncoproteins E6 and E7, which are critical to the virus's ability to transform host cells to malignant types. Vaccination of adolescents before the onset of sexual activity not only aims at lowering infection rates but also has an ultimate goal of precluding the subsequent development of HPV-induced cancers, demonstrating the critical interplay between vaccine and cancer prevention in public health measures. Moreover, new vaccine approaches continue to expand the platform of utilizing immunization against DNA viruses, particularly through the application of vector-based systems. Hepatitis B surface antigen (HBsAg), for instance, has been explored as a vector for delivering foreign antigens, augmenting cytotoxic T-lymphocyte responses. This approach holds promise not only to the prevention of hepatitis B infection but also to the attention of other viruses, as it demonstrates the potential to elicit immune responses against multiple epitopes of interest to various malignancies. Such research underscores the need for broad-spectrum vaccine platforms with the potential to target multiple viral-associated diseases, optimizing resources and response capacity. Accordingly, ongoing discovery of novel vaccine technologies, including DNA and viral vector-based vaccines, is poised to broaden therapeutic options against oncogenic infection, thereby improving patient outcomes (Gould et al., 2008). Beyond routine preventive therapy, research on therapeutic vaccines against established viral infections is a top oncology and virology innovation. Therapeutic vaccines having the capacity to stimulate immune responses against oncoviral antigens, including those from HPV and Epstein–Barr virus (EBV), are undergoing clinical effectiveness trials. Against oncogenic antigens like HPV E6/E7 and EBV-expressed proteins, the therapeutic vaccines are engineered to stimulate the immune system to selectively kill cancer cells. Promising first-in-man trials have proved safety and suggested effectiveness against HPV-related or EBV-related cancers. Ongoing research to enhance these therapeutic vaccines is ultimately poised to enhance the quality and duration of affected individuals while investigating mechanisms that can optimize immune responses (Broseghini et al., 2025). Ongoing research supports the case for ongoing investment in vaccination strategies as an effective approach against viral infection and associated malignancies (Figure 2.16).

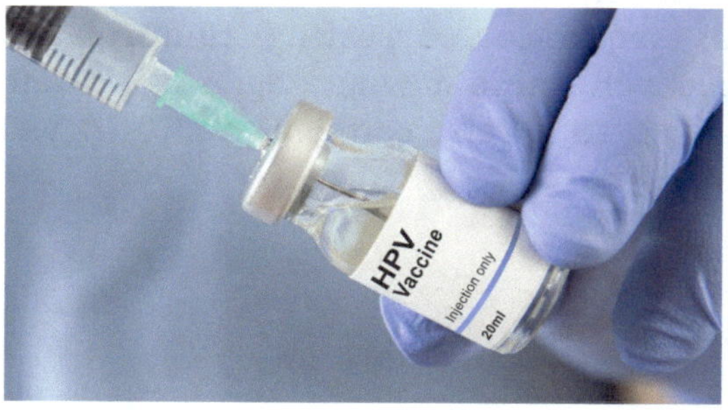

Figure 2.16. HPV vaccine.

Source: https://akm-img-a-in.tosshub.com/indiatoday/images/story/202402/hpv-vaccine-035539599-16x9_0.jpg?VersionId=929UCQf_tV6UR8VeCRXJtvaZFnAzdMJv.

2.6.3. Public Health Measures to Control Outbreaks

Successful public health interventions are critical in the management of DNA virus outbreaks because of the complexity of transmission dynamics and episodic epidemiological patterns of such pathogens. Detection and surveillance are critical components of an effective public health response. Systems of surveillance must be instituted and maintained in a manner to enable early outbreak detection. For instance, qualitative assessment of surveillance systems among five European countries indicated the importance of region-specific approaches taking into consideration local epidemiological and ecological context to enable early detection. Such flexibility is extremely important in the management of DNA virus outbreaks where environmental determinants play a role in disease transmission. Moreover, communication between public health officials and researchers and the general public can be crucial in playing a role in enhanced early detection and prompt proactive rather than reactive public health approaches towards the management of outbreaks (Chyba, 1998). Vaccination is also important in the management of DNA virus outbreaks, particularly preventable ones such as human papillomavirus (HPV) and hepatitis B virus (HBV). Public health interventions towards increased vaccination coverage have been critical in preventing the spread of infection related to these viruses. It is important to implement interventions that ensure equitable access to vaccines among different populations since inequalities in access to healthcare contribute to increased infectious disease transmission. Vaccination policies must be accompanied by education programs that create awareness among populations regarding the importance of vaccination in preventing outbreaks. Moreover, the availability and distribution of vaccines can be greatly influenced by information exchange among states and organizations, enhancing global preparedness against potential DNA virus outbreaks. This underscores the interconnectedness of global public health systems and the necessity of collective action in achieving high vaccination coverage (Chyba, 1998). In addition to vaccination and surveillance, public health interventions must include effective control and treatment measures for outbreaks once they have occurred. Isolation of infected patients and contact tracing are key practices that can limit the spread of DNA viruses during outbreaks. This technique was highly effective in preventing viral infection outbreaks in healthcare facilities, underscoring the importance of strict adherence to infection control protocols. Additionally, public health administrators must strive towards real-time data collection and analysis to inform tailored interventions in the event of an outbreak. Community awareness through campaigns and accessible health services can empower communities to take constructive action in the protection of their health and reporting of symptoms on time. Lastly, a multi-dimensional approach that integrates surveillance, vaccination, treatment, and public awareness is required in the prevention of DNA virus outbreaks and public health in general (Dórea et al., 2016).

Test Your Knowledge

1. What are some of the most commonly prescribed antiviral medications to treat DNA virus infections, and how do they function?
2. What DNA virus diseases are there good vaccines for, and what type are they?

Summary

In studying the vast canvas of DNA viruses, it is evident that these tiny entities have a profound impact on biological systems and shape evolutionary directions. Co-evolution of hosts and DNA viruses has been the driving force that has rendered life as we know it complex. Interestingly, the implications of this co-evolution challenge the traditional biological paradigms that seek to reserve a space for viruses only outside the Tree of Life. Instead, new models propose a more evolutionary, holistic view, where viruses are not only regarded as pathogens but as central players in the evolutionary process. The premise that viral interactions have led to landmark innovations, such as the evolution of non-coding DNA as a protection against viral devastation, is an indication of the enormous impact of these agents on genomic organization (Bandea, 2009). This new understanding emphasizes the pivotal role that DNA viruses have in shaping ecological and evolutionary processes. Additionally, the clinical significance of DNA viruses, particularly in the presentation of chronic infections, underscores the need for innovative approaches to therapy. The example of hepatitis B virus (HBV) co-infected with hepatitis D virus (HDV) illustrates the complexities involved with viral interactions that lead to more severe disease presentation, such as liver cirrhosis and hepatocellular carcinoma. Research has shown that chronic HBV + HDV infection is linked with increased liver fibrosis and other severe health outcomes compared to HBV mono-infection. The identification of conserved regions in the HBV surface antigen (HBsAg) and the hepatitis delta antigen (HDAg) provides important information on viral evolution that can be employed in designing targeted interventions (Andreoni et al., 2018). This demand for the identification of therapeutic opportunities thus becomes vital in the absence of current direct anti-HDV drugs, thereby raising a pivotal dichotomy in contemporary medicine. Lastly, a deep understanding of DNA viruses transcends characterization and delves into their multidimensional functions in microbial communities and human health. The intertwining of viral evolution with cellular life forms not only enhances our understanding of life's complexity but also impels scientific inquiry into new horizons of treatment for viral infections. With more studies, the confluence of knowledge from evolutionary biology and clinical medicine may offer revolutionary answers to the challenges posed by these viruses. The convergence of cellular and viral realms in biological inquiry is a paradigm shift that demands further exploration of the synergies between life forms and their viral counterparts, thereby enhancing our understanding of both health and disease (Bandea, 2009). Through further research, we are able to improve our preparations against the new threats of DNA viruses in a changing world.

In examining the universe of DNA viruses, there are some observations that play a pivotal role in understanding their structural as well as functional characteristics. Of particular note is the fact that icosahedral symmetry among these viruses is the norm, since it is required for stability as well as infectivity. Research has demonstrated that large DNA viruses are beset with challenges of structural stability, something which we observe in the fact that icosahedral protein capsomere packings may be unstable when pushed beyond optimal dimensions. The mechanism is reminiscent of buckling instability in two-dimensional crystals, suggesting a propensity for larger viral morphologies to adopt faceted morphologies. Such observations of elastic shell theory, as detailed in Blaurock et al. (2003), bring to the forefront the complexity of viral structure and the mechanical principles that underlie their development. Additionally, the location of G-quadruplexes (G4s) in DNA virus genomes has been of particular interest, namely their function in viral regulation and pathogenesis. These non-canonical nucleic acid structures, most typically formed in guanine-rich sequences, are increasingly being discovered linked to viral genomes, even epidemic pathogens such as Zika and Ebola. The targeting of G4s to viral regulatory elements suggests an advanced role in viral replication and latency processes. As detailed in Ruggiero & Richter (2018), the therapeutic application of G4 ligands presents promising pathways for antiviral development, with research into their mechanisms illustrating complex interactions at the genomic as well as the transcript levels, evidence of the multidimensional interaction of viral structure and function. Finally, bringing together observations on DNA viruses, we observe the delicate balance between structural stability and genomic regulation. The progress made in the understanding of how mechanical properties affect viral structure, as well as the effects of G4s on viral function, works to highlight the high-level nature of the microorganisms. These findings are of utmost importance, both to science and to therapeutic intervention designed to combat viral disease. Through the convergence of the fields of structural biology and virology, scientists are more able to take advantage of new methods of targeting these genetic units, resulting in more effective therapeutic modalities and greater insight into viral evolution. Taken as a whole, the salient points made in the course of the analysis of DNA viruses serve to shed light on areas of future scientific and therapeutic investigation.

KEY TERMS FROM THIS CHAPTER

- African swine fever virus
- Biological processes
- Co-infections
- Conservative viruses
- CRISPR/Cas9 system
- DDR pathways
- DNA virus replication
- Epstein–Barr virus
- Genetic makeup
- G-quadruplexes (G4s)
- Bioinformatics
- Cervical cancer
- Comparative genomics
- Conventional antiviral treatments
- Cytotoxic T-lymphocyte responses
- Disease transmission
- Epithelial cells
- Evolutionary biology
- Genomic sequencing
- Hepatitis B virus

Critical Thinking Questions

1. **Which of the following is a double-stranded DNA virus of the family Herpesviridae?**
   a. Parvovirus B19
   b. Human papillomavirus
   c. Epstein-Barr virus
   d. Hepatitis D virus
2. **Which structural feature is common among most DNA viruses (except Poxviruses)?**
   a. Enveloped, with single-stranded circular DNA
   b. Icosahedral capsid, replicating intracytoplasmically
   c. Helical capsid, replicating in the nucleus
   d. Icosahedral capsid, replicating in the nucleus
3. **During replication, what would be the first thing for a DNA virus to do when entering a host cell?**
   a. Integration into the host genome
   b. Host RNA polymerase viral RNA synthesis
   c. Assembly of new virions in the cytoplasm
   d. Release through budding using the Golgi apparatus
4. **Which of the following DNA viruses is most commonly associated with cervical cancer?**
   a. Human papillomavirus (HPV)
   b. Adenovirus
   c. Hepatitis B virus
   d. Cytomegalovirus
5. **What is the most commonly used method for a diagnosis of cytomegalovirus (CMV) infection?**
   a. Gram stain
   b. Blood agar viral culture
   c. PCR for CMV DNA
   d. Ziehl-Neelsen stain

Short Answer Questions

1. What are the major families of DNA viruses, and on what grounds are they divided according to the structure of their genomes?
2. How is the structure of enveloped DNA viruses different from non-enveloped DNA viruses?
3. What is the importance of the icosahedral capsid structure being prevalent in DNA viruses?

4. Where within the host cell is replication typically located in most DNA viruses, and what are the exceptions?
5. In what ways is the double-stranded DNA (dsDNA) virus replication process different from single-stranded DNA (ssDNA) viruses?
6. What are the general steps in the pathogenesis process of a DNA virus from entry to host cell damage?
7. How do DNA viruses escape the host immune response after infecting?
8. What are the normal laboratory tests to diagnose infections caused by DNA viruses?

Answer to Critical Thinking Questions

1. (c); 2. (d); 3. (b); 4. (a); 5. (c)

REFERENCES

1. Dórea, F. C., Elbers, A. R., Hendrikx, P., Enoe, C., Kirkeby, C., Hoinville, L., & Lindberg, A. (2016). Vector-borne disease surveillance in livestock populations: A critical review of literature recommendations and implemented surveillance (BTV-8) in five European countries. *Preventive veterinary medicine, 125*, 1–9. https://doi.org/10.1016/j.prevetmed.2016.01.005 (accessed on 13th June 2025).
2. Allander, T., Altschul, S., Cunningham, A. A., Antia, R., Baker, M., Chu, D. K. W., Holmes, C. E. G., et al. (2013). *Metagenomic Study of The Viruses of African Straw-Colored Fruit Bats: Detection of A Chiropteran Poxvirus and Isolation of A Novel Adenovirus.* https://core.ac.uk/download/16458337.pdf (accessed on 13th June 2025).
3. Anders, H. J., Patole, P. S., Pawar, R. D., Zecher, D., et al. (2005). *Molecular Mechanisms of Autoimmunity Triggered by Microbial Infection.* https://core.ac.uk/download/pdf/3779125.pdf (accessed on 13th June 2025).
4. Andreoni, M., Angelico, M., Barlattani, A., Battisti, A., et al. (2018). *HDV Can Constrain HBV Genetisc Evolution in HBsAg: Implications for the Identification of Innovative Pharmacological Targets.* https://core.ac.uk/download/160649117.pdf (accessed on 13th June 2025).
5. Bandea, C. I. (2009). *A unifying Scenario on The Origin and Evolution of Cellular and Viral Domains.* https://core.ac.uk/download/pdf/288874.pdf (accessed on 13th June 2025).
6. Bandea, C. I. (2009). *The Origin and Evolution of Viruses as Molecular Organisms.* https://core.ac.uk/download/pdf/288872.pdf (accessed on 13th June 2025).
7. Jon R. Cavicchi, Stanley P. Kowalski, et al, "Patent Landscape of Influenza A Virus Prophylactic Vaccines and Related Technologies" (2012).(accessed on 13th June 2025).
8. Barzon, L., Berto, A., Desole, G., Pacenti, M., et al. (2015). *Modeling Viral Infectious Diseases and Development of Antiviral Therapies Using Human Induced Pluripotent Stem Cell-Derived Systems.* https://core.ac.uk/download/53523165.pdf (accessed on 13th June 2025).
9. Barzon, L., Palù, G., & Trevisan, M. (2017). *Genome Editing Technologies to Fight Infectious Diseases.* https://core.ac.uk/download/141699794.pdf (accessed on 13th June 2025).
10. Ben-Shaul, A., Egecioglu, D. E., Gelbart, W. M., Gopal, A., et al. (2014). *Viral RNAs are Unusually Compact.* https://core.ac.uk/download/323067057.pdf (accessed on 13th June 2025).
11. Blanc, S., Fereres, A., Garzo, E., Gutiérrez, S., et al. (2012). *Circulating Virus Load Determines the Size of Bottlenecks in Viral Populations Progressing Within a Host.* https://core.ac.uk/download/195732308.pdf (accessed on 13th June 2025).
12. Blaurock, A. E., Lobkovsky, A. E., Lobkovsky, A. E., Murzin, A. G., Bausch, A. R., Caspar, D., Smith, D. E., et al. (2003). *Virus Shapes and Buckling Transitions in Spherical Shells.* http://arxiv.org/abs/cond-mat/0306741 (accessed on 13th June 2025).
13. Bordignon, V., Cavallo, I., Di Domenico, E. G., D'Agosto, G., et al. (2017). *How Human Papillomavirus Replication and Immune Evasion Strategies Take Advantage of the Host DNA Damage Repair Machinery.* https://core.ac.uk/download/188832163.pdf (accessed on 13th June 2025).
14. Braeckmans, K., De Smedt, S., Rejman, J., Remaut, K., et al. (2012). *Intracellular Partitioning of Cell Organelles and Extraneous Nanoparticles During Mitosis.* https://core.ac.uk/download/55801726.pdf (accessed on 13th June 2025).

15. Broseghini, E., Ferracin, M., Filippini, D. M., Gallerani, G., et al. (2025). *Vaccine-Based Immunotherapy for Oropharyngeal and Nasopharyngeal Cancers*. https://core.ac.uk/download/654518362.pdf (accessed on 13th June 2025).

16. Cannon, C., Dunsford, T. H., Hosie, M. J., Jarrett, O., et al. (2002). *Evolution of Replication Efficiency Following Infection with A Molecularly Cloned Feline Immunodeficiency Virus of Low Virulence*. https://core.ac.uk/download/87928.pdf (accessed on 13th June 2025).

17. Caspar, D. L. D., Bancroft, J. B., Elliot, J. P., Landau, L. D., Rochal, S. B., Flint, S. J., et al. (2006). *Density Waves Theory of The Capsid Structure of Small Icosahedral Viruses*. http://arxiv.org/abs/cond-mat/0611623 (accessed on 13th June 2025).

18. Thaker, S. K., Ch'ng, J., & Christofk, H. R. (2019). Viral hijacking of cellular metabolism. *BMC biology*, *17*(1), 59. https://doi.org/10.1186/s12915-019-0678-9(accessed on 13th June 2025).

19. Chen, Y. C., Liu, F., Sheng, J., Trang, P., et al. (2018). *Potential Application of the CRISPR/Cas9 System Against Herpesvirus Infections*. https://core.ac.uk/download/323080891.pdf (accessed on 13th June 2025).

20. Chiu, C. Y. (2013). *Viral Pathogen Discovery*. https://core.ac.uk/download/323063718.pdf (accessed on 13th June 2025).

21. Chiu, C. Y., & Miller, S. A. (2019). *Clinical Metagenomics*. https://core.ac.uk/download/323062552.pdf (accessed on 13th June 2025).

22. Chyba, C. F. (1998). *Biological Terrorism, Emerging Diseases, And National Security*. https://core.ac.uk/download/71349580.pdf (accessed on 13th June 2025).

23. Coben, R. M., Conn, M. I., DiMarino, A. J., Hann, H. W., et al. (2019). *Persistent Risk for New, Subsequent New and Recurrent Hepatocellular Carcinoma Despite Successful Anti-Hepatitis B Virus Therapy and Tumor Ablation: The Need for Hepatitis B Virus Cure*. https://core.ac.uk/download/220159115.pdf (accessed on 13th June 2025).

24. Cole, B., Lambrechts, L., Rutsaert, S., Trypsteen, W., et al. (2020). *Emerging PCR-Based Techniques to Study HIV-1 Reservoir Persistence*. https://core.ac.uk/download/287941778.pdf (accessed on 13th June 2025).

25. Costa, E. N. O. Q. (2011). *Viral Modulation of Interferon (IFN) Responses to African Swine Fever Virus (ASFV)*. https://core.ac.uk/download/12424877.pdf (accessed on 13th June 2025).

26. Cuestas, M. L., Eguibar, N., Gonzalez, R. H., Nusblat, A., et al. (2015). *Hepatitis B Virus (HBV) and S-Escape Mutants: From the Beginning Until Now*. https://core.ac.uk/download/159295712.pdf (accessed on 13th June 2025).

27. Drew, W. L. (1987). *Diagnostic Virology*. https://core.ac.uk/download/323074452.pdf (accessed on 13th June 2025).

28. Du, L., Jiang, S., Ojcius, D. M., Pan, C., et al. (2020). *Measures for Diagnosing and Treating Infections by A Novel Coronavirus Responsible for A Pneumonia Outbreak Originating in Wuhan, China*. https://core.ac.uk/download/323063844.pdf (accessed on 13th June 2025).

29. Mensaert, K., Van Criekinge, W., Thas, O., Schuuring, E., Steenbergen, R. D., Wisman, G. B., & De Meyer, T. (2015). Mining for viral fragments in methylation enriched sequencing data. *Frontiers in genetics*, *6*, 16. https://doi.org/10.3389/fgene.2015.00016(accessed on 13th June 2025).

30. Fang, F., Le Calvez, H., & Yu, M. (2004). *Biochemical Prevention and Treatment of Viral*

Infections–A New Paradigm in Medicine for Infectious Diseases. https://core.ac.uk/download/pdf/3550099.pdf (accessed on 13th June 2025).

31. Gentile, G., & Micozzi, A. (2016). *Speculations on the clinical Significance of Asymptomatic Viral Infections.* https://core.ac.uk/download/98344656.pdf (accessed on 13th June 2025).
32. Gould, A., Chen, D., Kattenbelt, J., Barnes, M., Mather, M., Haigh, O., Tindle, R. R., et al. (2008). *HBsAg-Vectored DNA Vaccines Elicit Concomitant Protective Responses to Multiple CTL Epitopes Relevant in Human Disease.* https://core.ac.uk/download/pdf/287837.pdf (accessed on 13th June 2025).
33. Hahn, C. S., Lenches, E. M., Rice, C. M., Strauss, J. H., et al. (1989). *Sindis Virus ts103 Has a Mutation in Glycoprotein E2 That Leads to Defective Assembly of Virions.* https://core.ac.uk/download/4871600.pdf (accessed on 13th June 2025).
34. Hanson, L. A., Montgomery, R. D., Rudis, M. R., Vasquez-Lee, M., et al. (2006). *A Broadly Applicable Method to Characterize Large DNA Viruses and Adenoviruses Based on the DNA Polymerase Gene.* https://core.ac.uk/download/pdf/3953291.pdf (accessed on 13th June 2025).
35. Heim, A., Kistler, A., Manning, A., Piralla, A., Wisdom, A., Kutkowska, A. E., Wisdom, A., et al. (2009). *Genetics, Recombination and Clinical Features of Human Rhinovirus Species C (HRV-C) Infections; Interactions of HRV-C with Other Respiratory Viruses.* https://core.ac.uk/download/9649254.pdf (accessed on 13th June 2025).
36. Kohl, A., Blomström, A. L., Delhaye, S., Dunn, G., Schnettler, E., Geerts-Dimitriadou, C., Hampsey, M., et al. (2013). *Non-Structural Proteins of Arthropod-Borne Bunyaviruses: Roles and Functions.* https://core.ac.uk/download/16462466.pdf (accessed on 13th June 2025).
37. Lošdorfer Božič, A., Šiber, A., Šiber, A., Šiber, A., Šiber, A., Šiber, A., Šiber, A., et al. (2012). *How Simple Can a Model of An Empty Viral Capsid Be? Charge Distributions in Viral Capsids.* http://arxiv.org/abs/1207.3188 (accessed on 13th June 2025).
38. Fiscon, G., Weitschek, E., Cella, E. *et al.* MISSEL: a method to identify a large number of small species-specific genomic subsequences and its application to viruses classification. *BioData Mining* **9**, 38 (2016). https://doi.org/10.1186/s13040-016-0116-2 (accessed on 13th June 2025).
39. Needham, J. M. (2023). *Manipulation and Dependence on Host Cell Cycle by Human RNA and DNA Viruses: Human Coronavirus OC43 and BK Polyomavirus.* https://core.ac.uk/download/640967912.pdf (accessed on 13th June 2025).
40. Ogbu, S. C. (2019). *Role of Topoisomerase II Alpha in DNA Topology and T Cell Responses During Chronic Viral Infections.* https://core.ac.uk/download/270040740.pdf (accessed on 13th June 2025).
41. Orlova, E. (2012). *Bacteriophages and Their Structural Organization.* https://core.ac.uk/download/19509491.pdf (accessed on 13th June 2025).
42. Ruggiero, E., & Richter, S. N. (2018). G-quadruplexes and G-quadruplex ligands: targets and tools in antiviral therapy. *Nucleic acids research, 46*(7), 3270–3283. https://doi.org/10.1093/nar/gky187(accessed on 13th June 2025).
43. Sankovski, E. (2018). *Papilloomiviiruse Transkriptsiooni Ja Regulaatorvalgu E2 Uurimine.* https://core.ac.uk/download/154745865.pdf (accessed on 13th June 2025).

44. Voet, D., Drake, J. W., Eigen, M., Schuster, P., et al. (2004). *Host-Parasite Co-Evolution and Optimal Mutation Rates for Semi-Conservative Quasispecies.* http://arxiv.org/abs/q-bio/0401026 (accessed on 13th June 2025).

45. Witzany, G. (2008). *Bio-Communication of Bacteria and Its Evolutionary Interrelations to Natural Genome Editing Competences of Viruses.* https://core.ac.uk/download/pdf/287751.pdf (accessed on 13th June 2025).

RNA VIRUSES

3

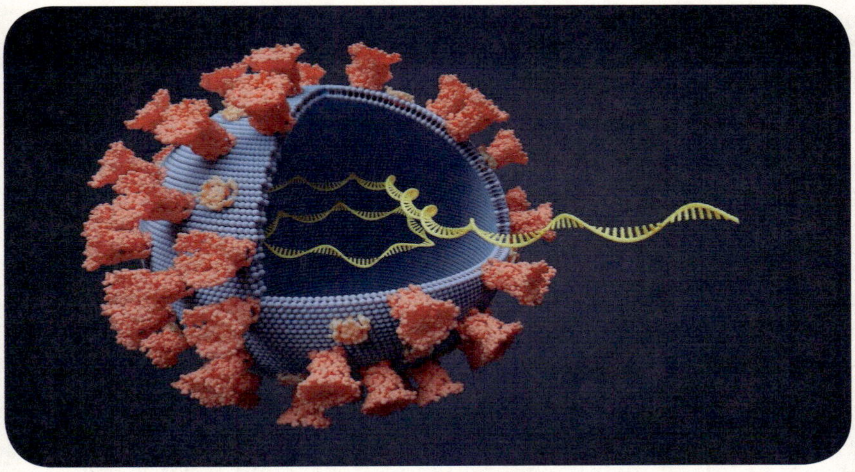

LEARNING OBJECTIVES

After studying this chapter, you will be able to:

1. Understand the classification of RNA viruses;
2. Explain the structure and function of RNA viruses;
3. Explain the replication cycle of RNA viruses;
4. Focus on RNA viruse pathogenesis;
5. Describe the RNA virus transmission dynamics and epidemiology;
6. Discuss treatment and prevention of RNA viruses.

Introduction

In virology, RNA viruses constitute a heterogeneous and widespread family that poses daunting challenges to global public health. With single or double-stranded RNA genomes with high mutation rates, the viruses are extremely variable. The genetic plasticity enables them to fit well into new environments, to evade host immune detection, and to develop resistance to antiviral therapy. With variability, RNA viruses constitute a heterogeneous group of pathogens that includes the highly prominent influenza, HIV, and recent SARS-CoV-2. With the significance of understanding their molecular biology and pathogenesis, effective management and therapeutic approaches must be developed. Since RNA viruses continually emerge and re-emerge, they constitute a leading research area that is concerned with understanding the intricate mechanisms whereby they interact with vectors and hosts. The role played by advances in technology cannot be overstated in the case of RNA viruses. Availability of high-throughput sequencing (HTS) has revolutionized viral genomics because it is now simple and cheap to rapidly sequence many viral genomes. The genomic explosion not only facilitates the detection of known and novel viruses from a broad set of sources but also sheds light on viral diversity and quasispecies dynamics. The ability to investigate intra-host variations constitutes a centerpiece of investigating key biological processes such as viral transmission and host adaptation. Furthermore, bioinformatics plays an increasingly significant role in this field because sophisticated algorithms and bioinformatics software tools must be employed to process and analyze the high levels of data produced by HTS technologies. Integration of these tools into RNA viral research is now yielding a more advanced understanding of viral biology. The interaction of RNA viruses and vector hosts is a highly interesting field in their biology. For example, arboviruses, a subgroup of RNA viruses, are able to provoke persistent infections within insect vectors with little effect on their physiology. Such infections are typically controlled by the RNA interference (RNAi) mechanism, an antiviral defense in the host. Recent studies have indicated that arboviral genomes do not contain major viral suppressors of RNAi, suggesting a delicate balance of their interaction with the immune system of the hosts. Furthermore, these viruses can be employed as viral silencing vectors, which can facilitate the study of gene function by reverse genetics. Nevertheless, safety concerns regarding pathogen status limit the practical application of these findings. Thus, exploration of alternative mosquito-specific viruses inducing equivalent RNAi responses might be an effective solution in deciphering and regulating RNA virus dynamics (Davison et al., 2016; Liu et al., 2019).

Definition of RNA Viruses

RNA viruses are a diverse collection of pathogens characterized by the genetic material, which is ribonucleic acid (RNA) rather than deoxyribonucleic acid (DNA). Such a basic variation allows RNA viruses to possess unusual replication strategies and a general pattern of pathological behavior compared to their DNA counterparts. The RNA genome is typically between positive-sense single-stranded RNA (+ssRNA), negative-sense single-stranded RNA (−ssRNA), and double-stranded RNA (dsRNA). All of these types have implications for the virus's life cycle, transmission mode, and interaction with the host organism. Such information is crucial in the development of successful antiviral strategies and treatments because the structural and functional features of RNA viruses tend to dictate their pathogenicity and mode of infection. From the biological and ecological function, RNA viruses infect a wide range of hosts, ranging from animals, plant hosts, and bacteria, reflective of their ubiquity in the biosphere. For example, some RNA viruses are members of the order *Picornavirales* that include a diverse collection of plant viruses classified into families such as *Comoviridae* and *Sequiviridae*. These viruses are characterized by their positive-strand RNA genomes and unique replication proteins that allow their transmission between host plants, reflective of the adaptability of RNA viruses in different environments. Furthermore, the division of this order into these families establishes the similarities that RNA viruses possess in relation to each other while pointing to unique features that are able to affect their ecological functions. Mechanisms like RNA interference are employed by certain hosts to combat viral infections, as has been the case with research conducted on the Israeli acute paralysis virus (IAPV). Interestingly, studies have documented that IAPV infection is able to optimize the RNA interference mechanisms of bumblebees instead of suppressing them, revealing complex interactions between RNA viruses and the immune mechanisms of the hosts (Cappelle et al., 2016). Furthermore, the structural characteristics common to most RNA viruses, including envelopment and non-envelopment forms, regulate their transmissibility and stability under various environments. Thus, the evolution of RNA viruses and their ongoing co-evolution with host organisms remain central themes of study, impacting extensively the areas of agriculture, veterinary medicine, and public health policy (Figure 3.1).

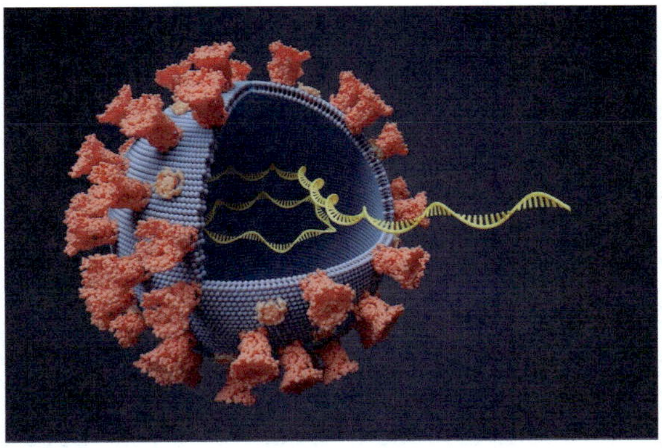

Figure 3.1. Illustration of an RNA virus.

Source: https://www.news-medical.net/image-handler/ts/20220606094803/ri/950/src/images/news/ImageForNews_715802_16545232836643164.jpg.

Importance in Virology and Medicine

The significance of understanding RNA viruses in medicine and virology cannot be overemphasized, given their contribution to global health crises. RNA viruses, including the influenza virus and coronaviruses, have demonstrated an unprecedented ability to adapt, mutate, and evade the immune system to cause mass infection and overwhelm the health system. On the rise are increasing outbreaks due to RNA viruses that necessitate a thorough understanding of their pathogenesis mechanisms. For example, studies have revealed how flaviviruses, such as dengue and Zika, develop mechanisms to evade host immune responses, more importantly, the type I interferon pathway, to become effective pathogens (Clark et al., 2017). Such an understanding is vital in the design of therapeutics and vaccines, illustrating the significance of an in-depth understanding of RNA viruses to combat their resultant diseases. Another significant feature of RNA viruses is that they can be models in research to understand virus evolution, pathogenesis, and viral-host interactions. The outstanding genetic features of RNA viruses, i.e., their high mutation rates, offer scientists the leverage of observing evolutionary processes in real time. Such a feature has been invaluable in research on virus evolution in new host tissues and resistance to antiviral drugs. Most relevant is the research on coronaviruses, which has revealed that various members encode for proteins counteracting host antiviral defense, e.g., the OAS-RNase L pathway (Chen et al., 2017). By demystifying such mechanisms, scientists can come up with ways of disrupting viral replication and enhancing the development of vaccines. The recurring outbreak of novel RNA viruses highlights the significance of adaptive research approaches in virology in an attempt to contain evolving pathogens. The field of RNA virology is not merely of personal health interest but also of public health policy and pandemic preparedness. The worldwide response to SARS-CoV-2 outbreaks demonstrates the interconnectedness of virology, epidemiology, and health care. Understanding RNA viruses informs public health policymakers with the data necessary to implement sound surveillance, control, and vaccine distribution policy. Furthermore, viral pathogenic and genetic research has facilitated the development of therapy for viral diseases. As is exemplified by how quickly mRNA vaccines were developed for COVID-19, information provided by RNA viruses offers new potential for preventing emergent infectious diseases. A comprehensive understanding of RNA viruses is thus required because it informs medical and public health initiatives for preventing future viral risk in populations.

3.1. Classification of RNA Viruses

Learning Outcome

1. Talk about the RNA viruses;
2. Identify significant RNA virus families;
3. Explain the methods of RNA virus classification.

RNA virus taxonomy is a fundamental branch of virology that enables their comprehension of structure, replication, and pathogenicity. RNA viruses are generally categorized based on their genomic nature, specifically the nature of RNA they possess, either single-stranded (ssRNA) or double-stranded (dsRNA). Subclassification is further based on the nature of ssRNA, with positive-sense RNA viruses being able to directly act as mRNA and negative-sense RNA viruses needing conversion to a complementary structure before translation. This system of classification not only serves scholarly research but also has real-world implications, such as vaccine development and antiviral therapeutic production, as seen in recent research on influenza vaccines and their technological innovations in response to pandemic issues (Cavicchi et al., 2012). Taxonomically, various methodologies assist in classifying RNA viruses. Utilization of genomic sequencing technology has been revolutionary, and scientists can now clearly define RNA viral species based on their genetic content. Ongoing advancements in next-generation sequencing enable large sets of genomic sequences, generating a vast amount of data that needs to be computationally filtered to identify and classify various viral strains. As noted, classification protocols are generally directed by phylogenetic analyses, which investigate evolutionary relationships among viruses. Such biological classification has considerable implications, as it allows for the prediction of epidemic outbreaks and formulation of public health policies in response to emerging infectious diseases (Fiscon et al., 2016). Further, classification of RNA viruses is dynamic; it changes with the emergence of new strains and the genetic mutation of old ones. For example, the rapid mutation of RNA viruses tends to lead to some species being reclassified, something that must be reviewed periodically to make certain that the systems of classification are up to date. This RNA virus fluidity makes one pay attention regularly to advances in the science of virology and the ensuing classification systems. Familiarity with the genetic variation that typifies such viruses can assist in the identification of emerging threats to public health and stimulate innovation in vaccine development. As research centers on the several technologies surrounding influenza, for example, the classification issues are symptomatic of wider trends affecting global health programs (Cavicchi et al., 2012).

3.1.1. Types of RNA Viruses (Single-Stranded vs. Double-Stranded)

The division of RNA viruses is primarily into two families: single-stranded RNA (ssRNA) and double-stranded RNA (dsRNA). Single-stranded RNA viruses are further divided into two families based on their polarity: positive-sense and negative-sense. Positive-sense ssRNA viruses are directly translatable into protein by the host ribosomes and are, therefore, highly efficient in their replication. Negative-sense ssRNA viruses, on the other hand, require transcription into a complementary positive strand for protein synthesis. This affects the viral life cycle and is the reason for the pathogenicity of most ssRNA viruses. This distinction is vital in the design of targeted antiviral therapy and therapeutic intervention against these viral entities, resulting in the cure of diseases caused by them. Double-stranded RNA viruses, on the other hand, are comparatively less prevalent and have unique structural and functional characteristics. The viral genome consists of two complementary strands, and the process of replication is complex and requires the use of RNA-dependent RNA polymerases. This feature makes the overall viral replication process complex and makes the host immune response complex. Despite being less prevalent, dsRNA viruses have important roles in various ecosystems, especially as plant pathogens. They can cause various types of responses in host organisms and have a beautiful interplay between viral infection and plant resistance mechanisms. The study of these mechanisms also points towards the possibility of biocontrol application, as in the case of certain mycoviruses, which have been explored for their role in forest pathology, indicating a greater ecological role of dsRNA viruses (Díez Casero et al., 2016). The epidemiological significance of single-stranded as well as double-stranded RNA viruses is enormous, owing to their influence on human, animal, and plant health. ssRNA viruses are notorious for hosting such disease-inducing agents as the flu virus, HIV, and coronaviruses, which exhibit high mutation rates and facile transmissibility. This plasticity tends to defy vaccine and public health intervention measures in outbreak control. dsRNA viruses, while less studied, can influence agriculture and forestry and impact forest and crop quality. Describing transmission patterns and evolutionary histories of the ssRNA and dsRNA viruses expands the knowledge base, facilitating better control and management of viruses. Study of the genetics and charge distributions of these viral capsids reveals new research fields, advancing virology and facilitating environmental sustainability in agriculture and forestry (Lošdorfer Božič et al., 2012) (Figure 3.2).

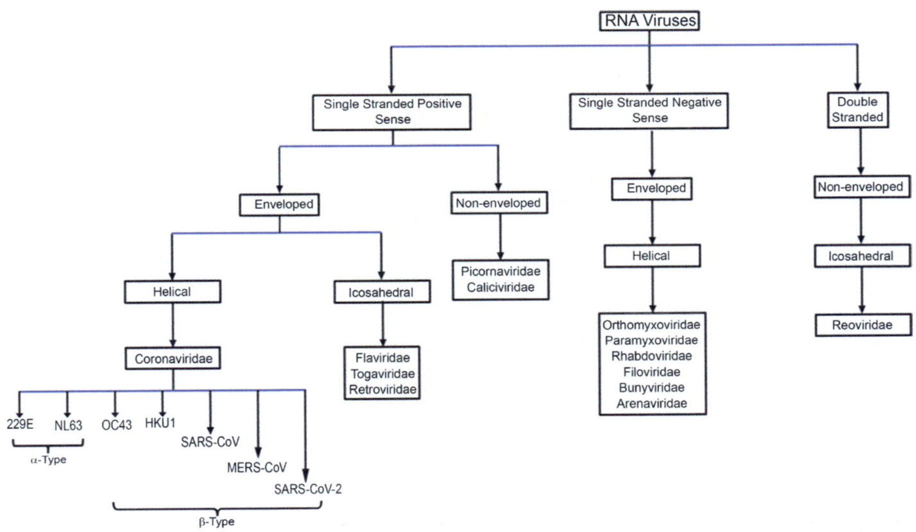

Figure 3.2. Classification of RNA-based viruses and a flow-chart showing the belongingness of Coronavirus and other closely related RNA viruses.

Source: https://www.researchgate.net/profile/Prabhu-Mishra-2/publication/344532922/figure/fig4/AS:961891643957271@1606344247896/Classification-of-RNA-based-viruses-and-flow-chart-showing-the-belongingness-of.png.

3.1.2. Major Families of RNA Viruses (e.g., Picornaviridae, Orthomyxoviridae)

The RNA virus structure is characterized by a richness of families with specific structural and genomic features, which influence their infection and transmission profile significantly. Among them, the family *Picornaviridae* stands out as one of the most significant in public health in terms of impact, with the notable pathogens being the poliovirus and rhinoviruses. They possess a non-enveloped capsid, which is accountable for conferring stability against the environment, thereby facilitating transmission through the fecal-oral route or respiratory droplets. The viral respiratory pathogens have been researched to emphasize the high morbidity of the viruses, especially in children and immunocompromized patients. Specifically, viral diversity in respiratory samples was studied, where detection of multiple strains of *Picornaviridae* was observed, which emphasizes its significance and prevalence in respiratory tract infections (Djikeng et al., 2012). Hence, learning about the characteristics of this family is significant to formulate effective prevention and treatment strategies against viral infections. However, the *Orthomyxoviridae* family is renowned for being represented by the influenza viruses, which are characterized by their segmented RNA genome and the presence of an envelope derived from the host cell membrane. This family encompasses notable strains like H1N1 and H3N2, with major implications for seasonal epidemics and pandemics. The segmented genome facilitates the reassortment during co-infection, which enhances their ability to evade host immunological mechanisms and complicate vaccine development (Figure 3.3).

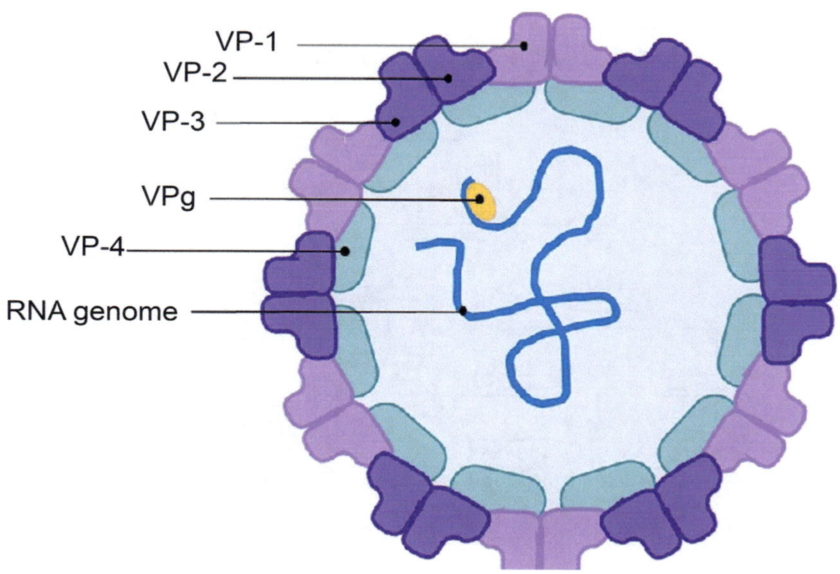

Figure 3.3. General structure of the *Picornaviridae* family.

Source: https://www.researchgate.net/profile/Jesus-Lujan-Montelongo/publication/357470377/figure/fig6/AS:1121095864320005@1644301491095/General-structure-of-*Picornaviridae*-family.png.

The relevance of influenza to public health is profound, with respiratory viruses in this family causing considerable morbidity and mortality worldwide, especially during epidemic seasons. Comprehensive virome studies demonstrate that *Orthomyxoviridae* viruses constitute a high proportion of respiratory pathogens, indicating their relevance in global health debate on viral transmission and epidemic readiness (Djikeng et al., 2012). Understanding the *Orthomyxoviridae* family is, therefore, at the core of understanding their potential for rapid mutation and transmission. Studies on large RNA virus families also demonstrate the intricate interaction between viral diversity and host biology, as seen in specialized ecosystems. For instance, virome studies on the Great Barrier Reef fish demonstrate deep variations in viral populations among fish families. This indicates the importance of host diversity in viral emergence and evolution, as highly diverse host communities may create barriers to cross-species transmission. Such findings demonstrate the intricacy of RNA virus dynamics in ecological systems and the importance of integrating virological studies with host interaction understanding. By advancing our understanding of interactions of families of RNA viruses, e.g., *Picornaviridae* and *Orthomyxoviridae*, and their respective hosts, future studies can better cope with viral emergence and the associated public health challenges (Figure 3.4).

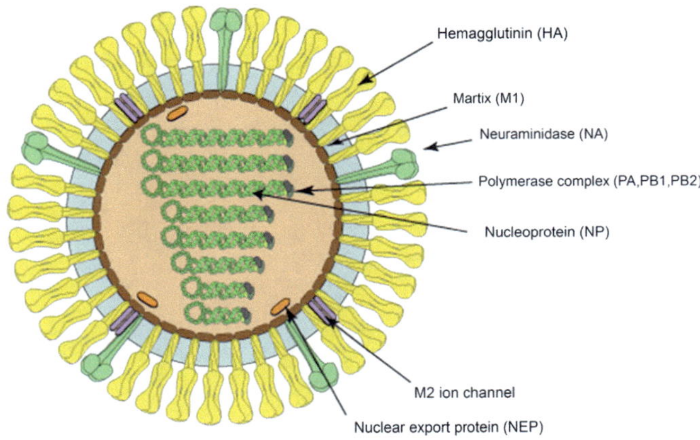

Figure 3.4. *Orthomyxoviridae.*

Source: https://viralzone.expasy.org/resources/InfluenzaA-virion.png.

3.1.3. Methods of Classification (Genomic Structure, Replication Strategy)

The genomic organization becomes relevant in the classification of the RNA viruses, i.e., the form their nucleic acid takes. RNA viruses are classified into two broad categories based on their genome type: single-stranded RNA (ssRNA) and double-stranded RNA (dsRNA). The ssRNA viruses are further classified into positive-sense and negative-sense viruses. Positive-sense ssRNA viruses act as direct templates for protein translation, as in the case of the poliovirus, whereas negative-sense ssRNA viruses need to be first transcribed into a complementary positive-sense RNA, which can be translated into proteins, as in the case of the influenza virus. This distinction in genomic organization plays a very crucial role in not just the lifecycle of the virus but also in the mechanism of the virus propagation, with each group showing very characteristic interactions with the host cellular machinery for successful viral replication. Replication mechanisms in RNA viruses are closely linked with their genomic organizations, regulating different patterns of infection and replication. For instance, in positive-sense ssRNA viruses, the virus RNA is able to hijack the host's ribosomes directly upon entry, compelling the host to synthesize viral proteins as a preliminary step in defense, whereas negative-sense ssRNA viruses are forced to utilize RNA-dependent RNA polymerase to synthesize the positive-sense intermediates required for protein synthesis. These distinctions in mechanisms play a very crucial role in understanding the behavior and adaptability of the pathogen, as different viruses use complex mechanisms to coordinate replication processes and evade host defenses. The significance of replication mechanisms illustrates the forces of evolution that operate on RNA viruses, leading to immense diversity among the different families and genera, making their classification perplexing and fascinating. Recent studies have also elucidated the interaction between RNA viruses and the host cellular machinery, particularly about gene expression and RNA stability. Viruses have been found to possess a mechanism for hijacking the host's RNA turnover process to maximize their replication and survive in an adverse environment. For example, positive-sense RNA viruses have been found to hijack the eukaryotic RNA stabilization machinery to extend their half-life in the cell, while negative-sense viruses have been found to suppress the host antiviral mechanisms to facilitate an efficient replication event. The interaction between RNA viruses and host cellular processes is essential to their survival and poses significant questions towards an understanding of the viral strategy evolution against host defense. Understanding such modes of interaction not only aids in the classification of RNA viruses but also aids in the identification of potential therapeutic interventions against viral infections (Gaglia et al., 2010; Beren et al., 2020) (Figure 3.5).

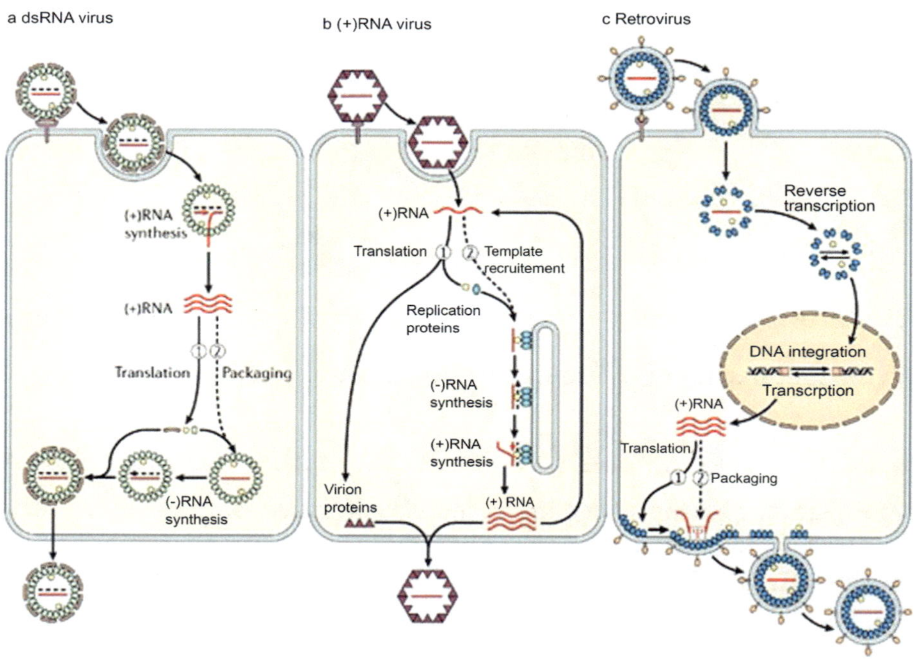

Figure 3.5. Replication strategies of different kinds of RNA viruses are shown: (a) replication of dsDNA virus; (b) replication of +ssRNA virus; and (c) retroviruses.

Source: https://www.researchgate.net/profile/Pathmanaban-Ramasamy/publication/288827106/figure/fig5/AS:312556980850692@1451530799693/Replication-strategies-of-different-kinds-of-RNA-viruses-are-shown-a-replication-of.png.

Test Your Knowledge

1. What are the main classifications of RNA viruses based on their genome structure?
2. Identify at least three general families of RNA viruses and describe one characteristic of each family.

3.2. Structure and Function of RNA Viruses

Learning Outcome

1. Describe viral genome organization;
2. Explain capsid structure and function;
3. Identify envelope presence and use.

The structural characteristics of RNA viruses are vital to understanding their function and virulence. Most RNA viruses possess single-stranded (ssRNA) or double-stranded (dsRNA) genomes that have specific replication strategies and mechanisms of interaction with the host cell. ssRNA viruses are further classified into positive-sense and negative-sense viruses, with positive-sense RNA being directly translatable into protein and negative-sense RNA requiring first to be transcribed into complementary strands. This is a critical consideration for the design of antiviral interventions, as it can be used to inform targeted therapeutic interventions. For example, picornaviruses have developed internal ribosome entry sites (IRES) that enable cap-independent translation of viral proteins to circumvent host cellular translation machinery for viral replication (Lozano et al., 2015). Understanding these structural characteristics is possible for scientists to determine new targets for antiviral drug development. The function of the characteristic structural features of RNA viruses is an important consideration in their ability to hijack the host cell machinery for replication. The capsid, composed of protein subunits, protects the RNA genome and plays a central role in initiating infection by facilitating host cell attachment. In addition, the nucleocapsid protein, particularly in negative-strand RNA viruses, is an encapsulating protein that protects viral RNA but also facilitates extensive interactions with viral polymerases required for transcription and replication (Gumpper, 2018).

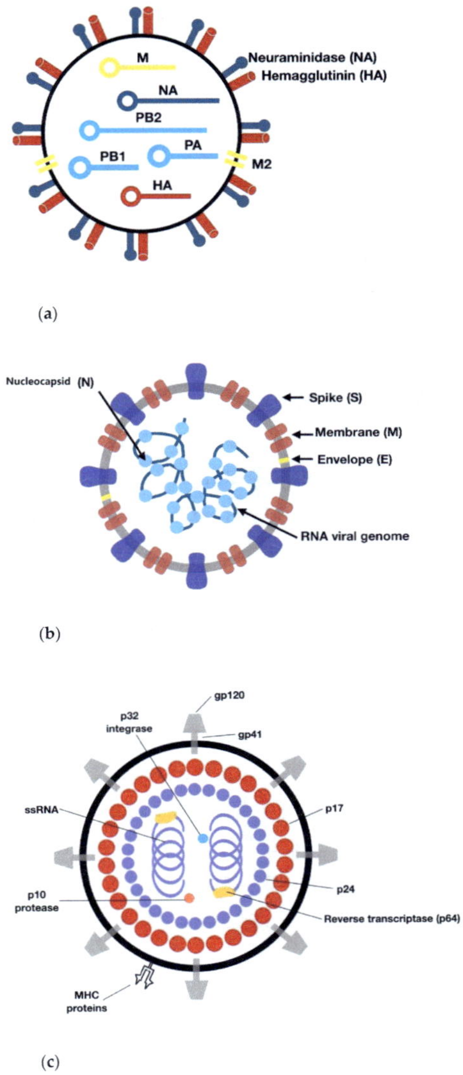

Figure 3.6. Structure of the three RNA viruses. (a) IV is an RNA virus 90–100 nm in diameter; (b) SARS-CoV-2 contains one single-stranded positive-sense RNA; and (c) HIV contains two single-stranded RNAs and two reverse transcriptase enzymes. In its membrane, there is a gp41 glycoprotein and a gp120 protein, as well as host cell-derived major histocompatibility (MHC) molecules.

Source: https://www.researchgate.net/publication/359492357/figure/fig1/AS:11431281365077061@1744213740152/Structure-of-the-three-RNA-viruses-a-IV-is-an-RNA-virus-90-100-nm-in-diameter-The.tif.

These interactions are often complex and require structural flexibility to allow the protein to bind a variety of cellular environments and viral requirements. This multifunctionality underscores the importance of structural integrity and function, as loss can result in a loss of infectivity and replication efficiency. As science advances, knowledge of RNA virus function in relation to structure is more crucial to public health. After outbreaks of highly pathogenic viruses such as those within the negative-strand RNA family, including Ebola and Influenza, there is an even greater need to investigate their biological processes (Gumpper, 2018). Detailed discovery of specific structural components enabling these viruses to replicate effectively within host cells can open the door to novel antiviral therapies. For example, drug discovery can be informed by targeting the nucleocapsid protein necessary for viral replication. With initial research suggesting changes to the nucleocapsid protein influence polymerase activity, future research is sure to provide significant findings that can enhance our understanding of RNA virus biology and inform global health interventions against viral outbreaks (Figure 3.6).

3.2.1. Viral Genome Composition

Viral genome composition is an important determinant of RNA virus pathogenicity and host interaction. In general, RNA viruses possess nucleotide compositions that are strategically advantageous for infection and replication. For instance, RNA viruses that infect mammals exhibit a significant suppression of CpG and UpA dinucleotide frequencies. Experiments with echovirus 7 (E7) mutants have shown that alterations of these nucleotide frequencies significantly influence replication kinetics. Specifically, viruses with enhanced CpG and UpA frequencies have compromised replication capabilities compared to their respective counterparts without these dinucleotides, which have better replication and infectivity. These findings suggest forces of evolution influencing viral genome composition and suggest that nucleotide sequence changes have strong influences on host-pathogen interaction and viral transmission effectiveness (Atkinson et al., 2014). In addition to dinucleotide frequency, the nucleotide composition per se is an important factor in the evolutionary strategies of various RNA viruses. A classic case is the variation in nucleotide ordering in the genomes of human immunodeficiency virus (HIV-1) and human T cell leukemia virus (HTLV-1). HIV-1 is characterized by high purine A enrichment, and HTLV-1 is pyrimidine C-preferent. This variation, suggested to have originated from a common ancestor, is a strategy for evading homologous recombination between the viruses. As the viruses evolved, HIV-1 evolved with low GC content and structured its genome to evade competition, while HTLV-1 evolved a divergent pathway. This variation in nucleotide composition demonstrates how forces of evolution influence the RNA virus genome structure, resulting in alterations of pathogenicity and host interaction (Forsdyke, 2013). In addition, competition between encoding functional proteins and maintaining crucial nucleic acid structures further demonstrates the complexity involved in viral genome composition. Prioritizing structural integrity over coding potential can be a major factor in viral recombination and adaptation abilities. When sequence divergence is extreme, the structural integrity required for effective recombination can be lost, resulting in the establishment of new viral species. This model emphasizes the necessity of RNA viruses to balance functional protein encoding against the maintenance of strong structural elements within their genomes. Through the processes, scientists can establish insight into the evolutionary trajectory of RNA viruses and develop novel solutions for combating viral infection, such as vaccine design and therapeutic treatments (Forsdyke, 2013).

3.2.2. Capsid Structure and Its Role

The capsid of the RNA virus plays a critical role in the structural integrity of the viral genome and the viral life cycle. Composed largely of protein subunits known as capsomers, the capsid encapsulates and protects the viral RNA from assault by the environment and enzymatic degradation. The protective function is particularly critical in the context of the lability of RNA to rapid enzymatic degradation by ribonucleases in host cells. Capsid structure also plays an active role in the mechanism of entry of the virus into cells. For example, during infection, the capsid must allow conformational change to facilitate fusion of the viral envelope with the host cell membrane, a process critical to the release of the genome. The architectural critical functional characteristics of the capsid therefore regulate not only the stability of the virus but its capacity to infect and replicate in the host. Uncoating, the release of the viral RNA from protective capsid, has been the subject of extensive research in recent years. What has been determined is that a range of mechanisms regulate this critical step, with varied implications for viral families. For example, the dengue virus proved that degraded capsid is mediated by the ubiquitin-proteasome system; however, it does not simply rely on complete degradation to facilitate uncoating of the genome. Rather, this release of the viral genome necessitates a nondegradative ubiquitination step, indicative of a sophisticated interplay between capsid proteins and host cellular machinery. Such sophisticated molecular interactions reinforce the dual function of the capsid as a protective vessel and active player in the viral life cycle, regulating how RNA viruses hijack host cellular pathways. Explanation of such processes is of potential interest for the design of novel antiviral strategies towards capsid dynamics and uncoating pathways (Byk et al., 2016). Moreover, knowledge of capsid organization is not only beyond its protective role but also as a therapeutic target. The organization and composition of the capsid proteins can determine the efficacy of antiviral therapy, which can act towards destabilizing the viral particle or blocking its assembly. For RNA viruses such as those of the Alphavirus genus, the nature of certain capsid protein interactions is crucial not only for the entry of the host cell but also for the success of replication. Modulation of capsid interactions, i.e., capsid protein palmitoylation, can influence virus fitness and its ability to evade the host immune system. Thus, enhancing our knowledge of capsid structure and function can open the way to new strategies in viral therapeutics, enabling the development of more effective treatments of RNA viral infections (Karo-Astover, 2013).

3.2.3. Envelope Presence and Its Significance

The envelope of the RNA virus is a crucial mediator of viral entry into host cells and greatly influences their infectivity and replication. This lipid bilayer envelope of host cell origin covers the viral nucleocapsid and contains viral glycoproteins required for the initiation of infection. Such glycoproteins, e.g., the HIV envelope protein, interact with specific cell surface receptors to enable fusion and entry into the host cell cytoplasm. The existence of an envelope not only optimizes the virus's ability to evade host immune systems but also determines the virus's tropism, e.g., in HIV infections. The complexity of envelope interactions, e.g., co-receptor usage, necessitates phenotypic analysis of viral tropism in specific strains, which is often crucial for the successful therapeutic interventions such as maraviroc acting on specific entry routes (da Silva et al., 2013). Furthermore, biochemical characteristics of envelope proteins are crucial to the pathogenesis of RNA viruses. For instance, the pattern of glycosylation of envelope proteins can vary significantly between viral strains, influencing the stability and functionality of such proteins. In viruses like mouse hepatitis virus (MHV), the glycoprotein gp65 is a prime example, where various glycosylation patterns influence its response during viral maturation and transport in the host cell. Investigations have demonstrated that factors such as carbohydrates play a crucial role in viral protein maturation, an influencing on their assembly and inclusion into new virions. The existence of envelope proteins like gp65 can also be attributed to secondary functions beyond structural integrity alone, such as enzymatic functions facilitating viral replication, thus defining the multifunctional role of envelope components in RNA viruses (Yokomori et al., 1989). The understanding of the presence of envelopes extends beyond the simple realm of virology. The structure, composition, and interactions with host cell processes of the envelopes are critical to the formulation of antiviral interventions. The targeting of envelope proteins continues to be a hopeful avenue in the formulation of vaccines and therapeutic intervention, as manipulation of the interactions can potentially cause prevention of virus entry and subsequent infection. Furthermore, the difference in envelope composition among various viral strains defines the challenge of formulating a universal intervention. The functionality of the envelopes is not structural but functional, and this influences the evolution of viral strategies in evading therapeutic interventions. With research ongoing to prove the complexity involved in RNA virus envelopes, the success of interventions will increasingly depend on the understanding of the critical roles these membranes play in viral life cycles and against host defense mechanisms (Yokomori et al., 1989; da Silva et al., 2013) (Figure 3.7).

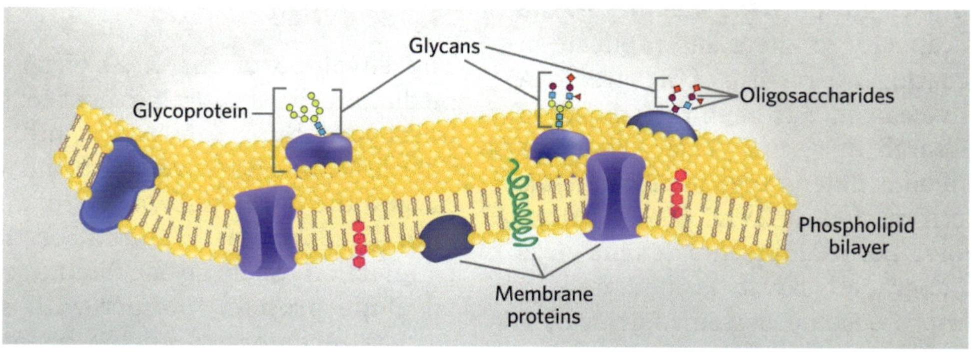

Figure 3.7. Glycoproteins infographic.

Source: https://cdn.the-scientist.com/assets/image/48344/glycoproteins-infographic-x.webp.

Test Your Knowledge

1. What is the overall organization of the viral genome in RNA viruses, and how does it differ in different families of RNA viruses?
2. Describe the capsid structure of RNA viruses and list its primary functions.

3.3. Replication Cycle of RNA Viruses

Learning Outcome

1. Describe the invasion of host cells by RNA viruses;
2. Identify replication and transcription processes of RNA viruses;
3. Explain how assembly and release of new virions are crucial processes in the life cycle of RNA viruses.

The replication cycle of RNA viruses is a complex array of steps that is very dependent on the interaction of the virus with host cell machinery. The process begins with viral particle attachment to host cell surface receptors, causing cell entry. Once inside, the viral RNA genome must be released into the host cytoplasm. The process usually consists of uncoating, where the protective protein shell is removed, exposing the viral RNA to translation and replication. Curiously, RNA viruses utilize a range of mechanisms to do so, including direct penetration or endocytosis, depending on the virus. The second key step is the translation of viral proteins, needed for subsequent replication, which attests to the diversity of RNA viruses to harness the host cellular machinery to facilitate their replicative processes. Following the release of viral RNA and translation, the replication phase ensues, which involves the synthesis of complementary strands of RNA. The primary enzyme responsible for this process is the RNA-dependent RNA polymerase (RdRp), which makes copies of the viral genome and produces messenger RNA (mRNA) that codes for structural proteins necessary for the assembly of new virions. This phase is essential for the spread of the virus, as a robust replication system must be available for explosive viral particle number increases in the host. The non-structural protein NS1 of a number of RNA viruses has been shown to be important in determining the replication cycle, not just by regulating viral RNA production but also by blocking host immuneresponses, thus increasing overall viral fitness and persistence within the host (Hale et al., 2012). This association between the host and the virus further complicates managing RNA virus outbreaks. Eventually, the assembly and release of the new virus particle finalize the replication cycle. Novel viral proteins and RNA genomes produced are encapsidated into capsids, allowing progeny virion formation. This assembly tends to take place at certain intracellular locations, for instance, the endoplasmic reticulum or Golgi apparatus. Fission or budding then results in the release of new virions into the extracellular medium, where they infect adjacent cells, spreading the infection. Host factors are also essential in this process of assembly as they can either facilitate or hinder viral replication and spread, affecting the virus's overall pathogenicity. For instance, certain host proteins have been shown to display proviral activity, taking part in essential processes of the replication cycle, such as translation of viral RNA and assembly of virions, testifying to the fine balance existing between viral success and host defenses (Garcia-Ruiz, 2018). Understanding these mechanisms gives one a sense of probable targets for therapy in managing RNA virus infections (Figure 3.8).

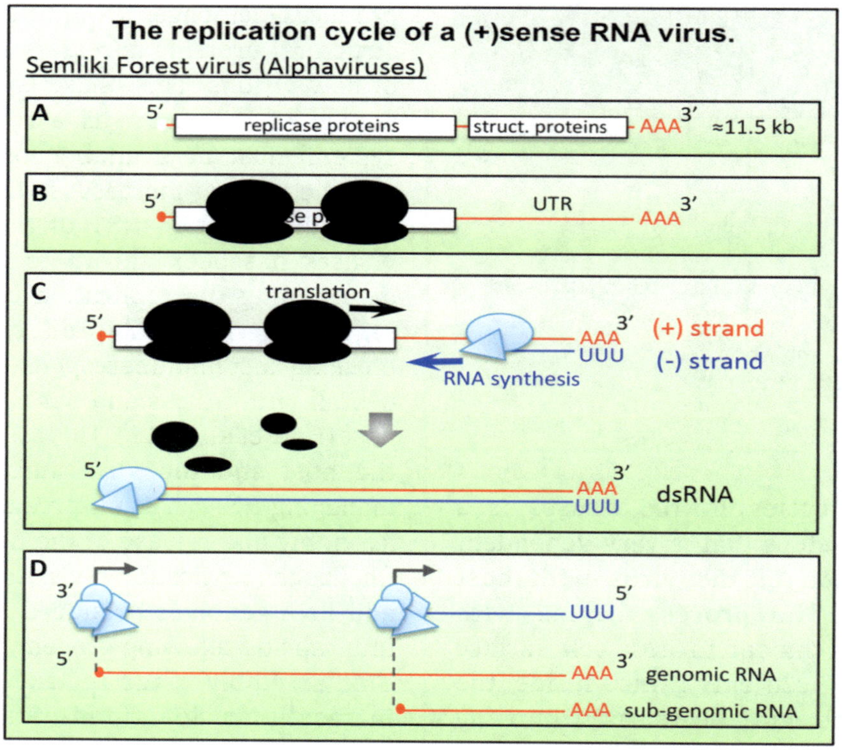

Figure 3.8. The replication cycle of a positive-stranded RNA (+)RNA virus.

Source: https://www.researchgate.net/publication/312647278/figure/fig3/AS:1143128121206193 9@1702524843611/The-replication-cycle-of-a-positive-stranded-RNA-RNA-virus-A-The-bi-cystronic.tif.

3.3.1. Entry Into Host Cells

Invasion of host cells by RNA viruses is a complex process that typically involves specific interactions between viral proteins and host receptors. The interaction is a prerequisite for successful invasion and subsequent virus replication in host organisms. For instance, arenaviruses use various cellular receptors, for instance, α-dystroglycan for Old World strains and human transferrin receptor 1 for New World strains, to invade permissive cells. The binding step is a critical requirement, as it will dictate the virus's ability to infect the host, leading to the establishment of viral replication. Moreover, the virus adsorption to the cell surface is typically followed by endocytosis, where the host's cellular machinery is exploited to internalize the viral particles. The intricacy of the mechanism speaks volumes about the necessity of a full understanding of entry pathways in the design of antiviral strategies. Subsequent to host cell invasion, RNA viruses must negotiate a series of intracellular barriers to establish productive infection. Following entry, some RNA viruses use endosomal pathways, where viral particles are subjected to the action of host cell factors such as cathepsins B and L, implicated in the uncoating of the viral genome. The uncoating is critical in delivering the viral RNA into the cytoplasm, where it can interact with the host's translational machinery. For hepatitis C virus (HCV), chronic infections have demonstrated that viral variants can adapt over time to be more replication competent. Based on studies, adaptation can be achieved through mutations in viral envelope proteins that will enhance receptor binding or immune evasion. These evolutionary dynamics emphasize the perpetual tension between viral persistence and host defense mechanisms that are crucial to both the etiology of pathogenesis and the design of effective therapy. Active examination of viral entry mechanisms suggests that interference with such processes can be of therapeutic value. Interference with the specific viral protein-host cell receptor interactions can potentially enable researchers to prevent viral infection from taking root. Monitoring of the critical cellular factors that have been implicated in productive entry by arenaviruses and HCV can guide new approaches to antiviral drug development. For example, therapeutic interventions that disrupt the interaction between viral glycoproteins and their cellular receptors can prevent the virus from establishing an infection. As the breadth of viral entry mechanisms increases, the synthesis of knowledge across a large spectrum of RNA viruses is necessary to build a unifying strategy for limiting the public health burden of these pathogens, and specifically in the context of emerging viral threats (Figure 3.9).

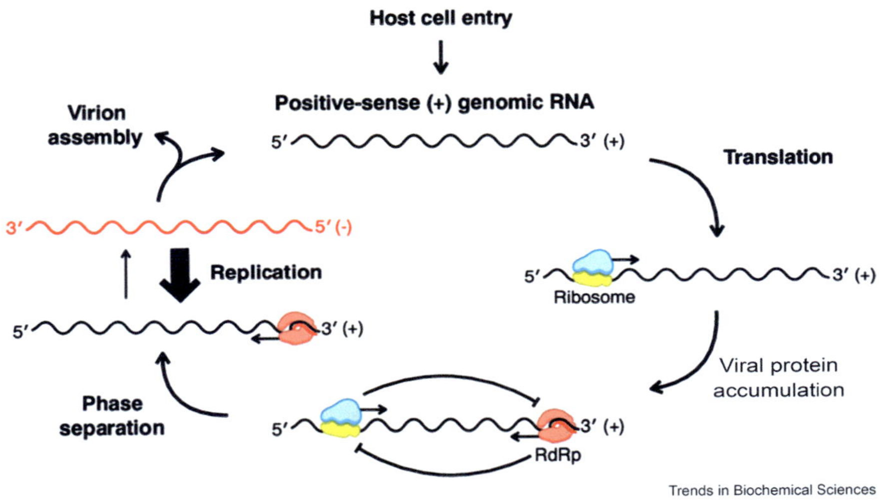

Figure 3.9. Phase separation may mediate the switch from translation to replication in positive-sense RNA viruses. After host cell entry, positive-sense RNA viruses can immediately serve as templates for translation by host cell ribosomes.

Source: https://www.researchgate.net/publication/364409439/figure/fig3/AS:11431281091017706@1666280360411/Phase-separation-may-mediate-the-switch-from-translation-to-replication-in-positive-sense.png.

3.3.2. Replication and Transcription Processes

RNA virus replication and transcription are critical to their ability to replicate and co-opt host cellular machinery. RNA viruses typically employ their RNA-dependent RNA polymerase (RdRp) to replicate their genome and generate mRNA. This polymerase begins replication by copying the viral RNA template as complementary strands of RNA to generate new viral genomes. This includes viral gene translation to mRNA, which is used as a template to generate proteins. RdRpc fidelity and the kinetics of these enzymatic processes control the efficiency of viral replication and, in turn, influence virus virulence and evolutionary fitness, as mutations can arise during RNA replication as a result of the lack of proofreading mechanisms inherent in these enzymes. Research into the interaction of RNA viruses with host cellular processes has revealed complex networks of regulation that facilitate viral replication and sustain infection. For instance, research into the Zika virus (ZIKV) has revealed far-reaching alterations in the transcriptomic profile of various human cell lines upon infection (Tiwari et al., 2017). These changes result in the downregulation of genes associated with the adaptive immune response, ensuring that the virus evades defense and enhances replication. These evasions illustrate how RNA viruses co-opt host cellular processes, including metabolic functions, to fuel their replication activities. ZIKV's ability to reprogram host resources illustrates the intricate schemes employed by RNA viruses in sustaining their life cycles, reflecting the significance of in-depth knowledge of these mechanisms in the design of effective antiviral therapies. In addition, more recent studies using fungal models, i.e., *Neurospora crassa*, have emphasized the function of RNA interference (RNAi) in regulating viral replication and transcription mechanisms (Aulia et al., 2020). In the model, viral infection elicits an immune response to upregulate the components of RNAi to suppress viral replication. The presence of Dicer proteins and Argonaute enzymes confirms interaction between virus replication systems and antiviral defense systems. The model not only displays the rudimentary mechanisms of viral replication but also the hosts' efforts to resist such mechanisms. Through the application of such models, scientists can appreciate the subtleties of host-virus relationships, leading to novel approaches in antiviral drug development and therapeutic interventions (Figure 3.10).

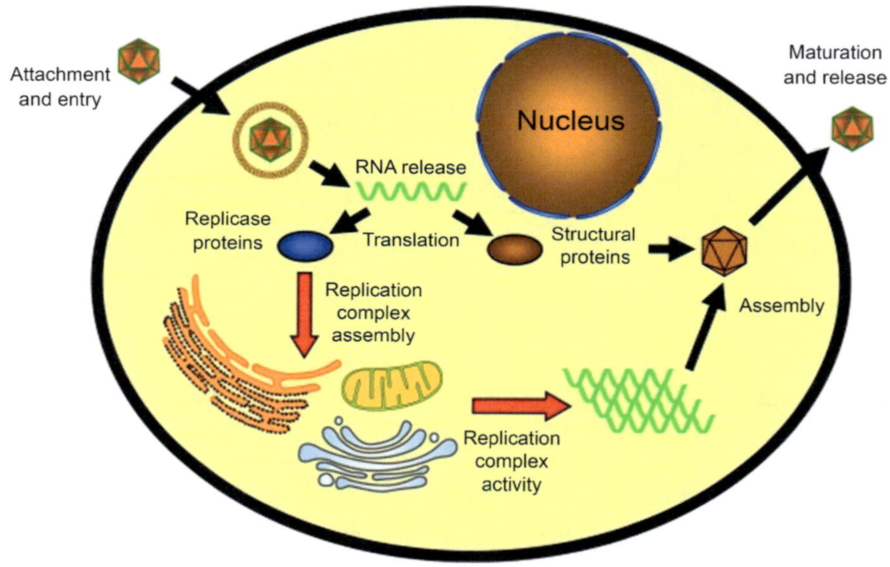

Figure 3.10. Schematic of positive-sense RNA virus replication cycle. General steps include: (i) attachment and entry; (ii) release of genome into cytoplasm; (iii) translation of genomic viral RNA into replicase or structural proteins; (iv) assembly of replication complex on host intracellular membrane; (v) amplification of viral genome via dsRNA intermediate; (vi) genome encapsidation; and (vii) maturation and release.

Source: https://www.researchgate.net/publication/51712002/figure/fig1/AS:202793873874960@1425361235971/Schematic-of-positive-sense-RNA-virus-replication-cycle-General-steps-include-i.png.

3.3.3. Assembly and Release of New Virions

Assembly and release of new virions are pivotal processes in the life cycle of RNA viruses, especially for influenza viruses. Morphogenesis of such viruses depends on the coordinated coordination of viral elements to the apical plasma membrane of polarized epithelial cells, where budding starts and virions mature. Central to this coordination is the viral envelope, which is made of lipids from the host cell membrane and studded with transmembrane proteins such as hemagglutinin (HA), neuraminidase (NA), and M2. Matrix protein (M1) plays a pivotal role as a nexus that connects the lipid envelope to the viral ribonucleocapsid (vRNP), providing structural stability in effect. This complex viral protein interaction is essential, as the efficiency of assembly directly affects the production of infectious particles and, hence, the viral pathogenesis (Balogun et al., 2009). 7Viral elements are directed to the assembly site by specialized routes, namely through exocytic pathways and lipid rafts, and thereby concentrate specific lipids and proteins at the budding site location. HA and NA possess intrinsic apical sorting signals, facilitating selective transport to the cell surface, where they aid budding initiation by distorting the lipid bilayer. The interactions of M1 proteins with the cytoplasmic tail of glycoproteins and the vRNP bring necessary elements to the budding site and, in effect, exclude most host proteins from this microenvironment. The cholesterol of lipid rafts and glycosphingolipids also plays a role in forming the required membrane curvature necessary for the mechanical process of budding. This coordination of viral and host proteins controls the critical transition from assembly to release, mirroring the fine balance in viral life cycles (Barman et al., 2004). The terminal process in virion release entails not only the finalization of budding but scission of mature particles from the cell membrane. This is an energy-requiring, finely regulated process that requires a subtle interaction between viral proteins like M1, NA, and M2, and host cellular elements. Scission is facilitated through the disruption of cortical actin microfilaments, allowing for efficient separation of the bud. The viral neuraminidase also plays a crucial role in this process by cleaving sialic acid residues on the host cell surface, inhibiting re-attachment and allowing spread to adjacent cells. Aberrations in any one of these processes, through mutations in M1, M2 itself, or NA, can have profound implications on the morphology of resulting virions and overall viral infectivity. Understanding these processes can provide a window of opportunity for targeted therapeutic interventions to influenza and other RNA viruses (Balogun et al., 2009).

Test Your Knowledge

1. By what mechanisms do RNA viruses typically gain entry into host cells, and how does the viral capsid or envelope facilitate such entry?
2. In what ways do positive-sense and negative-sense RNA viruses differ in how they proceed to transcribe viral mRNA within the host cell?

3.4. Pathogenesis of RNA Viruses

Learning Outcome

1. To comprehend viral infection mechanisms;
2. Explain how the host immune response against RNA viruses;
3. To give examples of RNA virus-causing diseases.

Pathogenesis of RNA viruses is a very complicated process involving complex interactions between viral architecture and host cellular mechanisms. RNA viruses, in contrast to DNA viruses, typically possess high rates of mutation, which result in effective evolution and adaptability. This genetic variability enables the RNA viruses to evade host immune responses and, thus, the development of vaccines and antiviral drugs is difficult. A good example of such viruses is the bunyaviruses, a family of Bunyaviridae viruses, which have tri-segmented genomes encoding various proteins like structural and non-structural proteins. These not only aid in viral replication but also in immunomodulation of the host immune response. By their interaction with the host's innate immune response, bunyavirus non-structural proteins can enhance pathogenicity and illustrate their function in controlling disease severity and transmission patterns (Kohl et al., 2013). Lastly, it is known that unraveling these viral-host interactions is crucial to developing a successful therapeutic strategy against RNA viruses. Another fascinating example of RNA viral pathogenicity is the Zika virus (ZIKV), which has been linked with severe neurological disorders. ZIKV possesses unique mechanisms to leverage host cellular processes, such as immune suppression and resource repurposing, for enhanced viral replication. Experiments have shown that ZIKV infection leads to differential gene expression in various human cell types, affecting those that participate in the adaptive immune response and cellular metabolism. In particular, ZIKV infection inhibits immune response genes within microglia cells and thereby facilitates the virus persistence within the central nervous system (Tiwari et al., 2017). This immune evasion not only enhances the virulence of infection but also enables the virus to sustain high levels of replication in the host, pointing to the fine balance between viral replication and resistance of the host. Pathogenesis of RNA viruses is also beyond direct viral effect on host cells; in many instances, it is extremely intricate interactions with the host immune system, leading to damaging inflammatory responses. For example, viral infections can trigger unintended tissue damage in the form of cytokine storms, which are overactive and unregulated immune reactions. RNA viruses can hijack host signal transduction pathways in a manner that activates or inhibits immune responses, depending on their survival strategies. The successful hijacking of host cell resources, including metabolic machinery, underlines the necessity of an integrated understanding of the pathogenesis of RNA viruses. Through unraveling these complex dynamics, researchers are better able to demarcate possible antiviral targets and develop ways of reducing the impact of RNA viruses on human health (Kohl et al., 2013; Tiwari et al., 2017). As such, continued investigation into RNA viral pathogenesis is imperative for improving public health measures against viral outbreaks.

3.4.1. Mechanisms of Viral Infection

The mechanisms of viral infection are sophisticated processes that enable RNA viruses to successfully infect host cells and replicate. Central to the process is the virus's ability to employ cellular processes to its advantage. For instance, RNA viruses tend to employ host cellular machinery to hijack translational processes to avoid the innate immune system. Such manipulation not only ensures the efficient production of viral proteins but is also central to viral replication. Regulation of both cellular and viral gene expression cannot be overstated, as such fine-tuned control is essential to both the infection process and the host's ability to mount an effective response to the viral threat. Notably, viruses have evolved different mechanisms to counteract or evade host defense mechanisms to survive and transmit themselves in the host organism (Gaglia et al., 2010). In addition to the use of host cellular machinery, RNA viruses have sophisticated means of interfering with host responses to limit infection, such as the formation of stress granules (SGs). SGs are inducible cytoplasmic structures elicited by cellular stress, including viral infection, and serve as an immune defense against the virus through inhibition of viral replication. It has been found that viral proteins can interfere with the formation of such granules and facilitate the virus to counter this host immune response. For example, in Semliki Forest virus infection, viral nonstructural protein 3 (nsP3) sequesters G3BP, a crucial protein component of SGs, in a very efficient manner into viral replication complexes. In addition to inhibiting SG formation, this process also underscores the critical role of SGs in the host's antiviral defense against RNA viruses (Eng et al., 2012). The two-way dynamic interaction between RNA viruses and the host cells is what governs viral pathogenesis complexity. Since these viruses mutate continuously, they become progressively more sophisticated at manipulating host gene expression as well as impairing antiviral defense mechanisms. This virus-host defense arms race highlights the necessity of ongoing research endeavors to deconstruct these mechanisms, thereby furthering our understanding of viral infections and the effectiveness of therapy. The ability of RNA viruses to hijack and exploit cellular machinery not only presents challenges in the control of viral disease but also offers an intrinsic understanding of cellular processes. By studying these interactions, scientists can determine putative antiviral targets and push the field of virology more generally (Gaglia et al., 2010) (Figure 3.11).

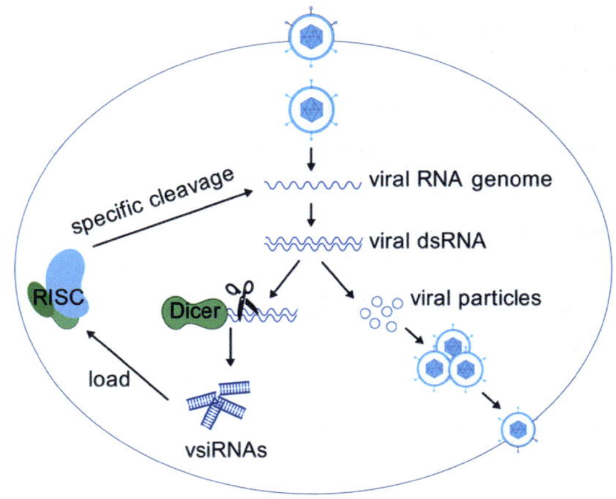

Figure 3.11. The mechanism of RNAi against viral infection.

Source: https://www.researchgate.net/publication/381264609/figure/fig1/AS:11431281250606604@1717916430018/The-mechanism-of-RNAi-against-viral-infection.ppm.

3.4.2. Host Immune Response to RNA Viruses

Host immune response to RNA viruses is a dynamic, complex process involving many cellular and molecular mechanisms. During infection, the innate immune system is the first line of defense that employs pattern recognition receptors (PRRs) to sense viral RNA. Stimulation of signaling pathways through these receptors results in the production of interferons and pro-inflammatory cytokines. Interferons play a crucial role in creating an antiviral milieu within infected cells and neighboring cells, inhibiting viral replication and facilitating the activation of adaptive immunity. Hence, the innate response not only reacts rapidly to RNA virus presence but also affects the related adaptive responses, testifying to the inseparable relationship between these two limbs of immunity in dealing with viral infections. As the disease progresses, adaptive immunity becomes increasingly important. The T and B cells specifically target the viral antigens, promoting the generation of viral-specific responses. B cells produce antibodies that neutralize the virus so it cannot infect additional cells. Or cytotoxic T lymphocytes (CTLs) recognize and kill infected cells, lowering the viral load. However, RNA viruses such as human immunodeficiency virus (HIV) and Zika virus (ZIKV) have evolved mechanisms that help suppress the immune system. For instance, ZIKV has been demonstrated to downregulate adaptive immune response-related genes in microglia, representing an immune evasion mechanism subsequent to central nervous system invasion. These approaches emphasize the ongoing arms race between host immune response and RNA viruses, key to understanding the pathogenesis of such infections. Recent advances, namely with next-generation sequencing (NGS), have contributed significantly towards significantly improving knowledge surrounding host immune response to RNA viruses. NGS allows for the unselected analysis of both the viral variants present in a host of infection and the host's antibody repertoire. Random peptide phage display library-based research (RPPDL) has provided insights into the antibody response elicited by various pathogens, including RNA viruses. Importantly, NGS not only accounts for the dynamics of the immune response but also unravels pivotal virus-host interactions responsible for the outcome of the infection. For instance, the high mutation rate of the RNA virus results in a heterogeneous viral population that complicates the immune response and permits persistent viral replication. These findings reveal the potential of NGS as a cost-effective tool to unveil the host-pathogen interaction complexity and develop effective antiviral therapies against RNA viruses (Gerasimov, 2017; Tiwari et al., 2017) (Figure 3.12).

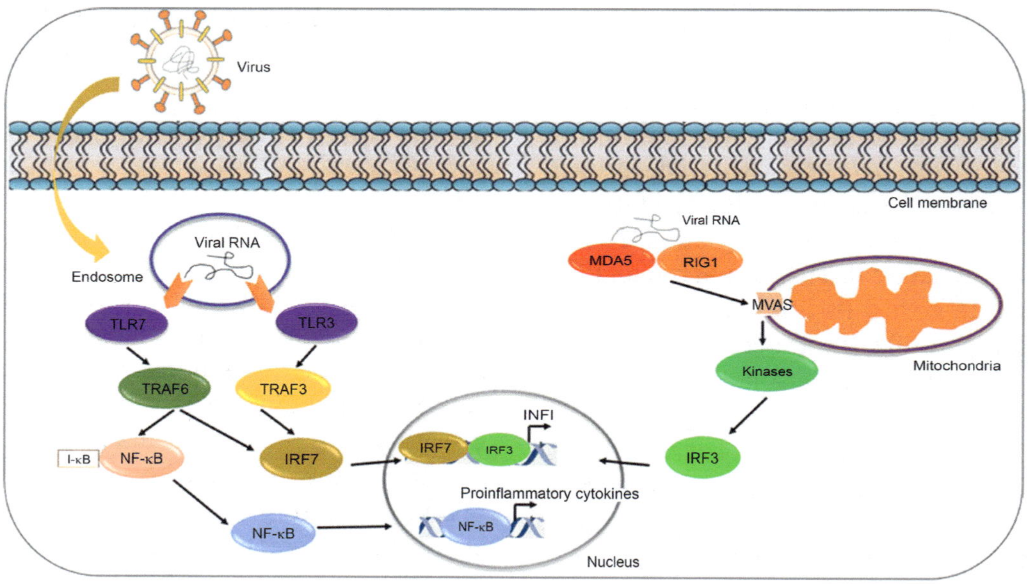

Figure 3.12. Innate immune response to RNA viruses. Innate immune response is activated after viral PAMPs (such as viral RNA) detection by host cells PRR including TLRs (TLR3, TLR7) and RLRs (MDA5 and RIG1).

Source: https://www.researchgate.net/publication/345145754/figure/fig1/AS:963553309765633@1606740419157/Innate-immune-response-to-RNA-viruses-Innate-immune-response-is-activated-after-viral.png.

3.4.3. Examples of Diseases Caused by RNA Viruses (e.g., Influenza, HIV)

RNA viruses are a diverse and significant group of pathogens that cause a wide range of diseases in animals and humans. Among these, the influenza virus is well noted for causing seasonal epidemics of high morbidity and mortality. The virus has high antigenic variation, and hence producing vaccines as well as carrying out public health measures is challenging. The impact of influenza extends beyond immediate health conditions, affecting health systems, the economy, and societal functioning in general. The historical record of influenza pandemics, such as the 1918 Spanish influenza, acts to underscore its potential as a disastrous global health risk. Scientific research indicates that the evolution of new strains necessitates continued surveillance and recasting of vaccines, which acts to highlight the indispensable role of international surveillance in making effective management of influenza epidemics possible (Flanagan et al., 2012). The second famous RNA virus is the human immunodeficiency virus (HIV), which induces acquired immunodeficiency syndrome (AIDS). Contrary to the seasonal nature of influenza, HIV becomes a lifelong illness that requires lifetime management. HIV largely infects CD4+ T cells, which causes progressive damage to the immune system, eventually rendering one susceptible to opportunistic infections and cancers. Despite significant advances made in antiretroviral treatment that have made HIV a chronic and manageable disease from its previous deadly state, drug resistance, stigma, and treatment adherence remain extremely prevalent.

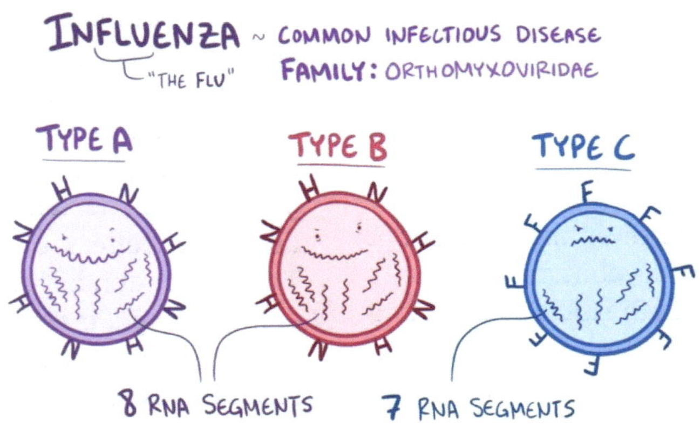

Figure 3.13. Influenza.

Source: https://d16qt3wv6xm098.cloudfront.net/l-f-CDnrQeCB_Iuzc9AQN7yiS4C_w5GS/_.jpg.

The socio-economic determinants of HIV infection among vulnerable populations underscore the need for comprehensive public health interventions directed at prevention, education, and access to care (Chiu et al., 2013). In addition to influenza and HIV, hepatitis C virus (HCV) and dengue virus are other prominent RNA viruses. HCV is a leading cause of liver disease and its chronicity, leading to cirrhosis and liver cancer, has a significant health burden across the globe. The invention of direct-acting antiviral drugs has revolutionized the treatment of HCV, giving hope to millions of individuals across the world. Conversely, the dengue virus is a major public health issue in tropical and subtropical regions, associated with high morbidity and mortality. The transmission of dengue fever is eased by increasing urbanization and climate change, which enhance the habitat of its mosquito vectors. Together, these illustrations point to the pressing need for ongoing research and public health initiatives to combat RNA virus-related illnesses and assist in the diminution of their contribution to world health (Flanagan et al., 2012) (Figure 3.13).

Test Your Knowledge

1. What are the key steps in entry and replication of RNA viruses into host cells?
2. How can RNA viruses avoid or suppress the host immune response during infection?

3.5. Transmission and Epidemiology

Learning Outcome

1. Describe transmission modes used by RNA viruses;
2. Explain factors that control RNA virus outbreaks;
3. Discuss global impact and figures on RNA virus infections.

The epidemiology and transmission dynamics of RNA viruses accentuate their ability to adapt and how hard they are to control for public health. RNA viruses such as the mumps virus and Oropouche virus exhibit complex transmission patterns that have a tendency to occur as outbreaks in specific communities. The mumps virus, for instance, experienced unusually large outbreaks across the United States during 2016 and 2017, indicating the nuanced relationship between vaccination activity and lingering viral circulation. Using epidemiological analysis supplemented by genomic evaluation, researchers concluded that despite high vaccine coverage, multiple independent introductions of the virus accounted for widespread undetected circulation. This is an example of how RNA viruses can become undetected and establish themselves as persistent in a population and hence prove challenging to contain. Beyond mumps, another RNA virus incurring significant public health concern is the Oropouche virus (OROV), and it particularly does so in Latin America. Studies have charted OROV as one of the leading etiologies of arboviral disease in Venezuela and Brazil. The transmission of the virus, primarily via insect vectors, highlights the relationship between environmental determinants and patterns of epidemiology. Evidence from the past reveals that OROV had triggered outbreaks that endured for decades, depicting a solid presence in the environment. As scientists analyze this virus, they gain significant information regarding its genetic makeup, evolutionary past, and pathogenesis pathways, all pertaining to its epidemiology and the effectiveness of vaccines and treatments. The integration of genomic data with traditional epidemiologic methods has revolutionized our understanding of RNA virus transmission. For instance, in the mumps virus, genomic sequencing made reconstruction of unseen transmission chains possible that were not visible from conventional surveillance practices. This is a demonstration of molecular epidemiology's power because the actual lineages of the virus can be determined and their evolutionary trends. Similarly, OROV research has shown that broad reviews of its epidemiological history are able to guide contemporary responses to the outbreaks. Merging genomic analysis with epidemiological data not only extends the knowledge of viral transmission but also equips public health authorities with tools critical for timely and informed intervention actions against RNA viruses, ultimately for controlling their impact on global health.

3.5.1. Modes of Transmission (Airborne, Vector-Borne, etc.)

The modes of transmission employed by RNA viruses play a pivotal role in their epidemiology, virulence, and control strategy. Airborne transmission is a powerful route, allowing viruses to transmit well through respiratory droplets. Flu and coronaviruses are good cases in point, where infected individuals emit viral particles that can be breathed in by other individuals, having a tendency to lead to rapid epidemics. The capability of aerosolizing these pathogens allows them to be more infectious, making them particularly hard to contain. Airborne transmission is not only responsible for person-to-person transmission but also poses issues of environmental stability, with viruses being able to survive on surfaces, thereby feeding into indirect channels of transmission. It is important to analyze the dynamics of airborne transmission in order to best develop effective public health interventions, particularly in the management of outbreaks and vaccination programs for high-risk individuals. Vector-borne transmission is another significant mechanism through which RNA viruses are spread, and the vectors are mosquitoes and ticks. Such transmission is often mixed with complex ecological processes that may disrupt the virus's life cycle and its pathogenic impact on host populations. The Zika virus and West Nile virus are examples in hand, highlighting how vectors can transmit RNA viruses from one geographic location to another. Environmental factors conducive to the sustenance of vector populations, such as climate and habitat, are of maximum significance in their optimization of transmission capabilities. Further, viral strain evolution may impact the vector competence of their vectors and, consequently, the epidemiological patterns of the infections they cause. The intricate interaction of vectors with pathogens demands integrated vector management approaches addressing both environmental and viral transmission aspects, providing an integrated framework essential in vector-borne disease control. It is important to comprehend the spatial dynamics of different transmission modes to fully understand the broader implications of RNA viruses in public health. Epidemic spaces are not fixed; they involve a continuum of forces that build up how diseases occur and propagate, as underscored in reports of cultural analyses and Actor Network Theory. The positioning of infected individuals, vectors, and environmental agents may create transmission patterns that obscure traditional epidemiological models. Understanding these spatial characteristics supports mapping risk areas, thereby guiding targeted interventions. For example, knowledge of the significance of index cases compared to general associations can assist in planning outbreak responses. With the constantly changing global scenario through urbanization and climate change, the mode of transmission research also needs to remain responsive, integrating both micro-level contacts and macro-level trends for effective disease control and management (Loon, 2010; Wilson et al., 2017).

3.5.2. Factors Influencing Outbreaks

Identification of determinants of RNA virus epidemics is critical to implement effective control and prevention measures. Among the principal determinants is the interaction between environmental components and virus genetics. An illustration is that the virulence of viruses such as the bluetongue virus (BTV) not only relies on the strain of the virus but also on the host species involved and their genetic make-up. Studies demonstrate that susceptibility varies among ruminant species as well as among breeds within a species, highlighting the host's influence on the course of viral infections. Additionally, the dynamics of viral transmission are affected by variability in environmental factors, such as temperature and humidity, which show the interaction between host and environmental parameters that allows outbreaks of RNA viruses like BTV and others to occur in comparable contexts (Caporale et al., 2014). Agricultural practice provides a valuable context in which RNA virus outbreaks could be affected. More intensified agricultural systems have the potential to alter the wildlife reservoir and livestock-hosting ecosystems, raising the chances of zoonotic spillover events. A systematic review indicated a direct link between agricultural intensification and the likelihood of increased zoonotic disease emergence because of the impact of human activities on the environment. Threats such as deforestation, land conversion, and animal concentration all make significant contributions towards habitat modification and increasing chances for human-wildlife interactions, which can promote RNA virus transmission. The agricultural environment is thus critical in regard to the comprehension and prediction of outbreaks and demands integrated responses that value the intricate interlinkages among agriculture, wildlife, and disease processes (Jones et al., 2013). The relationship between viral epidemics and behavior in human populations cannot be overemphasized, as it entails direct and indirect impacts on transmission risks. With population growth and expansion of urban areas, rising contact between humans, wildlife, and animals is bound to increase. The intensification of these contacts by a shift in behavior, such as greater movement, trade, and encroachment into habitats, contributes to the issue, allowing opportunistic RNA viruses to exploit new hosts. Moreover, public policy and health infrastructure are also essential to minimizing these risks of outbreak. Poor surveillance or response systems may lead to delayed outbreak detection, allowing viruses to spread uncontrollably. Hence, due to the multifaceted nature of the human impact, being aware of and reacting to it is paramount in forecasting and curbing RNA virus outbreaks and highlighting interdisciplinary cooperation in public health and environmental management policy (Jones et al., 2013) (Figure 3.14).

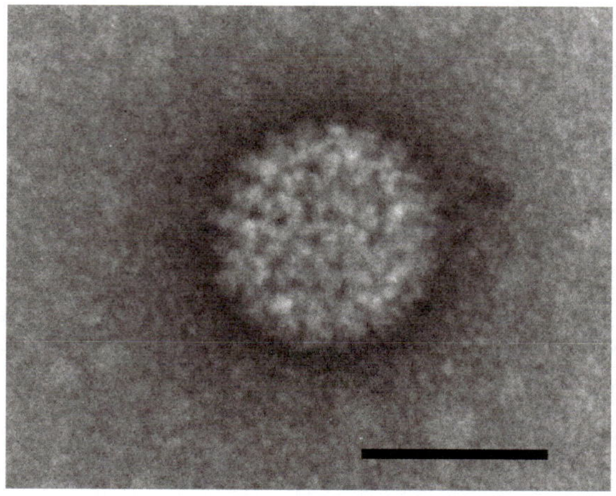

Figure 3.14. Electron micrograph of Bluetongue virus, scale bar = 50 nm.

Source: https://upload.wikimedia.org/wikipedia/commons/a/a5/Bluetongue_virus.gif.

3.5.3. Global Impact and Statistics on RNA Virus Infections

The global impact of RNA virus diseases is profoundly significant. The prevalence and multiplicity of such agents render their total impact broadly important. RNA viruses, including influenza, coronaviruses, and the diverse arboviruses, are responsible for causing the vast majority of infectious diseases on Earth. Influenza, to illustrate, imposes a heavy seasonal burden on the health of humankind, with its annual epidemics causing immense morbidity and mortality. Research in Italy from 2010 to 2016 pointed out that influenza B viruses were usually present during seasonal outbreaks, even surpassing influenza A in some years. This research pinpointed that the group of children up to 14 years was especially susceptible, identifying key data in terms of the age groups infected by these viruses. These statistics reinforce the need for ongoing monitoring and intervention practices to battle the high levels of medical burdens generated by RNA viruses across global populations (Alicino et al., 2018). Furthermore, the identification of RNA viruses that can cross species boundaries is an increasing public health risk. Specifically, zoonotic RNA viruses that undergo replication in animal reservoirs have led to numerous outbreaks, including most recently the COVID-19 pandemic caused by SARS-CoV-2. This demonstrates the interconnectedness of environmental, animal, and human health, and a One Health approach needs to be implemented to avoid and control disease. The ability of some RNA viruses to rapidly evolve complicates vaccine and treatment creation, with new strains evolving to evade immune systems continuously. Identification of these pathogens, particularly in cancer studies, has proved promising for their contribution to disease progression. For example, research showed the RNA virus HPV was present in the majority of cervical carcinomas examined, as evidence of the role such viruses play in the causation of cancer (Mensaert et al., 2015). Aside from their health effect, RNA viruses also create a massive economic cost to healthcare systems around the world. Direct treatment costs of infected individuals and general economic losses due to outbreaks are substantial. For instance, the flu pandemic alone costs the global economy billions annually in health care and lost production. In addition, the surprise emergence of viruses like Ebola and Zika has highlighted the capacity of RNA viruses to bring about the sudden collapse of societies and economies. With globalization spurring more human-animal contact and urbanization, the danger posed by emerging threats of RNA viruses is likely to grow. Hence, enhancing the global monitoring of RNA viruses and ensuring equitable access to vaccines and therapeutics is essential to address the public health challenges caused by RNA viruses and limit their worldwide diffusion (Alicino et al., 2018).

Test Your Knowledge

1. What are the principal mechanisms of transmission of RNA viruses, and how do they differ among airborne and vector-borne viruses?
2. What is the role of environmental and social factors in the transmission and epidemics of RNA virus infections?
3. Are you capable of describing the global implications of prevalent RNA virus infections in terms of morbidity, mortality, and public health concerns?

3.6. Treatment and Prevention

Learning Outcome

1. Identify antiviral treatments of RNA viruses;
2. Outline strategies of vaccination and how they work against RNA viruses;
3. Address public health interventions to curtail outbreaks from RNA viruses.

Treatment and prevention of RNA viruses have evolved significantly in recent decades, and vaccination remains the cornerstone approach to curbing viral infections. Immunologically based prevention strategies have been historically eclipsed by vaccination, which was developed to create immune responses that prepare the body to fight specific pathogens upon contact. However, the complexity of RNA viruses combined with their mutation rates presents major challenges to vaccine development. Moreover, some viruses have no effective vaccines, and the possibility of side effects in some portion of the population renders vaccination as a precaution for all an option of doubtful prudence. Thus, prevention and treatment options become a necessity, which gives rise to new strategies such as monoclonal antibodies, which can provide passive immunity and target viral dangers specifically, as in treatments for respiratory syncytial virus (RSV) (Fang et al., 2004). Considering the limitations of traditional vaccination methods, the researchers are exploring a novel approach called Biochemical Prevention and Treatment, which focuses on two main strategies. The first strategy involves the prevention of entry of viruses by passive transfer of antiviral proteins or blockers of host cell receptors, which can halt the stage of primary infection of RNA viruses. The second approach targets viral replication using advanced techniques such as RNA interference (RNAi) and anti-sense DNA, which interfere with viral mRNA and block replication. The measures demonstrate the potential of new therapeutic approaches to target RNA viruses more precisely and prevent the side effects of conventional vaccines and treatments. Such a paradigm shift is a critical development in our knowledge of viral infections and testifies to an imperative to move to comply with the sophisticated life cycle of RNA viruses (Fang et al., 2004). In addition, cell-to-cell transmission of RNA viruses is very challenging to treat, especially for the Hepatitis C virus (HCV). Research indicates that cell-to-cell transmission enables HCV to persist in the liver, thus evading neutralizing antibodies and rendering therapeutic interventions difficult. Understanding how intercellular communication is performed displays the requirement of utilizing dual strategies that entail the utilization of both host-targeting entry inhibitors (HTEIs) and direct-acting antivirals (DAAs). The strategy not only blocks the emergence of drug-resistant strains but also enhances the efficacy of treatment protocols. As exemplified in model systems of cutting-edge quality, inhibition of cell-cell transmission potently blocks the dissemination of resistant strains, predicting a potential means not only for curing established infections but also for preventing the emergence and spread of antiviral resistance in RNA viral infections.

3.6.1. Antiviral Therapies Targeting RNA Viruses

The discovery of antiviral treatments targeting RNA viruses has been of intense interest because of the specific features of these pathogens. RNA viruses such as influenza, hepatitis C, and coronaviruses are particularly difficult to target using traditional antiviral treatments due to high rates of mutation and multiple mechanisms of evasion. As the viruses are bound to become resistant to drugs, novel therapeutic approaches are needed. Direct-acting antivirals (DAAs) have been investigated, which target individual viral proteins to inhibit infection and transmission. Evidence shows that the efficacy of such therapies may be maximized by strategic combinations that have the ability to counteract resistance, and the importance of a combined strategy in antiviral design. Cell-to-cell transmission has been noted as significant in the persistence and spread of RNA viruses, with special emphasis on the hepatitis C virus (HCV). HCV utilizes conventional entry pathways in combination with direct cell-to-cell transmission, enabling it to escape neutralizing antibodies and render treatment difficult. There are indications that DAAs have reduced efficacy against viruses that utilize cell-to-cell transmission, as these viruses would be more resistant to antiviral agents. Inhibition of this mode of transmission has been a possible strategy, with evidence demonstrating that host-targeting entry inhibitors (HTEIs) can effectively inhibit the transmission of resistant mutants. With the synergistic effect of HTEIs and existing DAAs, the prevention of the emergence of drug resistance has been achieved, thereby improving the treatment outcome among infected individuals. Moreover, recent advances in biotechnology, i.e., the creation of induced pluripotent stem cells (iPSCs), are revolutionizing antiviral research. Using patient-specific iPSCs, researchers can create in vitro models with high similarity to human host-pathogen interactions, allowing for more precise investigation into viral replication modes and therapeutic responses. This method has proved critical to replicating a variety of viral diseases, advancing the understanding of genetic susceptibility and virus pathogenesis. By opening the door to genetic modification and genome editing of iPSC-derived cells, the potential for creating targeted therapies that confer antiviral resistance also grows. Such developments not only simplify drug testing but may also have the potential to generate new antiviral strategies, with customized interventions aimed at effectively countering specific RNA virus threats (Figure 3.15).

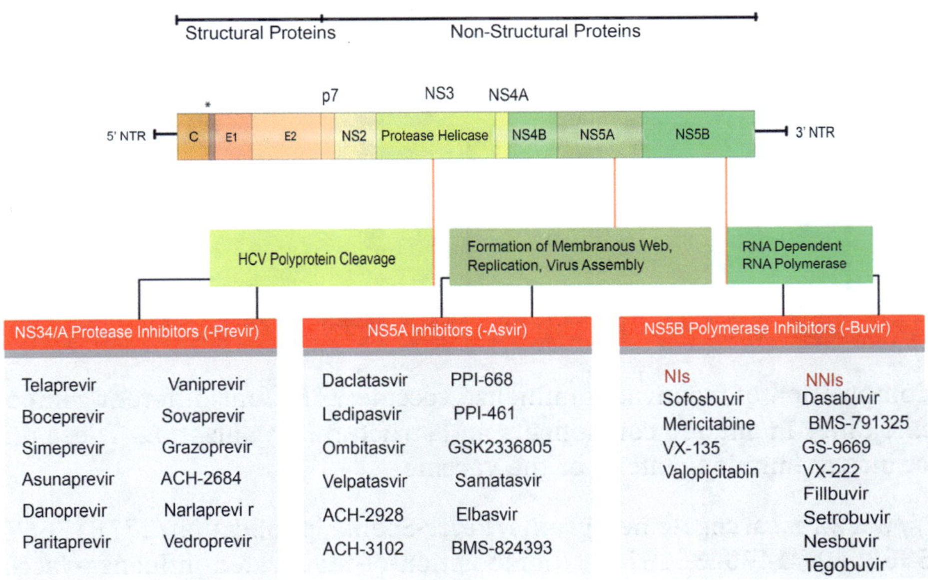

Figure 3.15. Direct-acting antiviral agents for treatment of hepatitis C virus infection.

Source: https://www.researchgate.net/profile/Seyed-Alavian-2/publication/305877907/figure/fig1/AS:391643644612615@1470386529847/Direct-Acting-Antiviral-Agents-for-Treatment-of-Hepatitis-C-Virus-Infection.png.

3.6.2. Vaccination Strategies and Their Effectiveness

Vaccination measures are currently a key component of public health, particularly in the fight against RNA viruses like influenza. The Centers for Disease Control and Prevention observes that annual influenza immunization is the best method to reduce incidence and disease severity, highlighting the necessity for comprehensive immunization programs (Coburn, 2018). However, implementation of such immunizations among such populations as high-risk students in colleges usually does not occur at desired levels. This disparity can be attributed to a variety of determinants, including misperceptions about vaccine safety, attitudes of invulnerability in young populations, and practical issues. As students usually reside in close contact and in close confines with each other, low vaccination coverage can lead to faster transmission, which in turn promotes enhanced public health issues in college communities.

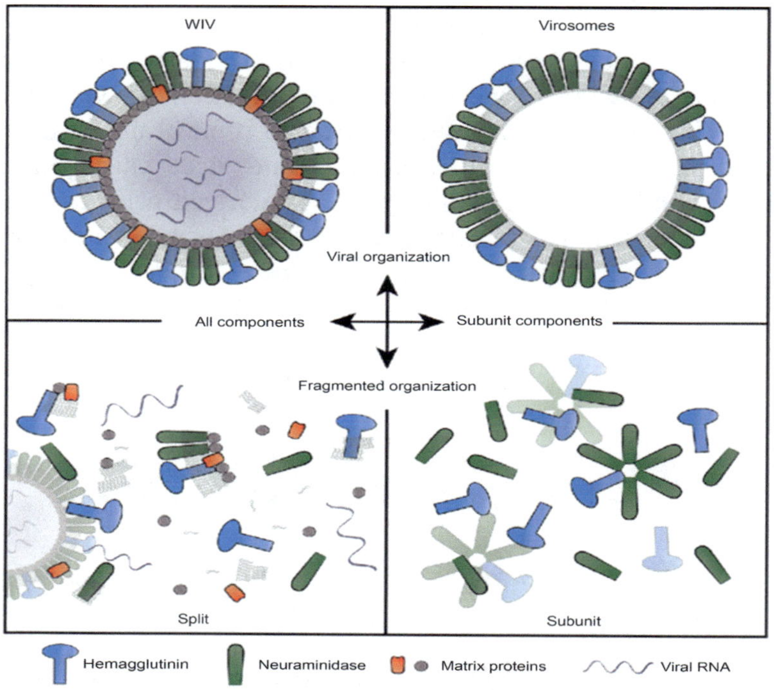

Figure 3.16. Composition of inactivated influenza vaccines. The four different compositions of the influenza vaccine differ in antigen components and structural organization. These differences also have an impact on the immunogenicity of the vaccine.

Source: https://www.researchgate.net/profile/Peter-Soema/publication/277817667/figure/fig2/AS:391851925360640@1470436187279/Composition-of-inactivated-influenza-vaccines-The-four-different-compositions-of.png.

3.6.3. Public Health Measures to Control Outbreaks

The control of outbreaks caused by RNA viruses requires a multi-faceted response to public health measures, specifically those for vector control and community awareness. A fine case in point is the response to the Zika virus, which has led to widespread advice aimed at minimizing human exposure to its principal vector, the Aedes aegypti mosquito. Through enforcing targeted insecticide spraying, community clean-up operations to eradicate standing water, and public campaigns of information about precautions to avoid contact, health authorities try to minimize the population of the mosquito and therefore cases of Zika. Of special importance, the World Health Organization (WHO) declared a global health emergency for the virus, emphasizing the necessity of immediate action to avert its spread and minimize its possible health consequences, particularly on pregnant women and their newborns (Ansari et al., 2016). Aside from vector control, there is a general public health communication system needed to effectively respond to outbreaks of RNA viruses. The dissemination of appropriate information regarding transmission, symptoms, and prevention can significantly alter community behavior, hence averting transmission of the virus. In this context, information sharing on the possible consequences of Zika virus infections, such as microcephaly in the fetus and neurological complications in adults, improves knowledge among at-risk groups. Public health authorities have made recommendations promoting the postponement of pregnancy in affected areas among women of childbearing age, which calls for strong, readily accessible public health messaging (Grazzini et al., 2016). This rapid response not only encourages individuals to take certain measures to safeguard their health but also generates a public reaction to the epidemic. Besides, deployment of diagnostic and surveillance interventions is a key element in controlling RNA virus outbreaks. Sensitive and specific rapid tests can aid the detection of infected individuals for the aim of intervening early by means of counseling and tailored public health interventions. In the case of the Zika virus, cross-reactivity issues between related viruses like dengue necessitate the creation of sensitive and specific assays (Ansari et al., 2016). In addition, national health authorities have been urged to apply strict surveillance measures to monitor Zika virus transmission and incidence levels precisely. Through the application of such stringent public health interventions, e.g., vector control, good communication, and robust diagnostics, health authorities are able to better control RNA virus outbreaks as well as their influence on public health.

Test Your Knowledge

1. What are the principal types of antiviral drugs used to treat RNA virus infections?
2. What is the impact of RNA virus mutation on the effectiveness of antiviral therapy and how is resistance addressed?

SUMMARY

As RNA virus research proceeds, it is becoming more apparent that the complexity of RNA viruses is an enormous challenge and opportunity for scientific exploration. Through detailed explorations of the genetic organizations and replication modes of RNA viruses, we gain valuable information regarding their behavior and adaptations. Of interest is the universality of hairpin structures among RNA genomes, reflecting a high level of evolutionary conservation, as reflected by the greater-than-expected frequency of these structures in noncoding as opposed to coding sequences. This observation not only informs the outcomes of studies on a broad range of viral groups but also calls for further exploration of a role for these secondary structures in influencing viral function and pathogenicity and, therefore, disease control and prevention strategies in public health (Tuplin et al., 2008).

Comparative studies of various RNA viruses, on the other hand, show fascinating evolutionary relationships between otherwise unrelated viral species. For instance, the presence of shared domains of homology among the nonstructural proteins of the tobacco mosaic virus and related viruses underscores the significance of molecular homologies in the understanding of viral replication phenomena. Such observations challenge the conventional classifications and reveal that the RNA viruses share common ancestors, further revealing our understanding of viral evolution. Through the dissection of relationships among diverse viral strains, scientists can potentially reveal common vulnerabilities that can be exploited in the therapeutic intervention, paving the way for novel antiviral strategies that utilize these evolutionary relationships (Ahlquist et al., 1985).

Lastly, the multidimensional nature of RNA viruses dictates that virology be addressed on a holistic level that not only encompasses molecular biology but also evolutionary principles. The continuous exploration of their genetic landscapes and conserved architectures provides useful knowledge that can guide future research. As we disassemble the intricacies of RNA virus replication and virulence, we should continue to place great importance on interdisciplinary cooperation and data sharing among the scientific community. This is imperative for the development of effective vaccines and therapies, particularly in the context of an emerging age of viral peril. In the end, improving our knowledge of RNA viruses can make us better prepared against viral outbreaks, highlighting the foundational role of rigorous scientific inquiry in public health (Ahlquist et al., 1985).

RNA virus research has uncovered important mechanisms by which such pathogens replicate and achieve persistence in host organisms. For instance, recent research has reported the presence of a replication enhancer element (REE) in the capsid gene of the tick-borne encephalitis virus (TBEV). Such an REE, present as a long stable stem–loop structure referred to as SL6, is common to all tick-borne flaviviruses. Experimental manipulations showed that mutations in this structure resulted in moderate attenuation of the virus, while the engineered strains eventually reached wild-type virus levels late in the infection pathway. Such observation accounts for the subtle role of such genomic elements and suggests that such elements constitute the core of the adaptive success of TBEV in natural environments, particularly in the context of the virus's life cycle involving co-feeding among infected and uninfected ticks, shedding light on its evolution dynamics and transmission patterns (Buckley et al., 2011). The variations in the behavior of RNA viruses, particularly at various stages of infection, also play a significant role in their pathogenesis. The case of the Cricket paralysis virus (CrPV) illustrates how chronic infections may have differential metabolic impacts based on the type of host cell. In persistently infected silkworm Bm5 cells, glucose and glutamine significantly increased at early infection stages, while these metabolites plummeted drastically with infection progression. In acutely infected Drosophila S2 cells, however, metabolic signatures showed a spectacular decline in amino acids and carbohydrates before the onset of pathogenesis, followed by the normalization of these metabolites during the pathogen stages. This dichotomy not only emphasizes the perception that metabolic responses are infection-type sensitive but also points to the relevance of metabolic pathways in host-virus interactions (Meeus et al., 2020).

These findings emphasize the intricacy of RNA virus infections, defying the general perception of viral behavior. Unraveling the roles of structural genomic features and host metabolic responses is critical in formulating effective means to manage these pathogens. Thus, additional research on the molecular mechanisms governing viral replication and persistence is crucial. This should include the examination of the implications of host cell metabolic dysregulation, which could guide therapeutic interventions in mitigating the effects of viral infections. Through continued deconstruction of the intricacy of RNA viruses, scientists can better forecast viral behavior in diverse ecosystems and enhance our preparedness for emerging viral risk, ultimately contributing to global public health and disease control (da Rosa et al., 2017).

KEY TERMS FROM THIS CHAPTER

- Acquired immunodeficiency syndrome
- Arenaviruses
- Bunyaviridae viruses
- Cellular processes
- Cricket paralysis virus
- Disease severity
- Genetic mutation
- Host defense mechanisms
- Host-targeting entry inhibitors
- Immunological mechanisms
- Arboviral genomes
- Bluetongue virus
- Capsid protein interactions
- Cortical actin microfilaments
- Cytokine storms
- Double-stranded RNA genomes
- High-throughput sequencing
- Host diversity
- Human-wildlife interactions
- Internal ribosome entry sites

CRITICAL THINKING QUESTIONS

1. **Which of the following is a single-stranded RNA negative-sense virus?**
   a. Poliovirus
   b. Influenza virus
   c. Rotavirus
   d. SARS-CoV-2
2. **What is the main role of the RNA-dependent RNA polymerase in RNA viruses?**
   a. Replicating host DNA
   b. Synthesizing viral proteins
   c. Copying and duplicating viral RNA
   d. Host cell RNA degradation
3. **Where is most of the replication of RNA viruses occurring within the host cell?**
   a. Nucleus
   b. Cytoplasm
   c. Endoplasmic reticulum
   d. Mitochondria
4. **What is the most important factor affecting the pathogenesis of RNA viral infections?**
   a. Mitochondrial count of host cell
   b. Rate of host cell DNA replication
   c. Chloroplasts in host cells
   d. Viral load and tissue tropism
5. **What is one of the most widely applied strategies to prevent RNA virus infections?**
   a. Passive immunization with monoclonal antibodies
   b. Broad-spectrum antibiotics
   c. Antifungal agents
   d. Iron supplements

Short Answer Questions

1. What are the main criteria on which RNA viruses are classified, and how are they related to the Baltimore classification system?
2. Describe the overall structural features of RNA viruses and how their structure makes them infectious and viable.
3. How does the viral RNA genome determine the type of replication strategy and the viral proteins?
4. Outline the general process for the replication cycle of an RNA virus and compare key differences among positive-sense, negative-sense, and double-stranded RNA viruses.

5. What are the principal mechanisms by which RNA viruses cause disease in the host, and to what degree do host immune responses influence the severity of disease?
6. Describe the principal mechanisms of RNA virus transmission and determinants of transmission in populations.
7. Why does re-emergence and emergence of RNA viral diseases occur due to zoonotic reservoirs and mutation rates?
8. How are RNA viral infections treated today, and how are they prevented by vaccines and public health measures?

Answer to Critical Thinking Questions

1. (b); 2. (c); 3. (b); 4. (d); 5. (a)

REFERENCES

1. Travassos da Rosa, J. F., de Souza, W. M., Pinheiro, F. P., Figueiredo, M. L., Cardoso, J. F., Acrani, G. O., & Nunes, M. R. T. (2017). Oropouche Virus: Clinical, Epidemiological, and Molecular Aspects of a Neglected Orthobunyavirus. *The American journal of tropical medicine and hygiene*, *96*(5), 1019–1030. https://doi.org/10.4269/ajtmh.16-0672 (accessed on 13th June 2025).
2. Owuor, D. C., Ngoi, J. M., Otieno, J. R., Otieno, G. P., Nyasimi, F. M., Nyiro, J. U., Agoti, C. N., Chaves, S. S., & Nokes, D. J. (2020). Genetic characterization of influenza A(H3N2) viruses circulating in coastal Kenya, 2009-2017. *Influenza and other respiratory viruses*, *14*(3), 320–330. https://doi.org/10.1111/irv.12717 (accessed on 13th June 2025).
3. Ahlquist, P., Haseloff, J., Rice, C. M., Strauss, J. H., et al. (1985). Sindi's virus proteins nsP1 and nsP2 contain homology to nonstructural proteins from several RNA plant viruses. https://core.ac.uk/download/4870733.pdf (accessed on 13th June 2025).
4. Alicino, C., Ansaldi, F., Calamusa, G., Canepa, P., Colomba, G. M. E., Orsi, A., Pojero, F., et al. (2018). Trends of influenza B during the 2010–2016 seasons in 2 regions of north and south Italy: The impact of the vaccine mismatch on influenza immunization strategy. https://core.ac.uk/download/287859184.pdf (accessed on 13th June 2025).
5. Loon, J. van. (2005). Epidemic space. *Critical Public Health*, *15*(1), 39–52. https://doi.org/10.1080/09581590500048374(accessed on 13th June 2025).
6. Andrus, A. F., Borisevich, S. V., Sizikova, T. E., Pantyukhov, V. B., & Lebedev, V. N. (2017). Molecular-biological peculiarities of arenavirus reproduction in sensitive cells. https://core.ac.uk/download/440670279.pdf (accessed on 13th June 2025).
7. Ansari, A., Chang, C., Gershwin, M. E., Ortiz, B. L., et al. (2016). The Zika outbreak of the 21st century. https://core.ac.uk/download/323068480.pdf (accessed on 13th June 2025).
8. B.A. Jones, D. Grace, R. Kock, S. Alonso, J. Rushton, M.Y. Said, D. McKeever, F. Mutua, J. Young, J. McDermott, & D.U. Pfeiffer, Zoonosis emergence linked to agricultural intensification and environmental change, Proc. Natl. Acad. Sci. U.S.A. 110 (21) 8399-8404, https://doi.org/10.1073/pnas.1208059110 (2013).(accessed on 13th June 2025).
9. Atkinson, N. J., Evans, D. J., Simmonds, P., Witteveldt, J., et al. (2014). The influence of CpG and UpA dinucleotide frequencies on RNA virus replication and characterization of the innate cellular pathways underlying virus attenuation and enhanced replication. https://core.ac.uk/download/29188749.pdf (accessed on 13th June 2025).
10. Aulia, A., Eusebio-Cope, A., Honda, S., Kondo, H., et al. (2020). Establishment of Neurospora crassa as a model organism for fungal virology. https://core.ac.uk/download/361937255.pdf (accessed on 13th June 2025).
11. Balogun, R. A., Barman, S., Nayak, D. P., Yamada, K., et al. (2009). Influenza virus morphogenesis and budding. https://core.ac.uk/download/323080192.pdf (accessed on 13th June 2025).
12. Bankamp, B., Barreira, P., Burns, M., Byrne, N., et al. (2020). Combining genomics and epidemiology to track mumps virus transmission in the United States. https://core.ac.uk/download/323081935.pdf (accessed on 13th June 2025).

13. Tiwari, S. K., Dang, J., Qin, Y., Lichinchi, G., Bansal, V., & Rana, T. M. (2017). Zika virus infection reprograms global transcription of host cells to allow sustained infection. *Emerging microbes & infections*, *6*(4), e24. https://doi.org/10.1038/emi.2017.9(accessed on 13th June 2025).
14. Barman, S., Hui, E. K. W., & Nayak, D. P. (2004). Assembly and budding of influenza virus. https://core.ac.uk/download/323079119.pdf (accessed on 13th June 2025).
15. Jon R. Cavicchi, Stanley P. Kowalski, et al, "Patent Landscape of Influenza A Virus Prophylactic Vaccines and Related Technologies" (2012).(accessed on 13th June 2025).
16. Barzon, L., Berto, A., Desole, G., Pacenti, M., et al. (2015). Modeling viral infectious diseases and development of antiviral therapies using human induced pluripotent stem cell-derived systems. https://core.ac.uk/download/53523165.pdf (accessed on 13th June 2025).
17. Bellwood, D. R., Costa, V. A., Geoghegan, J. L., Harvey, E., et al. (2023). Limited cross-species virus transmission in a spatially restricted coral reef fish community. https://core.ac.uk/download/590879441.pdf (accessed on 13th June 2025).
18. Beren, C., Chakravarty, A., Cui, Y., Gelbart, W., et al. (2020). Genome organization and interaction with capsid protein in a multipartite RNA virus. https://core.ac.uk/download/323308724.pdf (accessed on 13th June 2025).
19. Buckley, A., Evans, D. J., Gould, E. A., Gritsun, T., et al. (2011). Replication enhancer elements within the open reading frame of tick-borne encephalitis virus and their evolution within the *Flavivirus* genus. https://core.ac.uk/download/107770.pdf (accessed on 13th June 2025).
20. Flanagan, M. L., Parrish, C. R., Cobey, S., Glass, G. E., Bush, R. M., & Leighton, T. J. (2012). Anticipating the species jump: surveillance for emerging viral threats. *Zoonoses and public health*, *59*(3), 155–163. https://doi.org/10.1111/j.1863-2378.2011.01439.x(accessed on 13th June 2025).
21. Byk, L. A., de Maio, F. A., Gamarnik, A. V., Gebhard, L. G., et al. (2016). Dengue virus genome uncoating requires ubiquitination. https://core.ac.uk/download/159288331.pdf (accessed on 13th June 2025).
22. Caporale, M., Di Gialleonorado, L., Di Ventura, M., Janowicz, A., et al. (2014). Virus and host factors affecting the clinical outcome of bluetongue virus infection. https://core.ac.uk/download/42354692.pdf (accessed on 13th June 2025).
23. Cappelle, K., Dhaenens, M., Meeus, I., Smagghe, G., et al. (2016). Israeli acute paralysis virus infection leads to an enhanced RNA interference response and not its suppression in the bumblebee *Bombus terrestris*. https://core.ac.uk/download/84042020.pdf (accessed on 13th June 2025).
24. Chen, A. I., Elliott, R., Goldstein, S. A., Jha, B., et al. (2017). Lineage A beta coronavirus NS2 proteins and the homologous Toro virus Berne pp1a carboxy-terminal domain are phosphodiesterase's that antagonize activation of RNase L. https://core.ac.uk/download/80495056.pdf (accessed on 13th June 2025).
25. Cheng, G., Chisari, F. V., Chung, J., Gastaminza, P., et al. (2006). Persistent hepatitis C virus infection *in vitro*: Coevolution of virus and host. https://core.ac.uk/download/pdf/19070.pdf (accessed on 13th June 2025).
26. Chiu, C. Y. (2013). Viral pathogen discovery. https://core.ac.uk/download/323063718.pdf (accessed on 13th June 2025).

27. Clark, J. J., Cumberworth, S., Donald, C. L., Kohl, A., et al. (2017). Inhibition of type I interferon induction and signaling by mosquito-borne flaviviruses. https://core.ac.uk/download/80697084.pdf (accessed on 13th June 2025).

28. Coburn, H. (2018). Vaccine epidemiology and decision-making: A Bryant student focus. https://core.ac.uk/download/158246439.pdf (accessed on 13th June 2025).

29. da Silva, E. S., Lemaire, M., Lie, Y., Mulinge, M., et al. (2013). HIV-1 tropism determination using a phenotypic Env recombinant viral assay highlights overestimation of CXCR4-usage by genotypic prediction algorithms for CRRF01_AE and CRF02_AG. https://core.ac.uk/download/55802258.pdf (accessed on 13th June 2025).

30. Davison, A., Gu, Q., Hughes, J., Maabar, M., et al. (2016). Bioinformatics tools for analyzing viral genomic data. https://core.ac.uk/download/42372609.pdf (accessed on 13th June 2025).

31. Díez Casero, J. J., Fernández Fernández, M. M., Muñoz Adalia, E. J. (2016). The use of mycoviruses in the control of forest diseases. https://core.ac.uk/download/323366858.pdf (accessed on 13th June 2025).

32. Djikeng, A., Lindberg, A. M., Smit, A. F. A., Wetterbom, A., Bjerkner, A., Chevreux, B., Persson, B., et al. (2012). Characterization of the viral microbiome in patients with severe lower respiratory tract infections, using metagenomic sequencing. https://core.ac.uk/download/pdf/8683019.pdf (accessed on 13th June 2025).

33. Eng, K. E., Karlsson Hedestam, G. B., Lulla, A., McInerney, G. M., et al. (2012). Sequestration of G3BP coupled with efficient translation inhibits stress granules in Semliki Forest virus infection. https://core.ac.uk/download/46559852.pdf (accessed on 13th June 2025).

34. Mensaert, K., Van Criekinge, W., Thas, O., Schuuring, E., Steenbergen, R. D., Wisman, G. B., & De Meyer, T. (2015). Mining for viral fragments in methylation enriched sequencing data. *Frontiers in genetics*, *6*, 16. https://doi.org/10.3389/fgene.2015.00016(accessed on 13th June 2025).

35. Fang, F., Le Calvez, H., & Yu, M. (2004). Biochemical prevention and treatment of viral infections–A new paradigm in medicine for infectious diseases. https://core.ac.uk/download/pdf/3550099.pdf (accessed on 13th June 2025).

36. Forsdyke, D. R. (2013). Role of HIV RNA structure in recombination and speciation: Romping in purine A, keeps HTLV away. http://arxiv.org/abs/1305.2132 (accessed on 13th June 2025).

37. Gaglia, M., & Glaunsinger, B. (2010). Viruses and the cellular RNA decay machinery. https://core.ac.uk/download/323081353.pdf (accessed on 13th June 2025).

38. Gall, O. L., Karasev, A., Sanfacon, H., et al. (2009). *Secoviridae*: A proposed family of plant viruses within the order *Picornavirales* that combines the families *Sequiviridae* and *Comoviridae*, the unassigned genera *Cheravirus* and *Sadwavirus*, and the proposed genus *Torradovirus*. https://core.ac.uk/download/pdf/29249560.pdf (accessed on 13th June 2025).

39. Garcia-Ruiz, H. (2018). Susceptibility genes to plant viruses. https://core.ac.uk/download/215159745.pdf (accessed on 13th June 2025).

40. Gerasimov, E. (2017). Analysis of NGS data from immune response and viral samples. https://core.ac.uk/download/84927082.pdf (accessed on 13th June 2025).

41. Grazzini, G., Liumbruno, G. M., Marano, G., Pupella, S., et al. (2016). Zika virus and the never-ending story of emerging pathogens and transfusion medicine. https://core.ac.uk/download/54532486.pdf (accessed on 13th June 2025).

42. Gumpper, R. (2018). Structure-function relationships of the nucleocapsid in vesicular stomatitis virus. https://core.ac.uk/download/215176301.pdf (accessed on 13th June 2025).

43. Hale, B. G., Jackson, D., Ortin, J., Randall, R. E., et al. (2012). The multifunctional NS1 protein of influenza A viruses. https://core.ac.uk/download/9821699.pdf (accessed on 13th June 2025).

44. Karo-Astover, L. (2013). Semliki Forest viiruse replikaasivalgu nsP1 auramine. https://core.ac.uk/download/16393680.pdf (accessed on 13th June 2025).

45. Kohl, A., Blomström, A. L., Delhaye, S., Dunn, G., Schnettler, E., Geerts-Dimitriadou, C., Hampsey, M., et al. (2013). Non-structural proteins of arthropod-borne bunyaviruses: Roles and functions. https://core.ac.uk/download/16462466.pdf (accessed on 13th June 2025).

46. Liu, J., Swevers, L., Kolliopoulou, A., & Smagghe, G. (2019). Arboviruses and the Challenge to Establish Systemic and Persistent Infections in Competent Mosquito Vectors: The Interaction With the RNAi Mechanism. *Frontiers in physiology*, *10*, 890. https://doi.org/10.3389/fphys.2019.00890(accessed on 13th June 2025).

47. Yokomori, K., La Monica, N., Makino, S., Shieh, C. K., & Lai, M. M. (1989). Biosynthesis, structure, and biological activities of envelope protein gp65 of murine coronavirus. *Virology*, *173*(2), 683–691. https://doi.org/10.1016/0042-6822(89)90581-3(accessed on 13th June 2025).

48. Lošdorfer Božič, A., Šiber, A., et al. (2012). How simple can a model of an empty viral capsid be? Charge distributions in viral capsids. http://arxiv.org/abs/1207.3188 (accessed on 13th June 2025).

49. Lozano, G., & Martínez-Salas, E. (2015). Structural insights into viral IRES-dependent translation mechanisms. https://core.ac.uk/download/80861230.pdf (accessed on 13th June 2025).

50. Meeus, I., Smagghe, G., Swevers, L., Van Meulebroek, L., et al. (2020). Metabolomic analysis of cricket paralysis virus infection in *Drosophila* S2 cells reveals divergent effects on central carbon metabolism as compared with silkworm Bm5 cells. https://core.ac.uk/download/322827688.pdf (accessed on 13th June 2025).

51. Fiscon, G., Weitschek, E., Cella, E. *et al.* MISSEL: a method to identify a large number of small species-specific genomic subsequences and its application to viruses classification. *BioData Mining* **9**, 38 (2016). https://doi.org/10.1186/s13040-016-0116-2(accessed on 13th June 2025).

52. Owsianka, A., Sigal, A., Siddiqui, A., Patel, A. H., Lok, A. S., Tarr, A. W., Bartolini, B., et al. (2014). Hepatitis C virus cell-cell transmission and resistance to direct-acting antiviral agents. https://core.ac.uk/download/9649232.pdf (accessed on 13th June 2025).

53. Tuplin, A., Thurner, C., Chew, D. S. H., Lillo, F., Ratcliff, F., et al. (2008). Statistical properties of thermodynamically predicted RNA secondary structures in viral genomes. http://arxiv.org/abs/0803.2608 (accessed on 13th June 2025).

54. Wilson, A. J., Longdon, B., Okamura, B., Brem, D., Centers for Disease Control, Kallio, E. R., Ewald, P. W., et al. (2017). The evolution of transmission mode. https://core.ac.uk/download/74236453.pdf (accessed on 13th June 2025).

EMERGING AND RE-EMERGING VIRAL INFECTIONS

4

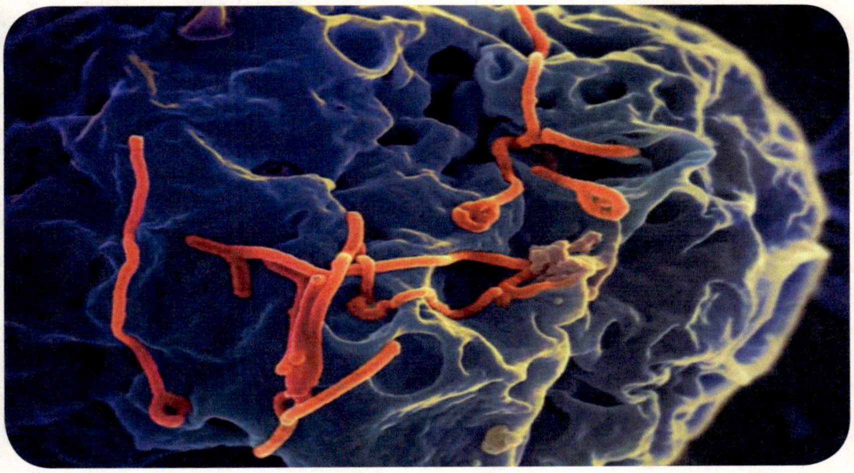

LEARNING OBJECTIVES

After studying this chapter, you will be able to:

1. Describe the historical context of emerging and re-emerging viral infections;
2. Explain the mechanisms of viral emergence;
3. Discuss case studies of emerging viral infections;
4. Emphasize global health implications;
5. Address prevention and control measures of the emergence and re-emergence of viral infections.

Introduction

The epidemiologic profile of infectious diseases is still evolving and constitutes a monumental challenge to global health systems. As more populations increase and the rate of urbanization grows, man's interface with nature increases, and new virus agents have the potential to emerge. This is a scenario commonly referred to as emerging viral infections, in which the pathogens involved come from reservoirs not of human origin , such as animals and move to human populations via spillover. Such diseases have complex epidemiology and are shaped by environmental, ecological, as well as sociopolitical factors. For instance, the emergence of zoonotic diseases, which is triggered by environmental and behavioral aspects, underscores the need for public health surveillance and research in predicting and preventing impending outbreaks (Bozzette et al., 2006). The understanding of why the transmissions take place is at the center of proactive, preventive and control strategies against viral emergence. Re-emerging infectious viral diseases constitute another category of public health problems, where established pathogens re-emerge or mutate to evade available control measures. Measles and tuberculosis are touching reminders of the same, reappearing in situations when vaccination coverage wanes or when the public health infrastructure has been compromised. The re-emergence of the diseases is not only an indicator of breakdowns in healthcare delivery, but also confirms the ability of viruses to adapt to human actions, e.g., climatic and land use change. From the recent epizootics of such infections as hepatitis or HIV, it is clear that an effective response, as has been traditionally understood, largely relies on a balanced combination of scientific investigation, public health policy, and international cooperation. Emerging and re-emerging viral diseases are serious threats necessitating novel strategies to keep up with their evolving dynamics and arrange for adequate and timely surveillance apparatuses to effect timely and efficient epidemic control (Bozzette et al., 2006).

The complexities of emerging and re-emerging viral infections require an interdisciplinary science that unifies various disciplines, such as virology, epidemiology, ecology, and social sciences. With the world grappling with the harsh realities of pandemics, it is certain that the traditional means of handling infectious diseases will not be sufficient. Emerging technologies and methodologies, like advanced mathematical modeling and enhanced diagnostic powers, can assist in boosting our capacity for anticipating and controlling viral infections. The same technology and methodology can also facilitate focused surveillance, focusing on the detection of dangerous pathogens before they cause extensive damage. By facilitating collective research activity globally, research can also facilitate the shift of strategy from post-infection to prevention of infection, thus bolstering our defenses against the ever-changing virulence of viral infections (Morse et al., 2012).

Definition of Emerging and Re-Emerging Viral Infections

Emerging and re-emerging viral infections are a notional term at the edge of the science of global public health threats. Emerging viral diseases are the ones that are newly seen among a population or previously seen but now increasing in frequency or geographic distribution. They tend to reflect most often a new interaction between humans and zoonotic reservoirs, which can involve other animal species, thus the dynamic aspect of association within ecosystems. The rapid mutation of viral genotypes also makes it more difficult, emphasizing the ongoing evolution of viruses that can potentially cause outbreaks. For instance, the influenza viruses that spillover from animal reservoirs become infected with mutations that enable them to infect humans more effectively and become an immediate pandemic threat that requires constant monitoring and swift response. Conversely, re-emerging viral diseases refer to infections that previously declined in prevalence but are now re-emerging, often due to environmental, human, or public health causes. Infections may be due to causes , such as antimicrobial resistance, population migration, and disruption of vaccination coverage. Of particular interest, the recent upsurge of infections , such as measles and tuberculosis, is an age-old illustration of how social circumstances and public health policy are in a state of constant change, once again creating the infection risk previously thought to be contained. This is exacerbated by populations whose immunity is weakened, i.e., HIV-positive individuals, with increased vulnerability to re-emergent threats. Increase in incidence among susceptible populations also highlights the need for continued education and healthcare programs to stem the impact of such infections on public health (Clark et al., 2016). Differentiation between re-emerging and emerging infections is crucial in pandemic preparedness and response contexts. Incident outbreaks are more likely to prompt preemptive countermeasures based on genetic and biological research, , such as the description of influenza viruses with attention to characterization of strains of greatest possible human infectivity (Barclay et al., 2016). Public health agencies know how to target control and surveillance interventions based on characteristics that increase viral adaptation, e.g., receptor-binding specificity and polymerase efficacy. By recognizing the complex interdependence of hosts, pathogens, and externalities, stakeholders are able to create holistic frameworks for surveillance and management of these viral diseases. This multi-dimensional approach is at the core of addressing dynamic viral pathogen changes and safeguarding public health against emerging and re-emerging pathologies (Figure 4.1).

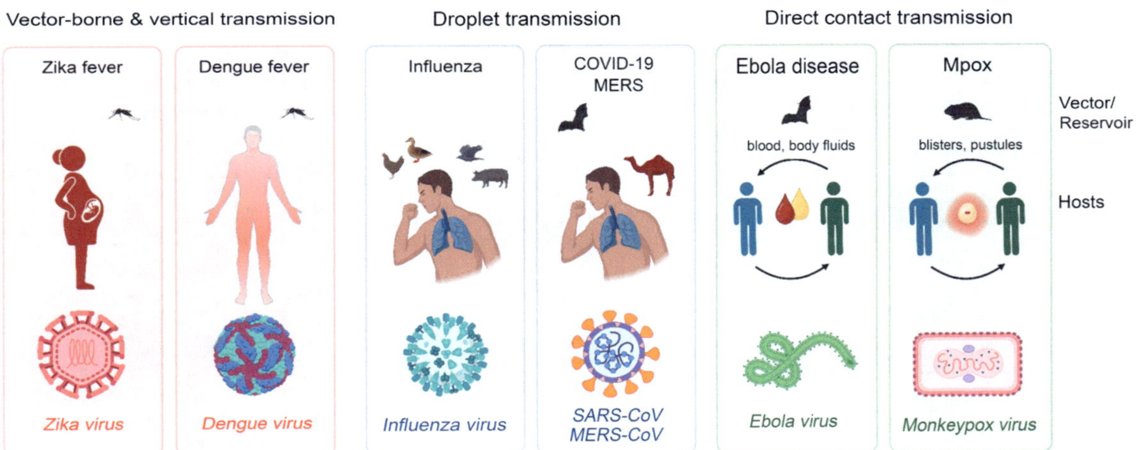

Figure 4.1. (Re)-emerging viral diseases: vectors, reservoirs, and routes of transmission.

Source: https://www.mdpi.com/microorganisms/microorganisms-11-02618/article_deploy/html/images/microorganisms-11-02618-g001.png.

Importance of Studying Viral Infections

There is a need to study viral infections because they are dynamic, fluctuating entities. While the rate of mutation in viruses and the development of new hosts occur, re-emerging or emerging infections caused by viruses have important implications for public health. For instance, ranaviruses that infect primarily amphibians, reptiles, and fish have been noted to be increasing as agents of biodiversity threats in certain regions of the world, resulting in catastrophic die-offs among the infected populations. The viruses' capability to adapt and spread indicates the need for ongoing observation and research. Studying these types of viral diseases is important not only for wildlife conservation but also as a way of researching potential spillover that may impact human populations. Whenever these types of viruses emerge in new areas, the implications for nature's balance and human health cannot be overstated, and research along this line is necessary for science and society as a whole (Brunner et al., 2014). In addition, interactions between wild animals and human beings make it problematic for epidemiology to cope with viral infections. Wild birds, especially migratory birds, may act as vectors of various microorganisms, including various viruses that are related to diseases in human beings. Although relatively less common, transmission from wild birds to human beings should not be downplayed for their reservoir potential of pathogens like the influenza A virus and West Nile virus. Understanding how such pathogens are being spread in the wildlife will be essential to successful public health measures.

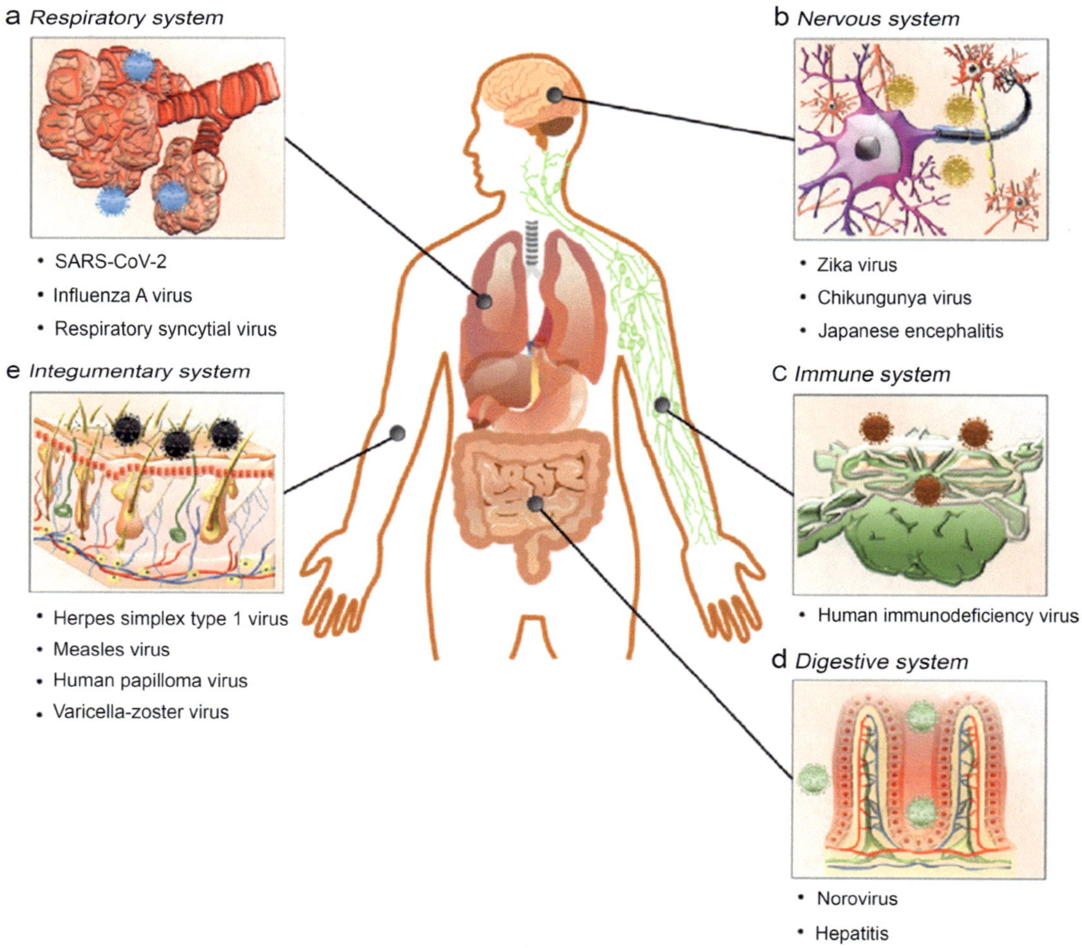

Figure 4.2. Schematic illustration of viral infection in organ systems.

Source: https://www.researchgate.net/publication/363775332/figure/fig1/AS:11431281088705685@1665246151709/Schematic-illustration-of-viral-infection-in-organ-systems-Viral-infection-in-human.png.

Continuing work in migratory behavior, habitat change, and environmental stress will give a broader epidemiological perspective within which to predict and prepare for probable outbreaks. Thus, an interdisciplinary research strategy to the inquiry of viral diseases and primarily those emerging from the wildlife reservoir is essential in maintaining public health interventions (Bauchinger et al., 2008). Going beyond ecological concerns is the place of viral infection studies that is experienced in public policy and global health security. As was seen in recent pandemics around the world, the ability of viral infections to cross species boundaries can lead to health crises of pandemic magnitude and economic uncertainty. Policymakers and public health managers need sound epidemiological studies upon which to base effective response and surveillance interventions.

Greater insight into the virological mechanisms of infection transmission allows it to design effective vaccines and treatment strategies and, ultimately, eradicate threats from new and re-emerging infections. Future epidemics are forecast on a solid scientific basis, taking into account both the biological characteristics of viruses and socio-economic disease determinants of transmission. Lastly, studying viral infections is not merely academic work but a worthwhile component of safeguarding humankind from the ever-present threat of infectious diseases (Figure 4.2).

4.1. Historical Context of Emerging and Re-emerging Viral Infections

Learning Outcome

1. Talk about noteworthy past viral outbreaks;
2. Explain the virus emergence factors;
3. Learn lessons from previous pandemics.

In trying to locate the re-emerging and emerging viral diseases' historical context, it is worth noting how public health responses and social conditions guide the course of disease. The HIV/AIDS pandemic, as it formed through the early 1980s, is an example of how virology is irretrievably intertwined with social conditions. Perceived initially in a narrow context related to high-risk groups, the response to HIV too frequently was liberal and facilitated its dissemination. Access gaps in health care and social stigmatization of illness added to pre-existing systemic gaps present in health care systems and broader society. This context is the background from which to see how public health programs adapt and grow around new impending infections, to be an outgrowth of different underlying issues and past injustices in society. As information about HIV increased, production of campaigns like the Getting to Zero campaign in San Francisco demonstrated a powerful shift in public health policy. From a once-postulated epicenter of the HIV epidemic in a city, this campaign is seeking not only zero infection but also the corresponding social determinants of health, including housing, that are most profoundly impacting public health. Despite its cutting-edge design, the campaign is a testament to shortcomings in knowledge of the interplay between socio-economic status and health. The exclusion of housing concerns in official interventions is a blanket shortcoming in managing health emergencies, meaning that public health interventions need an integrated process to be effective in preventing viral infections that are increasing (Zaragoza, 2019). The history of viral infections also contains precious lessons in reading the current global health crises. Intensities of zoonotic spillover, e.g., with viruses SARS and Ebola, suggest the impact of globalization and climate change on infectious disease dynamics. What happened in the past, i.e., the influenza pandemic of 1918, has shaped today's epidemiologic evidence and response, but the same trends persist with disease today. New viral infections tend to exploit society's weaknesses, fueled by drivers like climate change and urbanization. Against such multilateral challenges as societies are faced with meeting, examination of the previous histories of previous viral pandemics reveals the necessity for an integrated strategy that targets not only the pathogens themselves but also the socio-economic and political settings in which they thrive (Zaragoza, 2019).

4.1.1. Notable Past Viral Outbreaks

The previous history of viral epidemics is full of lessons regarding new and re-emerging infectious diseases as well as the politics around them. For instance, the 2014–2016 West African Ebola Virus Disease (EVD) epidemic is a painful reminder of the threat to public health caused by emerging agents. With mortality rates greater than 40% in affected regions, the epidemic only served to underscore collaborative global public health action as a necessity. Their exponential spread was facilitated by a chain of events that involved traditional burial rituals, poor health infrastructure, and cultural acceptability of intervention. The epidemic thus not only amplified the vulnerabilities of local healthcare systems but also demanded a reassessment of global surveillance and response strategy in efforts to put on the top agenda the need for preparedness against such emerging threats from zoonotic diseases. Another graphical representation is that of the Zika virus, which was initially discovered in the central and eastern regions of Africa in the 1940s but erupted into fame in the Americas in 2015. A localized disease began to rapidly transform into a pandemic public health crisis, one that came with serious birth defects , such as microcephaly in newborns. The pandemic was the most concerning because the mode of transmission via mosquito vectors that propagated its dissemination far and wide across continents was of concern. The experience raised concerns not only regarding the epidemiology of Zika but also regarding the implications for the health of mothers and children in general. After the pandemic, there was a compelling need for aggressive global collaboration and viral genomics and pathogen dynamics studies, adding further validation to the urgency of One Health in preventing future viral pandemics (Lewnard et al., 2019). Historical patterns of outbreaks have redefined infectious disease epidemiology with the relentless pathogen evolution and necessity for versatility in public health response. The COVID-19 pandemic illustrates the lessons of the past, showing that the interaction of human behavior, environmental processes, and virus biology presents complex challenges. As new epidemiology is increasingly embracing advances in the gathering of data and its analysis, there is an increasing recognition of the value of multidisciplinary approaches. By bridging knowledge between veterinary medicine, ecology, and epidemiology, public health systems are in a better position to respond to new infections, learning from previous outbreaks to maximize response and preparedness (Lewnard et al., 2019) (Figure 4.3).

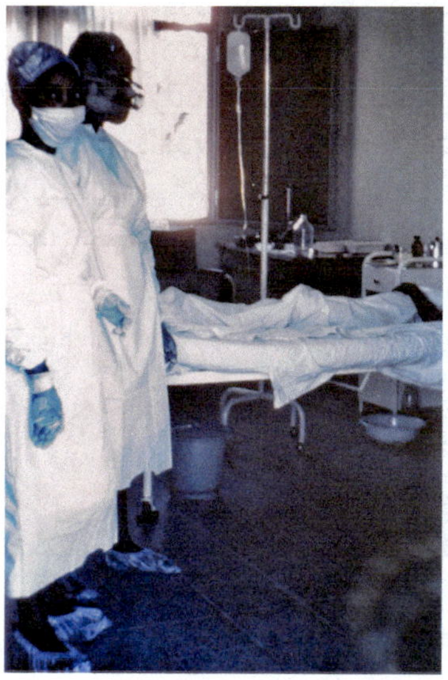

Figure 4.3. Two nurses standing near Mayinga N'Seka, a nurse with Ebola virus disease in the 1976 outbreak in Zaire.

Source: https://upload.wikimedia.org/wikipedia/commons/thumb/a/ab/7042_lores-Ebola-Zaire-CDC_Photo.jpg/800px-7042_lores-Ebola-Zaire-CDC_Photo.jpg.

4.1.2. Factors Contributing to the Emergence of Viruses

Emergence of viruses is an important public health concern worldwide, and it is important to be aware of the determinants of the phenomenon so that preventive measures can be formulated appropriately. The human-animal relationship, or the human-animal interface, is one of the determinants. As the world becomes more integrated, human contact with wildlife increases, and thus, there is more opportunity for zoonotic transmission. This interface is a major tipping point for animal-to-human disease spillover, and this is fueled by ecological drivers , such as habitat loss and climate change. Additionally, with urbanization spreading to natural and rural areas, disturbing animal groups can induce unexpected viral epidemics, thus the need for enhanced understanding and observation of such interactions in order to minimize risks of emerging infections (Djoko et al., 2010). Human activities highly promote the onset of new viral infections, most significantly through activities , such as deforestation, farming, and wildlife trade. As human activities expand into natural environments, they break ecosystems and offer windows of opportunity for viruses to spill over from animal reservoirs to human beings. The interactions are further controlled by modified climate regimes, which possess the ability to alter animals' migration ranges and habits, and therefore further increase disease transmission potentials. Mass agricultural activities also create conducive environments where viruses multiply and evolve very rapidly, especially in closely populated housing farms. Global trade in commodities and human movements can expedite the spread of both viral pathogens and contaminated individuals, leading to rapid development and re-emergence of diseases. Regulation and prevention of these industry and environmental drivers are hence essential to disease control and prevention strategies (Al-Tawfiq et al., 2018). Public health interventions and community behaviors make a significant contribution to viral emergence patterns. Public health education, social mobilization, and behavior change interventions play a key role in reducing the risk of outbreaks, particularly in highly impacted communities. Weak global disease surveillance systems for zoonotic diseases compromise preparedness and timely response, allowing viruses to burst uncontrolled. Suggested modifications involve enhancing communication measures to raise awareness of emerging health threats and community-based interventions that engage communities in monitoring and response. Additionally, understanding the socio-economic environments in which such viruses propagate can enable targeted prevention measures, hence the requirement for an inter-disciplinary approach integrating science research, public policy, and community engagement. Consequently, intervention of these socio-environmental determinants is the core in the mitigation of the impact of emerging and re-emerging viral diseases (Djoko et al., 2010).

4.1.3. Lessons Learned from Historical Pandemics

Historic pandemics provide valuable lessons in how to keep in check the spread of newly emerging and re-emerging viral infections. Pandemics , such as the 1918 flu pandemic and the recent COVID-19 pandemic provide valuable lessons on how to detect early and utilize rapid response mechanisms to curtail viral infection spread. For example, the early adoption of public health interventions, , such as social distancing, wearing face masks, and large-scale vaccination campaigns, helped to contain COVID-19 cases. Historical evidences show that nations that responded quickly, , such as Taiwan and South Korea, were able to contain their infection rates in comparison to nations that lagged behind. Along with this, the necessity of global collaboration has been put into the spotlight due to the fact that collective data and resources are the priority when surveillance and preparedness for potential future outbreaks are in question. With the outbreak of Mpox hanging over the horizon, such regulations are not recommendations but recommendations for ensuring future global health (Adebanjo et al., 2024). Evidence-based public health interventions and surveillance epidemiology are today major determinants in fighting viral infections. History in the guise of past pandemics can inform us that the response to epidemics is heavily dependent on surveillance and containment measures. In the West African Ebola epidemic, incomplete assemblages of data compromised responses and containment. Contemporary surveillance efforts, utilizing technological and bioinformatics advancements, can now transmit and process data in real time and produce useful data on viral evolution and transmission. This was brought out during the COVID-19 pandemic, where genomic sequencing became a central activity for tracking variant mutations. Therefore, investment in robust surveillance systems along with better healthcare infrastructure is required to control emerging pandemics effectively. The need for equitable access to such systems also has the effect of strengthening lessons learned and the identification of inequities that must be remedied in future public health planning (Akele et al., 2024). Finally, previous pandemics demonstrate the natural relationship between activity in society and the effect of public health intervention. Inequities in access to health care and vaccine coverage, as during the COVID-19 pandemic, are an expression of structural inequities that can amplify the transmission rate of infectious diseases. Cultural background is also a key determinant of how populations respond to health crises; extensive misinformation can undermine cooperation between the broader public and public health authorities. Empowering communities, open communication, and culturally sensitive health promotion efforts addressing community cultures are essential to maintaining compliance with health interventions. Health interventions, now experience-based, must draw on community input and prioritize recognizable local issues in order to gain public trust and effect. Lastly, the history of previous pandemics supports the imperative of an interdisciplinary solution with scientific knowledge, social engagement, and global solidarity to manage recrudescent and emerging viral disease effectively (Adebanjo et al., 2024) (Figure 4.4).

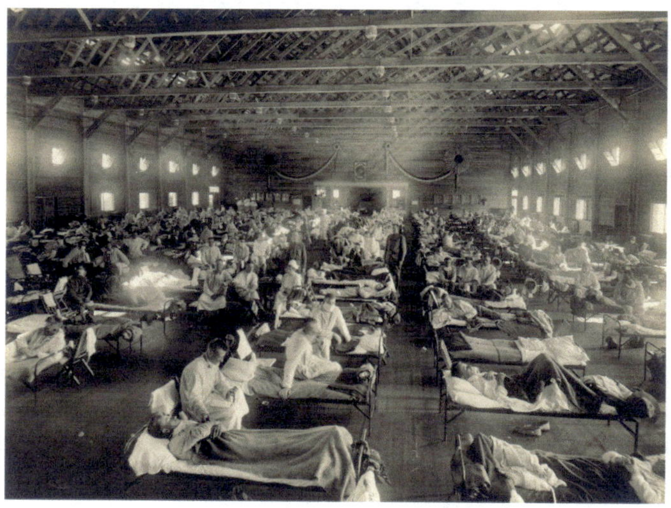

Figure 4.4. Influenza pandemic of 1918–19: temporary hospital A temporary hospital in Camp Funston, Kansas, during the 1918–19 influenza pandemic.

Source: https://upload.wikimedia.org/wikipedia/commons/2/20/Emergency_hospital_during_Influenza_epidemic%2C_Camp_Funston%2C_Kansas_-_NCP_1603.jpg.

Test Your Knowledge

1. What were the most impactful viral outbreaks in history and what was their impact on global public health?
2. What impact did the 1918 influenza pandemic have on today's approaches to pandemic readiness and response?

4.2. Mechanisms of Viral Emergence

Learning Outcome

1. Define Genetic mutations and recombination;
2. Explain zoonotic transmission and animal reservoirs;
3. Outline environmental changes and the effects on viral transmission.

Viral emergence is a complex phenomenon shaped by a range of causes, many of which are the result of zoonotic transmission, the viruses "jumping" from animals to humans. This process is of particular significance in accounting for pandemics, in light of the fact that most recent epidemics , such as HIV/AIDS and SARS reveal that animal reservoirs are significant sources of emerging human viruses. Ecological processes , such as habitat disruption and altered land use, contribute significantly to this process by increasing human contact with wildlife. Also, behavioral and socioeconomic factors, including poverty and urbanization, can potentially influence such interactions, resulting in spillover viruses into human populations. The challenge in predicting such outbreaks is our poor understanding of the dynamics of the complexities underlying the zoonotic pathways, and thus a multidisciplinary approach to generating enhanced knowledge of the viral emergence mechanisms and their effects on global public health (Morse et al., 2012). The search for predictive surveillance for potential viral outbreaks is increasingly regarded as crucial in the foretelling of human infections. Studies have reported that genetic and ecological data can be integrated to provide sharp insights into the detection of high-risk viruses before they develop the ability to infect humans. Workshops conducted by virologists, ecologists, and computational biologists have sought to explore the feasibility of such predictions. By researching the reservoir-host or vector species, scientists aim to gain more understanding of the biology of transmission of viruses. This involves not only finding endemic viruses but also developing systems that can successfully predict future species jumps. The importance of this predictive ability cannot be overstated because it offers a proactive approach to managing threats from newly emerging zoonotic diseases and could enhance public health preparedness significantly (Flanagan et al., 2012). Moreover, existing surveillance approaches are more reactive rather than anticipatory in nature, responding after the outbreak of disease, thus making a huge gap in current public health responses. To overcome this hurdle, increased efforts to screen domesticated animals as well as wildlife for potential zoonotic viruses need to be put in place. Research has established that wildlife, particularly rodents and bats, carry an extensive reservoir of viruses with the potential to jump to the human species. This necessitates an agreement between scientific disciplines and the government to come up with a strong, unified surveillance system. Employing cutting-edge technologies and techniques focusing on high-risk human-animal interfaces, we can design predictive models. These techniques not only accelerate our response to emerging viral threats but also allow us to switch from reactive to proactive prevention with the ultimate aim of minimizing the possibility of pandemics in the future (Flanagan et al., 2012; Morse et al., 2012).

4.2.1. Genetic Mutations and Recombination

The complexity of viral genomes is at the core of the emergence and re-emergence of viral diseases, predominantly through genetic mutation and recombination. During virus replication, error may occur in the genetic template, causing mutation that has the potential to alter viral behavior, transmissibility, and pathogenicity. Genetic heterogeneity may contribute to the generation of quasispecies, a diverse population of related viral variants. A classic example is HIV, which has demonstrated significant genetic diversity by mutations during replication in host infections. The continuously changing nature of such quasispecies enables the virus to adapt in response to immune pressures and makes it all the more susceptible for the virus to survive and exist among populations. Lastly, the interplay between host immune system selective pressures and gene mutation is the foundation on which genetic fluidity observed in emerging viral pathogens is based (Alvarez et al., 2012). In addition to mutation, recombination is the other dominant force in shaping viral diversity. Recombination refers to two different viral strains infecting a single host cell, causing the passing of genetic material and creating new viral genotypes. It can significantly enhance virulence and pathogenicity, , such as with many emerging viruses that have altered host ranges or increased virulence through recombination. Re-emerging and emerging viruses, , such as HIV-type viruses, provide important insights into how recombination is responsible for virus adaptation, with special reference to co-infection. An example of a discovery in plant viruses illustrates how genetic recombination enables viruses to shift hosts or break resistance, indicative of its greater evolutionary role (Acosta-Leal et al., 1995). Genetic recombination and mutations also have implications in public health management of emerging diseases, as well as in the evolution of viruses. Understanding the genetic dynamics of the virus is significant in designing effective antiviral drugs and vaccines. Identification of conserved genomic blocks in extremely variable viruses, for instance, can inform the development of a vaccine that generates broad immunity. Similarly, monitoring viral mutation can provide information on drug resistance against antivirals, enabling timely modifications of treatment modalities. As re-emerging and emerging virus populations are placed continuously under a challenge to global health, full knowledge of genetic mutations and recombination will be instrumental in initiating preventive measures in disease management and outbreak control (Acosta-Leal et al., 1995; Alvarez et al., 2012) (Figure 4.5).

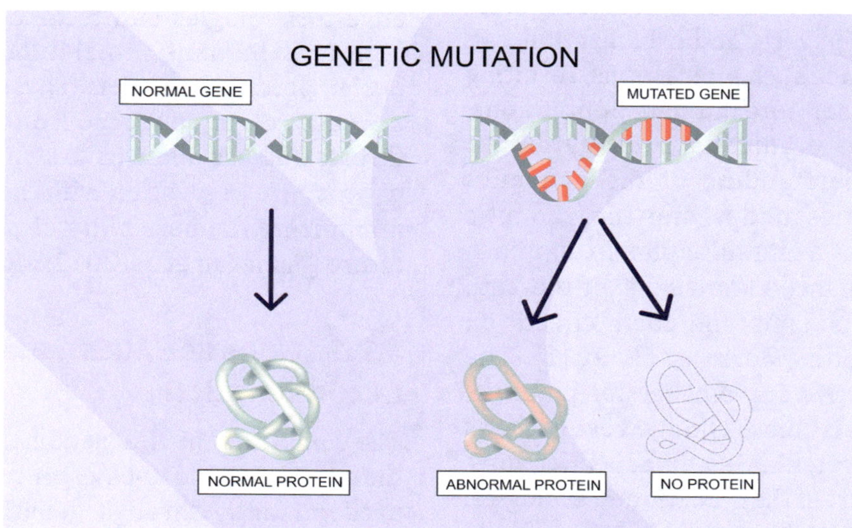

Figure 4.5. Genetic mutation.

Source: https://www.health.com/thmb/7UPmUcOC32y23eEXnKKjbbDzOjk=/1500x0/filters:no_upscale():max_bytes(150000):strip_icc()/Health-Genetic-Mutation-background-light-purple-a6ad7969c03e4780ae174b4c9f705c0c.jpg.

4.2.2. Zoonotic Transmission and Animal Reservoirs

The phenomenon of zoonotic transmission, where infectious agents are passed from animals to humans, is one of the leading causes of the emergence of viral diseases. It has been studied that zoonoses account for an astonishing 60% of new human pathogens emerging, with over 71% of these pathogens originating from wildlife. Such direct correlation points to the importance of having knowledge of animal reservoirs as potential incubators for new infectious diseases. As zoonotic diseases evolve, they can acquire new genetic properties and therefore enhance their potential for pathogenicity. Besides, varying ecological, behavioral, and socio-economic changes may influence the transmission of the pathogens, rendering it challenging for us to predict their emergence. Hence, recognition of the sophisticated dynamics between wildlife, domesticated animals, and human beings becomes imperative to proactive public health measures in preventing pandemics in the future, as demonstrated by historical viral disease patterns that have grown to broad epidemics (Morse et al., 2012). Animal reservoirs are central in the transmission pathway of emerging viruses. The environmental conditions and host behavior, and also changes that have been made in the environment, play a core role in the transmission of infectious diseases. Habitat destruction and climate change, for instance, increase more interfaces between humans and animals through their impact, , such as new opportunities for the spillover effect where pathogens transfer from wildlife to humans. Adaptation of species to such changes also results in new infections that affect human health. Analyzing such dynamics calls for an interdisciplinary strategy that brings together ecological information with public health paradigms. Enhanced systems for surveillance and mathematical modeling will increase our capacity to evaluate and forecast the onset of zoonotic pathogens, thereby guiding targeted strategies in the prevention of outbreaks ahead of time (Cutler et al., 2010). With these complexities, it is apparent that zoonotic transmission involves an extensive understanding of animal reservoirs and their role in viral infection. Pathogen and animal host dynamics are governed by numerous factors, including ecological disturbance and altered host behavior. To effectively regulate, the role of researchers is to chart the ecological niches where the emergence of zoonotic pathogens is likely.

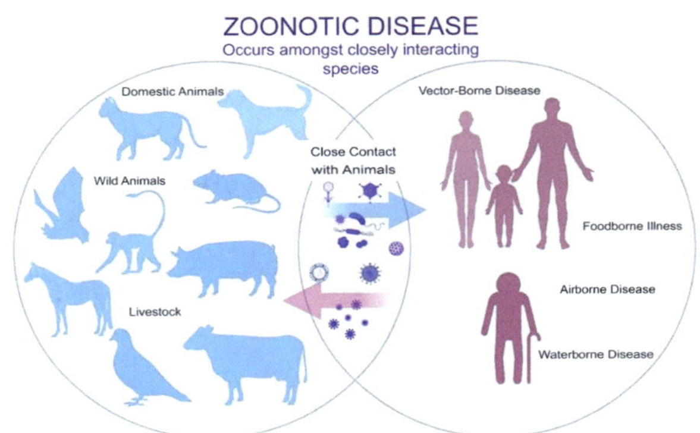

Figure 4.6. Zoonotic transfer of pathogens occurs when close contact encourages species-jumping transmission between animals , such as domestic, wildlife, or livestock-and humans.

Source: https://www.researchgate.net/profile/Abdullah-Channo/publication/377089354/figure/fig1/AS:11431281215539863@1704285706071/Zoonotic-transfer-of-pathogens-occurs-when-close-contact-encourages-species-jumping.jpg.

This involves not only monitoring wildlife populations but also addressing the broader socio-economic forces enabling zoonotic spillover. With the development of models that incorporate predictive analytics and dynamic monitoring of animal disease, we can significantly lower the risk posed by emerging infectious diseases. Such measures will transform our approach towards public health from passive responses to active, preventive steps that can save thousands of lives in the case of viral epidemics (Cutler et al., 2010; Morse et al., 2012) (Figure 4.6).

4.2.3. Environmental Changes and Their Impact on Viral Spread

The intricate dynamics between viral transmission and environmental changes are slowly emerging as ecological systems face unprecedented modification in the wake of climate change, deforestation, and urbanization. Environmental changes directly influence the habitats of animals, which are large reservoirs of both emerging viral and re-emerging viral pathogens. When animals migrate or lose their habitats, they inevitably come into contact with new ecological dynamics, which alter channels of virus transmission. For instance, the encroachment of human settlements into wildlife habitats can increase zoonotic spillover risks that result in viral transmissions like HIV/AIDS and SARS that have had a tremendous effect on public health. An understanding of the ecological drivers behind these viral transmissions is essential to come up with countermeasures to their spread and to inform targeted antiviral interventions and policies to minimize human-animal contact (Morse et al., 2012). Beyond habitat modification, human activities , such as land use shifts and agricultural intensification are key drivers of viral emergence patterns. These processes establish conditions that favor increased contact between wild animals, domesticated animals, and humans, thereby increasing the likelihood of spillover events.

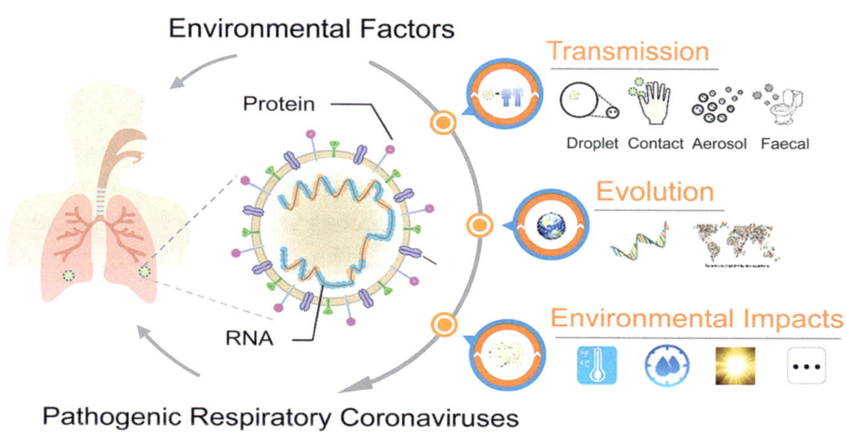

Figure 4.7. Environmental factors.

Source: https://ars.els-cdn.com/content/image/1-s2.0-S0269749120363090-fx1_lrg.jpg.

Agricultural intensification, for example, produces perfect environments for viral transmission through practices that disrupt natural ecosystems. Furthermore, worldwide climate change increasingly impacts vector-borne diseases by redistributing geographic ranges and altering the behavior of pathogens and vectors. This calls for the integration of ecological and virological research to counter the complexity of emerging infections to enable early surveillance and intervention activities across high-risk areas (Flanagan et al., 2012). More advanced surveillance and predictive models are required due to an awareness that many potential future viral outbreaks will be avoidable through forward-thinking measures. These need interdisciplinary solutions involving virology, ecology, and public health, necessary to identify high-risk sites for potential viral spillover before the event. Genetic and ecological studies, for instance, can determine species and habitats where the likelihood of zoonotic transmission is elevated. Such expectation holds the potential to re-model pandemic preparedness from a response to a pre-emptive one. By expanding our understanding regarding environmental determinants of viral transmission, we can develop overarching models that intensify our ability to anticipate and curb changing and re-emerging viral challenges, and ultimately protect international health in the context of changing ecosystems (Flanagan et al., 2012; Morse et al., 2012) (Figure 4.7).

Test Your Knowledge

1. What is the role of genetic mutations and recombination in emerging new viral strains?
2. What is the contribution of animal reservoirs to zoonotic virus transmission to man?

4.3. Case Studies of Emerging Viral Infections

Learning Outcome

1. Know about the Ebola virus outbreak in West Africa;
2. Describe the Zika virus and its implications globally;
3. Discuss about COVID-19 pandemic and its impact on society.

In recent decades, epidemics of viral disease outbreaks have posed significant global health issues, giving insight into the complex interactions of the pathogen biology, the environment, and human conduct. The case in point is the outbreak of the Zika virus, first isolated in the 1940s but now in the 2010s, to global renown. The Brazilian outbreak illustrated the extent to which urbanization and globalization could disseminate virus infections that were regionally limited previously. Higher tourist activities and global warming, which enhanced the size of the habitats for mosquitoes, were some of the critical factors that caused the rapid spread. It is critical to comprehend these dynamics since it demands novel surveillance and response systems that can anticipate and curtail subsequent outbreaks, emphasizing the demand for rigorous research into pathogen and vector emergence, as presented in the findings on new viral infections (Morse et al., 2012). Another appropriate case study is that of the 2014-2016 Ebola virus epidemic in West Africa, which emphasized the destructive impact of zoonotic transmissions. Originating predominantly from fruit bats and spreading across the population, it made the pivotal link between environmental change and human health more real. Social determinants of health, including poverty and poor healthcare infrastructure, exacerbated the crisis, implying that interventions have to address broader socioeconomic factors if they are to be successful. Flanagan et al. (2012) also support this premise by highlighting the necessity of predictive surveillance in identifying high-risk viruses before they can transmit to humans. By embracing pre-emptive strategies taking into account ecological data and wildlife behavioral patterns, health systems will be in a position to better predict future zoonotic spillovers, eventually with the aim of reducing the occurrence and impact of emergent infections. Finally, an understanding of surveillance as a pre-emptive strategy brings with it the possibility of improving global health security against emergent viral infections. As advancements are made in the analysis of genetic and ecological data, researchers can identify potential viral threats in reservoir animals and vectors and therefore provide early intervention. Nipah virus is a stark reminder of the degree to which health impacts are influenced by shifts in the environment as well as agriculture. As Flanagan et al. (2012) recognize, predictive surveillance workshops illustrate collaboration among ecologists, virologists, and computational biologists. This cross-disciplinary response can significantly enhance our capacity to forecast potential outbreaks, and thus the importance of a comprehensive health system that addresses both animal and human health. With such holistic surveillance approaches being welcomed, the global community can effectively deal with the complexities involved in the development of viral diseases.

4.3.1. Ebola Virus Outbreak in West Africa

The West African Ebola virus outbreak that emerged in 2014 is a good example of how a transmissible disease can gain global health crisis status in such a short space of time. Spurred by the zoonotic transmission of the Ebola virus from animal reservoirs to humans, this outbreak highlighted significant deficiencies in the healthcare infrastructure and response framework. Initially, the outbreak was confined to Guinea but soon spread to Sierra Leone and Liberia, where there were thousands of cases and deaths. The speedy geographic spread illustrated how weak public health systems could reinforce the effect of new viral infections. Furthermore, the incident illustrated the weakness of nations hitherto believed to be exempt from such devastating diseases, underlining the interdependence of global health security in fighting viral pandemics. Better surveillance and international cooperation became a necessity in preventing such a crisis from occurring in the future. Systemic healthcare readiness enhancements became crucial to note. At the heart of the response to the Ebola outbreak was the recognition of the global health community's necessity to act collectively. The active involvement of institutions like the World Health Organization and non-governmental organizations provided essential resources, but the response showed basic gaps in preparation and implementation. Countries less experienced with dealing with outbreaks in such a way were not able to implement proper methods of quarantine and healthcare protocol. This was most evident in the interaction of local healthcare personnel with international aid organizations, some of which caused communication hiccups and suspicion. There is a clear need for strong training and mobilization of health workers, as highlighted in calls for the setting up of enhanced screening and detection systems at airports and borderposts so that early detection of potential cases can occur and further transmission is avoided (Adu-Gyamfi, 2019).

In the Ebola outbreak response, there is a critical importance to be aware of adopting a One Health perspective, which is an appreciation for the interconnectedness of human, animal, and environmental health. The transmission of zoonotic diseases like Ebola shows how increasing the reach of human activities into wildlife realms can facilitate viral spillover events. This comprehensive response calls for inter-cooperation among several stakeholders, including public health experts, animal experts, and environmental experts, to facilitate an integrative understanding of zoonotic transmission patterns (Alagaili et al., 2016). Through multidisciplinary research collaborations, affected regions can adopt more effective surveillance and intervention methods, ultimately bridging the gap between emerging viral threats and public health responses. As evidenced by West Africa's Ebola outbreak, inter-system partnership is at the heart of building health security and preparedness for future viral epidemics (Figure 4.8).

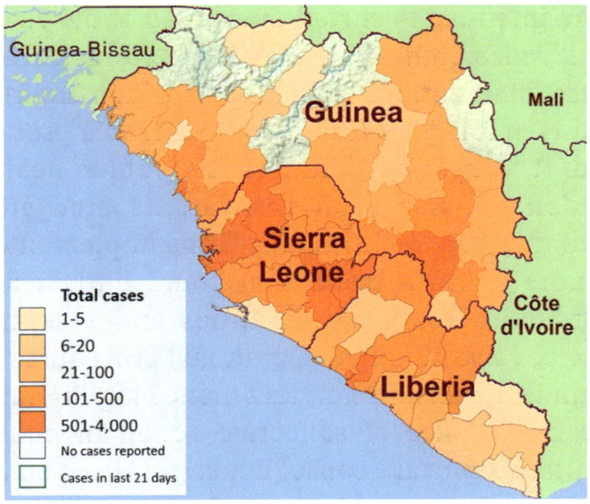

Figure 4.8. Ebola virus outbreak distribution map affected part of Western Africa.

Source: https://upload.wikimedia.org/wikipedia/commons/thumb/f/f3/2014_West_Africa_Ebola_virus_outbreak_situation_map.jpg/1024px-2014_West_Africa_Ebola_virus_outbreak_situation_map.jpg.

4.3.2. Zika Virus and Its Global Implications

The Zika virus outbreak presents a dramatic threat to international public health, primarily because of its rapid spread in pathogen-naïve areas. Initially identified in Africa, the virus gained notoriety following its outbreaks in the Pacific Island nations and later in Latin America, frightening for its potential causes of neurological diseases , such as microcephaly in children. The Zika virus is primarily transmitted by the Aedes mosquito, hence it can move very fast in susceptible communities. Hence, concerted efforts at global health have to be instituted to capture the full magnitude of Zika implications, including the need for effective surveillance systems to monitor its expansion and the development of preventive measures to cut its expansion in vulnerable locales where vector control remains a challenge (Grazzini et al., 2016) (Figure 4.9).

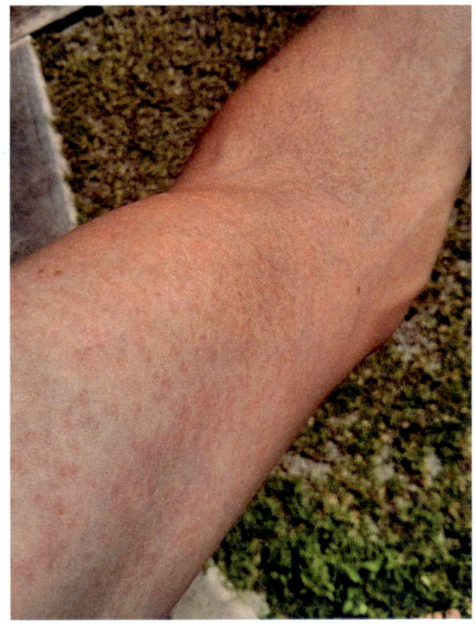

Figure 4.9. Rash on an arm due to Zika.

Source: https://upload.wikimedia.org/wikipedia/commons/thumb/b/b8/Zika.Virus.Rash.Arm.2014.jpg/800px-Zika.Virus.Rash.Arm.2014.jpg.

Countries which experienced large outbreaks disrupted their healthcare systems, with additional expenditure on child and maternal health programs. Also, the stigma associated with Zika-affected groups has further impeded efforts to treat the affected, thereby augmenting anxiety and public fear. As such, viral diseases re-surge as a looming threat, it becomes necessary for nations to adopt holistic strategies that involve vector control, public education, and health preparedness. Learning from experience with the Zika virus can help inform the improvement of global response to emergent viral dangers, framing resource distribution and research priority into emergent infectious diseases (Lewnard et al., 2019). Moreover, the Zika virus epidemic underlines the necessity for coordination among different disciplines in controlling new viral pandemics. The combination of epidemiological research with technological advancement can enhance disease monitoring capacity and allow for the exchange of real-time data among public health authorities. Furthermore, an understanding of social determinants of health perpetuating disease transmission is pivotal to the construction of effective interventions. International health organizations must focus on developing robust infrastructures that allow for interdisciplinary research, community engagement, and the development of local health capacities. Long-term attention and adaptive responses are needed to avert future epidemics of the Zika virus and other emerging infections in the future to ensure that efforts in global health are proactive rather than reactive in meeting health threats around the world (Grazzini et al., 2016) (Figure 4.10).

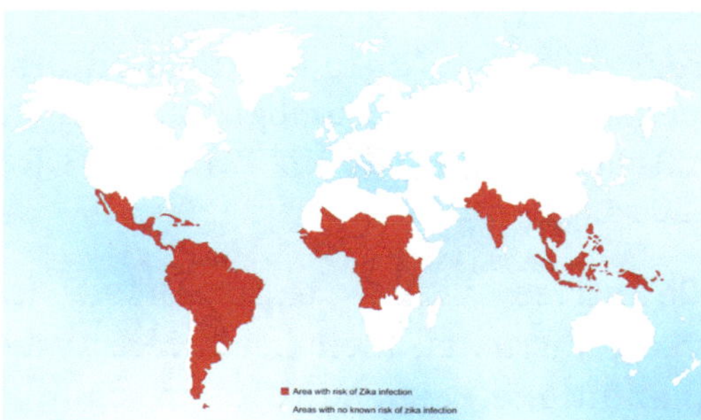

Figure 4.10. Global map of Zika virus infection.

Source: https://www.researchgate.net/profile/Morteza-Zaim/publication/330422906/figure/fig7/AS:716724374605824@1547891815243/Global-map-of-Zika-virus-infection-Content-source-Centers-for-Disease-Control-and.png.

4.3.3. COVID-19 Pandemic and Its Effects on Society

The COVID-19 pandemic has radically revolutionized societal norms, encouraging reform in public health practices and individual behaviors. The unprecedented emergence of SARS-CoV-2 triggered immediate responses in various sectors, including healthcare, education, and the economy. Lockdowns and social distancing regulations by the government were intended to curtail the spread of the virus, thus redesigning how societies interact. Also, these interventions highlighted health inequities and technology access since vulnerable groups had it tougher to adhere to public health guidelines. As social institutions struggled with this new reality, many firms implemented remote work, a trend that could outlast the pandemic. Healthcare facilities and essential services also modified operational procedures to minimize transmission risk, hence highlighting the importance of collective action in public health. The future consequences of these shifts reveal a society preoccupied with resistance against viral threats and the need to be prepared in the face of emerging infectious diseases. In response to the issues posed by the COVID-19 pandemic, scientists and policymakers have increased their focus on understanding the interactions of viruses and built environments.

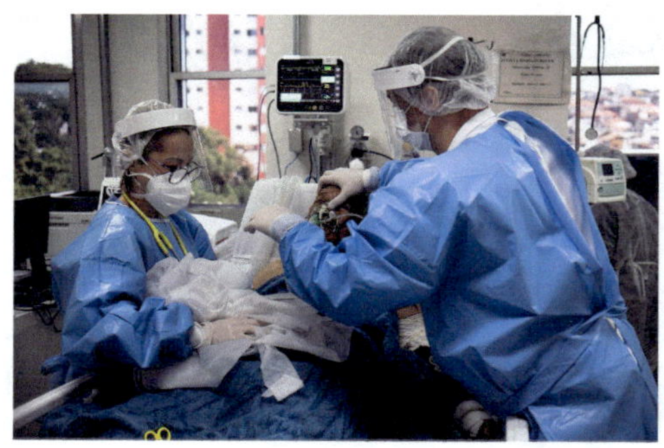

Figure 4.11. Medical professionals treating a COVID-19 patient in critical condition in an intensive care unit.

Source: https://upload.wikimedia.org/wikipedia/commons/thumb/f/f6/Covid-19_SP_-_UTI_V._Nova_Cachoeirinha.jpg/1280px-Covid-19_SP_-_UTI_V._Nova_Cachoeirinha.jpg.

As explained in recent research, the pandemic identified the necessity of minimizing transmission in indoor spaces and prioritized exploration of environmental factors that enhance or inhibit viral spread. With greater emphasis placed on airflow, surface properties, and sanitation practices, comprehension of microbiology in the built environment now guides corporate and public decision-making. This new body of knowledge encourages the creation of policies to reduce the risk of transmission, with an ongoing need for environmental monitoring and modifications to building design and operation (Figure 4.11).

As has been brought to the fore by the virus exposures of the pandemic, there is now a raw understanding of deficiencies in existing healthcare infrastructure and the need for comprehensive surveillance systems. Stakeholders in various industries have cited the need to enhance the safety of blood-derived products and healthcare practice, as noted by the innovation in recombinant technology that minimizes reliance on human plasma, thus increasing safety against potential viral threats (Bozzette et al., 2006). The evolving nature of viral diseases, combined with the lessons of the COVID-19 pandemic, has enabled an international debate on the imperative of early action, rapid-response mechanisms, and collaborative research efforts. The strategy of the future must be multisectoral in approach, with input from virology, public health, and ecology to build resilience against the inevitability of future pandemics (Figure 4.12).

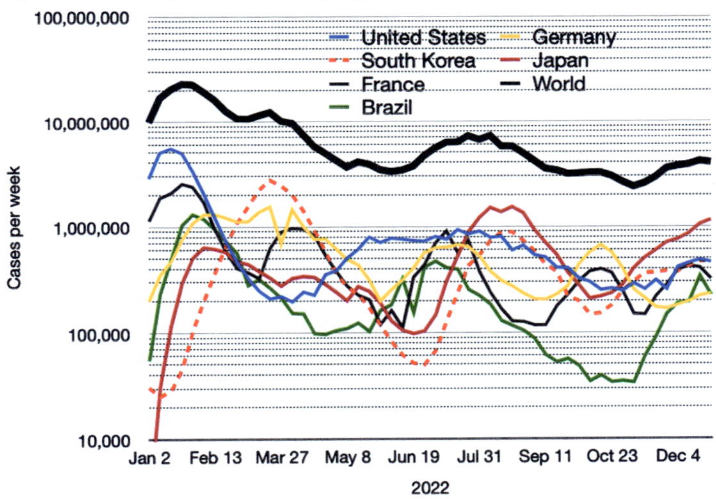

Figure 4.12. Semi-log plot of weekly new cases of COVID-19 in the world and the top six countries in 2022.

Source: https://upload.wikimedia.org/wikipedia/commons/4/4e/Covid-19_new_cases_in_top_5_countries_and_the_world.png.

Test Your Knowledge

1. What were the key causes of the widespread outbreak of the Ebola virus during the West African epidemic?
2. How did the Zika virus epidemic highlight the nexus between viral infections and birth defects?
3. How did the COVID-19 pandemic expose weaknesses in global public health systems?

4.4. Global Health Implications

Learning Outcome

1. Explain the implications for health systems;
2. Explain the economic cost of viral epidemics;
3. Value the importance of global surveillance and response.

The implications of emergent and re-emergent viral infections in global health are vast and manifold. The compound influence of globalization, urbanization, and climate change has led to an environment that fosters the transmission of infectious diseases. With populations on the move and coming into contact more than ever before, viruses discover new ways of being transmitted. The Hajj pilgrimage, which is one of the biggest mass gatherings globally, best illustrates this effect, with millions of travelers converging from all countries, requiring tight health measures to prevent the spread of disease. This event underscores the imperative for mandatory vaccinations, , such as the quadrivalent meningococcal vaccine, that are imperative to the protection of pilgrims and prevents outbreaks that could have potentially far-reaching effects globally, , such as disease outbreaks for diseases like cholera or MERS-CoV. With no adequate monitoring and increased vaccination schemes, the potential for extensive health crises still remains acute (Al-Tawfiq et al., 2019). Zoonotic disease emergence adds yet another complicated aspect to global health issues. An estimated 60% of recently emerging human pathogens are zoonotic, and the natural environment is often the primary reservoir of infection. Transmission of pathogens to humans can be through several routes, often facilitated by climate change, wildlife trade, and the intrusion of the human environment. These zoonotic infections usually undergo extreme genetic transformation, gaining their infectivity for new hosts or expressing increased pathogenicity. Hence, knowledge of the mechanisms underlying the emergence of zoonotic disease is significant for appropriate preventive and response strategies. The interdependence of animal health, human health, and the environment underscores the urgency to follow a One Health approach, which demands cross-sectoral work to address these complex interlinkages (Cutler et al., 2010).

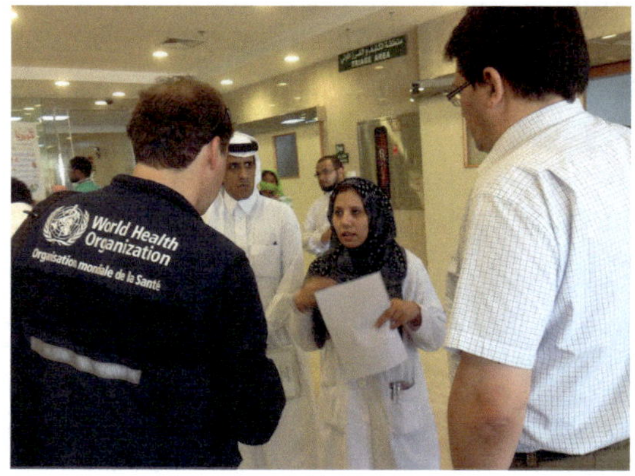

Figure 4.13. Training workers in health facilities can help to reduce health care-associated outbreaks of MERS-CoV.

Source: https://www.emro.who.int/images/stories/csr/mers_copy_copy.jpg.

Management of emerging and re-emerging viral threats should also integrate global public health with national healthcare systems. Sound health infrastructure involves strong surveillance, early reporting, and collaborative research. As global commerce and travel increasingly integrate the world, rapid outbreak detection and containment are necessary to prevent large-scale transmission. Initiatives , such as the Global Health Security Agenda seek to enhance countries' capabilities to detect and respond to infectious disease risks. Hearteningly, growing recognition of fair access to vaccines and medication treatment, particularly in low-resource settings, is required so that global efforts to combat viral diseases do not create a widening of existing health disparities.

Ultimately, establishing global cooperation and enhancing local capabilities are of most importance in safeguarding global health in the face of new virus emergence (Figure 4.13).

4.4.1. Impact on Healthcare Systems

The emergence and re-emergence of viral infections have serious implications for global health care systems, necessitating strong responses, which usually put tremendous pressure on available resources. With every new novel pathogen, healthcare infrastructures are forced to adapt rapidly to manage not only the immediate health implications but also the long-term public health policy and resource allocation impact. Emergent viral infection uncertainty can generate enormous economic burdens, with hospital admission, equipment, and human resource deficits as the origin of these expenditures. Furthermore, the economic constraint of health expenditure extends beyond treatment and includes preventive services, with a focus on the need for an effective surveillance system to enable early detection and reaction. The pressure underscores the sheer need for a One Health approach with human, animal, and environmental health integration for greater resilience against future pandemics (Dar et al., 2015). In addition to the expense that is directly attributable to treatment and management of emergent viral illness, healthcare systems around the world also face an issue in the form of antimicrobial resistance (AMR). The interplay between viral infection and AMR not only complicates the treatment regimen but also undermines the efficacy of existing antimicrobial medications that are required to handle secondary bacterial infections. As practitioners hasten to address these complexities, their impact can ripple across the system, leading to longer lengths of stay and increased mortality. Such issues are further exacerbated by the lack of standardization within treatment protocols and infection control measures, producing a strong imperative for regional solutions that chart regional health landscapes. Transnational collaboration that aims to enhance policy tools can be employed to increase knowledge of AMR dynamics, thereby enabling better practice (Cookson et al., 2002). Healing the weaknesses in healthcare systems demands innovative models that revisit screening and treatment practices. For instance, hospitals can employ low-cost laboratory-screening methods especially designed for high-risk wards, thereby creating better outcomes among patients bearing compounded viral as well as bacterial infections. These strategies require close examination: estimating the sensitivity and specificity of tests can significantly influence the course of infection control actions. Testing the cost-effectiveness of alternative clinical interventions, in addition, can allow health systems to reduce resource consumption with tailored responses to each new threat. Ultimately, fostering flexibility in health systems will prove crucial to the improvement of resilience against future viral epidemics and limiting their system impacts (Cookson et al., 2002).

4.4.2. Economic Consequences of Viral Outbreaks

The economic consequence of viral outbreaks extends far beyond immediate healthcare costs, impacting every sector and leading to long-term financial instability. During outbreaks, the healthcare systems are under tremendous strain, needing additional funds for treatment, research, and prevention. The economic burden of inflated healthcare expenses can result in resource mobilization problems in public health systems. Besides, viral outbreaks also have the impact of causing labor disruptions through infection and related quarantine, apt to decrease productivity. For instance, industries requiring a stable labor force, , such as agriculture and manufacturing, are likely to experience extreme operational disruptions, thereby hastening the overall economic slump resulting from an outbreak. Economic globalization causes the viral epidemics which erupt in a local area to have spreading effects, affecting trade and travel at the global scale and hence propelling the economic consequences. Apart from that, viral epidemics have very large indirect costs that add up to their economic effects.

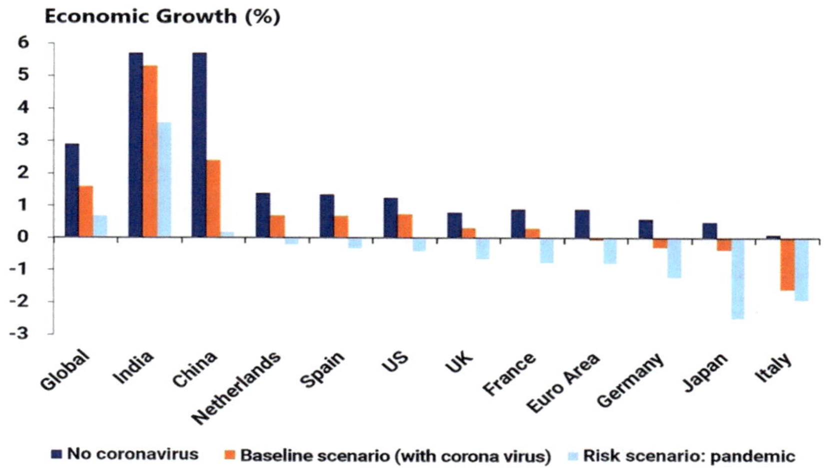

Figure 4.14. The economic impact on the world and different countries due to the COVID-19 outbreak.

Source: https://www.researchgate.net/publication/348106175/figure/fig1/AS:976152336293890@1609744261285/The-economic-impact-on-world-and-different-countries-due-to-COVID-19-outbreak-Source.png.

The perception of contagion can give rise to a decline in consumer confidence and this results in less spending and investment. For example, hospitality and tourism businesses can be hit hard by losses when travel restrictions and safety threats keep people away. Additionally, agricultural businesses can lose money when their animals get infected or die due to diseases or infections, necessitating prevention or extermination at a high cost. The financial cost is doubled when businesses have to change their safety protocols, adding more strain on their resources. Research has established that the cumulative effects of such indirect costs may be staggering and fully include the economic loss calculated in terms of both direct medical costs, but also the broader economic environment shaped by consumerism and market patterns. In controlling the economic blow of viral epidemics, effective surveillance and control strategies are necessary. The Bovine Viral Diarrhea Virus (BVDV) case illustrates the complexity of handling a widespread viral disease in agriculture. Despite its ruinous effect on the health and economic performance of cattle, there is a significant number of farms not even know their BVDV status, which underlines the pressing need for enhanced surveillance programs. Installation of robust monitoring programs not only ensures timely disease control but also serves as a preventive measure to protect economic interests. Along with preventive action, such as immunization and widespread testing, ensuring the economic viability of targeted industries in the long run is possible. Therefore, connecting health policies to economic models is capable of reacting strongly to the challenges posed by viral outbreaks, increasing resilience in public health as well as in economic systems (Figure 4.14).

4.4.3. Importance of Global Surveillance and Response

Increased rates of emerging and re-emerging viral infections necessitate robust systems for global surveillance and response. These systems are crucial for monitoring viral epidemics and identifying pathogens before gaining a niche among human populations. History shows that most pandemics, including HIV/AIDS and severe acute respiratory syndrome, have zoonotic pathogen causes that are traditionally brought about by ecological, behavioral, or socioeconomic changes. These changes highlight the importance of understanding the convergence of human, animal, and environmental health. Enhanced surveillance systems, therefore, not only detect potential threats but also feed inputs for timely interventions, which may prevent the implications for public health. Developing mathematical models, diagnostic procedures, and innovative communication technologies can help augment our ability to predict and respond to viral threats in a superior way, ultimately driving the transition from reactive control to proactive action in international health management (Morse et al., 2012). A crucial component of global surveillance is the early identification of high-priority viruses that have the potential to jump from animals to humans. Our current approach has a tendency to act once the virus has already been transmitted to humans, and this reflects a critical flaw in our capability. The importance of predictive surveillance is now universally recognized, and workshops assemble virologists, ecologists, and computational biologists to engage with plans for anticipating viral species jumps. Through integration of genetic and ecological information, scientists can identify potential viral risks before their occurrence in humans. Such an anticipatory strategy has the potential to minimize the occurrence of outbreaks by enabling public health authorities to undertake preventive interventions in more risk-prone areas and thus protect global health (Flanagan et al., 2012). More so, emerging viral infections present challenges necessitating global collaboration in surveillance (Flanagan et al., 2012). The global interconnectivity of our world allows an outbreak in one region to become a pandemic in a few days worldwide. Shared scientific knowledge and resources that are shared through collaborative systems are essential since they enable nations to respond rapidly and effectively. Standardized guidelines for surveillance practices, data sharing, and outbreak control will make the world more prepared. Such cooperative effort not only bolsters local capacity but it constitutes an overarching understanding of virus ecology and transmission dynamics. Through investment in these global efforts, we equip ourselves with the means necessary to address viral challenges in the future, eventually reducing the public health burden caused by emerging and re-emerging diseases (Morse et al., 2012).

Test Your Knowledge

1. How do emerging and re-emerging viral infections stress healthcare systems internationally?
2. In what ways can healthcare infrastructure investment improve readiness against subsequent viral infections?

4.5. Prevention and Control Strategies

Learning Outcome

1. Comprehend vaccination and prevention;
2. Emerging and re-emerging viral infection public health policies: discussion;
3. Antiviral drug research and development: focus.

The outbreak and re-emergence of viral infections need proper prevention and control measures to annihilate the danger caused by them to international public health. The framework for such interventions needs to incorporate strong surveillance systems that can detect and follow viral pathways. Such systems are the foundation of identifying outbreaks at their early phase so that a rapid public health response is possible. As seen through the implementation of tuberculosis (TB) during the COVID-19 pandemic, routine healthcare services were severely impacted, disrupting disease control and management interventions. Studies have shown that lockdown-induced disruptions of TB care resulted in increased levels of prevalence and mortality. It is therefore essential to reinstate normal services and reorient healthcare delivery to provide continuity, even in the event of pandemics, to effectively address high-burden diseases (Chaturvedi et al., 2023). Another prime determinant of successful prevention interventions is vaccine generation and deployment. Immunization programs can decrease the prevalence of epidemic viruses substantially, thus lessening the workload for the healthcare system. Past evidence indicates that vaccines have been instrumental in the control of diseases like influenza and Ebola, yet new approaches need to adapt in light of new threats. Scientists underscore the need to target viral reservoirs by implementing cross-species surveillance and realizing ecological determinants that enhance zoonotic transmissions. By bringing mathematical modeling and informatics technologies together, public health authorities can predict probable outbreaks and implement pre-emptive vaccination drives to shield vulnerable groups (Morse et al., 2012). Last but not least, formal education and public awareness campaigns are intrinsic to successful prevention and control strategies. Active population compliance with health measures—hand washing, mask wearing, and immunization—is vital to minimize the spread of viral infections. Communication approaches should be tailored so that they can reach various groups in a bid to ensure that all vulnerable groups have access to essential health information. Further, experience with the COVID-19 pandemic also sensitizes us to the importance of having clear and transparent messages that help manage public anxiety and adherence to health interventions. In the event of emerging and re-emerging viral diseases, educating an enlightened society can build resilience and provide for a coordinated response to impending health hazards (Chaturvedi et al., 2023).

4.5.1. Vaccination and Its Role in Prevention

The role of vaccination in the prevention of emerging and re-emerging viral diseases becomes increasingly vital with changing global health hazards. The last few decades have witnessed some of the viral pathogens that, heretofore, were believed to dominate, showing a resurgence now and thus creating severe threats to public health. The need for an effective vaccination strategy has grown due to the spread of these pathogens among populations with low immunity. Vaccination has proved to be a crucial defense mechanism through the generation of protective immunity, thereby reducing the incidence of disease and restricting outbreaks. The infectious disease epidemiology underscores that mass vaccination's achievement of herd immunity has the potential to safeguard the immunologically naive segments of society adequately, thereby limiting expansion and reducing the possibility of recurrence, as reiterated by recent public health summaries (Khalaf, 2022). Vaccine production for emerging viruses is even more challenging in view of the rapid mutations and plasticity of these pathogens. The traditional methods may be insufficient, and thus new vaccine technologies must be introduced. New avenues for vaccine manufacture have been opened by advances in molecular biology, , such as mRNA vaccines and viral vector platforms. Such advanced technologies allow for quicker responses to emerging threats and assist in the development of effective and producible vaccines. They also provide the chance to tackle not only emergent viruses but also to improve existing vaccines against re-emerging diseases. By employing various platforms as well as an improved understanding of viral biology, public health programs are well situated to prepare for probable future pandemics and epidemics. Therefore, it is required that modern technologies be merged with conventional methods to enhance our vaccination policy (Khalaf, 2022). Further, increasing appreciation for the complexity of viral epidemiology necessitates a focused approach to vaccine evaluation and use. Modern epidemiology has evolved to make amends for the deficiency between traditional chronic disease methods and infectious disease dynamics, acknowledging the specific challenge of new pathogens. This evolution calls for robust data-based analysis to contrast the effectiveness of vaccines, the transmission dynamics of the pathogens, and the widespread effect of public health measures. By integrating molecular and digital sources of data, surveillance is heightened and information on vaccine effectiveness across various populations is provided. Second, novel causal inference techniques are reshaping the future of vaccine research and enabling measurement of vaccine effects on public health endpoints. As the field advances, there remains huge potential in vaccines as a bulwark in re-emerging and emerging viral disease control (Figure 4.15).

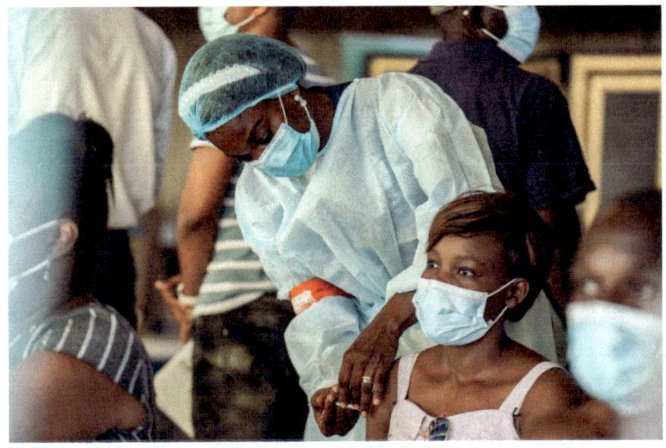

Figure 4.15. Vaccination for viral infection prevention.

Source: https://www.afro.who.int/sites/default/files/2022-05/vaccination_efficacy.jpg.

4.5.2. Public Health Policies and Education

Public health policies play a crucial role in controlling and minimizing re-emerging and emerging viral infections. The policies must be based on solid evidence and consider the unique socio-economic and cultural environments of every country, particularly low- and middle-income countries. A comprehensive policy development requires an evaluation of existing infection prevention and control measures, the use of resources, and surveillance systems. According to Dar et al. (2015), the complexity of implementing effective public health interventions across various sectors requires strategies tailored to meet the special needs and situation of each region. It is the duty of policymakers to make investments in developing standardized frameworks to evaluate the cost-effectiveness and generalizability of health interventions so that these policies remain responsive in the long run to the changing epidemiology of infectious diseases. Education is a critical component of public health policy, particularly about emerging viral infections. Education programs conducted within communities can enhance hygiene practice knowledge awareness, vaccination needs recognition, and transmission dynamics of new pathogens. Education programs ought to empower the people within the communities to protect themselves and their communities from health hazards by giving them the necessary knowledge and skills.

The collaboration of global research institutes and local institutions, as exhibited in Molia et al. (2012), indicates the potential for training modules being developed, ultimately resulting in an educated workforce that can address health problems. By leveraging existing networks of disease control and education, public health programs can foster a culture of preparedness and response and thereby improve community resilience against emerging outbreaks. Further, championing a One Health approach emphasizes the interconnectedness of environmental, animal, and human health in the fight against viral diseases. Joint cooperation between veterinary and public health systems is necessary for more effective monitoring of disease and risk assessment of zoonotic pathogens. For example, intensive training and research in zoonotic diseases like rabies can give substantial insight into pathogen transmission patterns and available control measures, as stated in Molia et al. (2012). The collaborative approach not only facilitates the sharing of information among disciplines but also enables the formulation of participatory policies that consider the complex dynamics between ecosystems and public health. Ultimately, a concerted effort to address health policy and education can significantly advance the effect of interventions against new and re-emerging viral infections, advancing global health security in an increasingly interconnected world.

4.5.3. Research and Development of Antiviral Treatments

The research and development environment for antiviral treatment is constantly evolving, especially considering emerging and re-emerging viral infections. One of the significant focus areas is on the mechanisms by which viruses evade the host immunity. Understanding these mechanisms allows scientists to design antiviral drugs that are effective in targeting viral replication and spread. Advances in molecular biology techniques have allowed scientists to chart out viral genes and pathways necessary for survival and transmission in host organisms. For instance, the mechanisms through which the feline infectious peritonitis virus (FIPV) evades immune detection target potential sites for therapeutic intervention. Aside from the progress, the pursuit for optimal treatments remains challenging, highlighting the need for an innovative approach in antiviral drug development (Pedersen et al., 2014). Aside from traditional antiviral treatment, the application of RNA interference (RNAi) as an antiviral therapy has also gained considerable attention. RNAi is a natural defense to viral infections that breaks down viral RNA and targets it. Exciting research has demonstrated that certain viruses can hijack and suppress the RNAi machinery, presenting a challenging problem for developing effective therapeutics. Antiviral research in species , such as bumblebees revealed unexpected findings, whereby infection by IAPV actually enhances the RNAi apparatus, contrary to established expectations of viral suppression. This finding emphasizes the importance of understanding the host-virus interactions at the molecular level and suggests that the disruption of the RNAi process may produce novel avenues for therapeutic approaches against viral infections (Cappelle et al., 2016). The complexity of viral infections and their interaction with the host systems necessitates a multidisciplinary approach in the development of antiviral therapies. New strategies, , such as combination therapy based on the use of direct antiviral agents and immunomodulators, are promising in the battle against viral threats. Furthermore, the use of high-throughput screening technologies coupled with bioinformatics approaches has accelerated the identification of new antiviral drugs. Since new viruses tend to develop ways to escape existing treatments, research must counter the ongoing development of these pathogens. Continuous investment in research and development will be critical in the formulation of a robust arsenal of antiviral drugs that will be able to counter present and emerging viral risks to public health in the context of greater interconnectivity worldwide.

Test Your Knowledge

1. What is the role of vaccination in the prevention and control of viral infection?
2. What is the role of public health policy and community education in the reduction of the spread of viral infections?

SUMMARY

The studies of the re-emerging and newly emerging viral diseases go on, and it is increasingly clear that the world environment is characterized by highly dynamic interaction among pathogens, hosts, and environmental determinants. The setting recognizes that pandemics are of the zoonotic virus type, the majority of which are animal-to-human transmission, and calls for an in-depth understanding of the ecological and behavioral etiology of viral emergence. While a lot has been done in detecting them and responding to epidemics, no pandemic was predicted before its infection of humans, highlighting significant gaps in preparedness and surveillance. They have to be transcended in the drive to increase public health attainment and will be achieved through a multi-disciplinary process with science and technological innovations (Morse et al., 2012). Surveillance efforts against viruses have emerged, particularly in predictive modeling, which indicates that blocking outbreaks should be intercepted before amplification. This is active and thus early detection methods and high-risk virus identification based on analysis of ecological and genetic data are important. Through understanding where and how these zoonotic transfers are occurring—most notably in wildlife animals, such as bats and rodents—risk assessment strategies can be developed by scientists that reliably predict future species jumps. Workshop discussion among virologists, ecologists, and computational biologists produces an action plan for the development of a virus surveillance system that can predict future infection (Flanagan et al., 2012). Such multidisciplinary coordination will be crucial as it balances scientific inquiry with effective public health. On balance, the risk of re-emerging and emerging viral pathogens constitutes an umbrella response of research, worldwide cooperation, and public policy. By integrating high-tech surveillance systems, founded on genetic data, and promoting multidisciplinary cooperation, the scientific community will better be able to anticipate and prevent viral danger. The imperative for new strategies and overall preparation plans is strengthened by the rising pandemics in the modern world. Future preventive care with a predictive model will not only help in managing continuous threats but can actually stop future epidemics from being formed at all, thereby ensuring global public health (Morse et al., 2012; Flanagan et al., 2012).

One of the matters that has characterized the discussions on emerging and re-emerging outbreaks of viral diseases has been the necessity for more comprehensive surveillance networks. The recent meetings highlighted the need to set up predictive systems that will identify high-risk viruses before they break out from reservoirs in animals to infect human beings. This forward-thinking approach relies on demystification of zoonotic disease processes, and in this section, what is being addressed is integrating genetic and ecological data for predicting specie jumps. The conclusions that arise from such workshops are to work with multidisciplinary teams of virologists, ecologists, and computational biologists in order to establish good schemes of surveillance. These proactive measures can potentially become a powerful tool in reducing the incidence of zoonotic spillovers and shaping public health policy in infectious disease control before an epidemic outbreak (Flanagan et al., 2012).

In addition to this, this interactive dynamic between animal physiology and viral transmission dynamics has also become a force driving the prediction of zoonotic infection. Bat studies, particularly where henipavirus dynamics are concerned, illustrate just how intricate such interactions might prove. Studies of antibody levels in captive groups have not only found persistence of maternal antibodies but have quantified the contribution of maternal factors to the modulation of viral transmission rates, especially in critical life events , such as pregnancy and lactation. These findings add to the understanding of persistent infection in reservoir hosts and shed light on how persistent environmental processes in each season could be sustaining infection transmission. With this information, public health scientists and policy makers can make more informed predictions of when and where spillover events will occur, ultimately optimizing outreach efforts and preparedness measures required in the event of novel viral outbreaks (Baker et al., 2014).

Finally, appreciation of ecological and behavioral pressures governing viral infections cannot be overemphasized. Habitat-animal interaction and human encroachment are likely to enhance infectious disease transmission from animals to humans. Careful attention should thus be placed on surveillance in reservoir habitats of newly evolving viruses. This entails examining under what circumstances these viruses are propagated and what role environmental pressure plays in their dynamics: data required for effective surveillance schemes. With the integration of ecological data with virological studies, scientists can create a more complete picture of how risks from what could be zoonotic diseases can be circumvented. An integrated plan that takes into consideration these factors will improve countermeasures to known as well as to unknown viral epizootics, resulting in enhanced public health security (Flanagan et al., 2012; Baker et al., 2014).

KEY TERMS FROM THIS CHAPTER

- Antimicrobial resistance
- Bacterial infections
- Blood-derived products
- Bovine Viral Diarrhea Virus
- COVID-19 pandemic
- Diagnostic procedures
- Ecology
- Epidemiology
- Feline infectious peritonitis virus
- Global health security
- Global health systems
- Global interconnectivity
- Health preparedness
- Healthcare infrastructure
- Healthcare protocol
- Human species
- Human-animal interfaces
- Infectious disease dynamics
- Measles
- Multilateral challenges

Critical Thinking Questions

1. **Which of the following is an emerging viral infection?**
   a. Measles
   b. Influenza (seasonal)
   c. Zika virus
   d. Rabies
2. **Which factor most contributes to re-emerge previously controlled viral infections?**
   a. Decrease in international travel
   b. Advanced diagnostic devices
   c. Urban green spaces increase
   d. Vaccine resistance and low immunity coverage
3. **Adherence of the Ebola virus to which of the routes mentioned?**
   a. Airborne route
   b. Direct contact via body fluids
   c. Contaminated water
   d. Mosquito bite
4. **Which of the following is an example of a re-emerging viral infection?**
   a. HIV/AIDS
   b.
   c. Smallpox
   d. Dengue fever
5. **Which of the following is NOT a cause of new viral infections?**
   a. Vector elimination
   b. Global warming
   c. Increased wildlife-human interaction
   d. Antiviral drug resistance

Short Answer Questions

1. What are the most common reasons for the emergence and re-emergence of viral diseases during the past decades?
2. Define an emerging and a re-emerging viral infection with an example of each.
3. What is the role of zoonosis in the emergence of new viral diseases? Give examples of zoonotic viruses.
4. Explain the role of international travel and trade in the spread of emerging viral diseases.
5. Explain the role of climate change in the epidemiology of the spread of vector-borne viral illnesses like dengue or Zika.

6. Explain the challenge in the diagnosis and management of emerging viral diseases in low-resource settings.
7. Describe the role of genomic surveillance and early detection in managing emerging viral diseases.
8. Critically evaluate the public health control measures utilized for a recent outbreak of an emerging or re-emerging virus.

Answer to Critical Thinking Questions

1. (c); 2. (d); 3. (b); 4. (d); 5. (a)

REFERENCES

1. Dar, O. A., Hasan, R., Schlundt, J., Harbarth, S., Caleo, G., Dar, F. K., Littmann, J., Rweyemamu, M., Buckley, E. J., Shahid, M., Kock, R., Li, H. L., Giha, H., Khan, M., So, A. D., Bindayna, K. M., Kessel, A., Pedersen, H. B., Permanand, G., Zumla, A., ... Heymann, D. L. (2016). Exploring the evidence base for national and regional policy interventions to combat resistance. *Lancet (London, England)*, *387*(10015), 285–295. https://doi.org/10.1016/S0140-6736(15)00520-6(accessed on 13th June 2025).

2. Acosta-Leal, R., Duffy, S., Xiong, Z., Hammond, R. W., et al. (1995). Advances in plant virus evolution: Translating evolutionary insights into better disease management. https://core.ac.uk/download/pdf/36058493.pdf (accessed on 13th June 2025).

3. Adebanjo, A. A., Adole, A. R., Ajayi, O. A., Ajayi, T., et al. (2024). Mpox resurgence: Preventing a potential pandemic through lesssons learned from COVID-19 experience and future research directions. https://core.ac.uk/download/651745471.pdf (accessed on 13th June 2025).

4. Adu-Gyamfi, S. (2019). Ebola hemorrhagic fever in Africa: A necessary highlight. https://core.ac.uk/download/480549437.pdf (accessed on 13th June 2025).

5. Akele, R. Y., Akinpelu, R. T., Dada, M. O., Edafetanure-Ibeh, E., et al. (2024). The role of travel medicine in managing future pandemics: Lessons learned from global infectious disease outbreaks. https://core.ac.uk/download/604373473.pdf (accessed on 13th June 2025).

6. Al-Tawfiq, J. A., & Memish, Z. A. (2014). Emerging respiratory viral infections: MERS-CoV and influenza. https://core.ac.uk/download/322846911.pdf (accessed on 13th June 2025).

7. Al-Tawfiq, J. A., & Memish, Z. A. (2019). The Hajj 2019 vaccine requirements and possible new challenges. https://core.ac.uk/download/322846916.pdf (accessed on 13th June 2025).

8. Al-Tawfiq, J. A., Benkouiten, S., & Memish, Z. A. (2018). A systematic review of emerging respiratory viruses at the Hajj and possible coinfection with *Streptococcus pneumoniae*. https://core.ac.uk/download/322846904.pdf (accessed on 13th June 2025).

9. Alagaili, A. N., Alagaili, A., Zumla, A., Arabi, Y., Arabi, R., Azhar, E., Briese, T., et al. (2016). Taking forward a 'One Health' approach for turning the tide against the Middle East respiratory syndrome coronavirus and other zoonotic pathogens with epidemic potential. https://core.ac.uk/download/45467901.pdf (accessed on 13th June 2025).

10. Alvarez, M., Batmanian, J., Bocharov, G., Brennan, C. A., Burgard, M., Buzon, M. J., Dahl, V., et al. (2012). HIV types, groups, subtypes and recombinant forms: Errors in replication, selection pressure and quasispecies. https://core.ac.uk/download/16432564.pdf (accessed on 13th June 2025).

11. Ansari, A., Chang, C., Gershwin, M. E., Ortiz, B. L., et al. (2016). The Zika outbreak of the 21st century. https://core.ac.uk/download/323068480.pdf (accessed on 13th June 2025).

12. Arrieta, G., Calderon, A., Figueiredo, L. T., Guzman, M. G., et al. (2016). Viral zoonoses that fly with bats: A review. https://core.ac.uk/download/77938854.pdf (accessed on 13th June 2025).

13. Baggaley, R. F., Ferguson, N. M., & Garnett, G. P. (2005). The epidemiological impact of antiretroviral use predicted by mathematical models: A review. https://core.ac.uk/download/pdf/3765667.pdf (accessed on 13th June 2025).

14. Baker, K. S., Barr, J., Boots, M., Broder, R., et al. (2014). Viral antibody dynamics in a chiropteran host. https://core.ac.uk/download/9357743.pdf (accessed on 13th June 2025).

15. Barclay, W., Beauchemin, C. A. A., Bedford, T., Belser, J. A., et al. (2016). Viral factors in influenza pandemic risk assessment. https://core.ac.uk/download/74230057.pdf (accessed on 13th June 2025).

16. Bauchinger, U., Falagas, M. E., Kelesidis, I., Kelesidis, T., et al. (2008). Human infections associated with wild birds. https://core.ac.uk/download/323062291.pdf (accessed on 13th June 2025).

17. Booth, R., De Vliegher, S., Deprez, P., Dewulf, J., et al. (2013). Assessment of two essential elements of BVDV control on selected Flemish dairy and beef farms. https://core.ac.uk/download/55761867.pdf (accessed on 13th June 2025).

18. Molia Sophie, Gaidet Nicolas, Bourhy Hervé. 2012. Mission to Indonesia to participate to the 1st Indonesia- France Seminar in Medicine & Public Health and investigate potential collaborations on animal health : 2nd - 9th of November 2012. s.l. : s.n., 33 p.(accessed on 13th June 2025).

19. Bozzette, S., Diamond, M., Koerper, M. A., Kulkarni, R., et al. (2006). Clinical perspectives of emerging pathogens in bleeding disorders. https://core.ac.uk/download/323066967.pdf (accessed on 13th June 2025).

20. Brunner, J. L., Duffus, A. L. J., Gray, M. J., Miller, D. L., et al. (2014). Second International Symposium on Rana viruses: A North American herpetological perspective. https://core.ac.uk/download/289166243.pdf (accessed on 13th June 2025).

21. Flanagan, M. L., Parrish, C. R., Cobey, S., Glass, G. E., Bush, R. M., & Leighton, T. J. (2012). Anticipating the species jump: surveillance for emerging viral threats. *Zoonoses and public health*, *59*(3), 155–163. https://doi.org/10.1111/j.1863-2378.2011.01439.x(accessed on 13th June 2025).

22. Cappelle, K., Dhaenens, M., Meeus, I., Smagghe, G., et al. (2016). Israeli acute paralysis virus infection leads to an enhanced RNA interference response and not its suppression in the bumblebee *Bombus terrestris*. https://core.ac.uk/download/84042020.pdf (accessed on 13th June 2025).

23. Morse, S. S., Mazet, J. A., Woolhouse, M., Parrish, C. R., Carroll, D., Karesh, W. B., Zambrana-Torrelio, C., Lipkin, W. I., & Daszak, P. (2012). Prediction and prevention of the next pandemic zoonosis. *Lancet (London, England)*, *380*(9857), 1956–1965. https://doi.org/10.1016/S0140-6736(12)61684-5(accessed on 13th June 2025).

24. Thaker, S. K., Ch'ng, J., & Christofk, H. R. (2019). Viral hijacking of cellular metabolism. *BMC biology*, *17*(1), 59. https://doi.org/10.1186/s12915-019-0678-9(accessed on 13th June 2025).

25. Chaturvedi, T., Gupta, S., & Rajput, S. (2023). Impact of the COVID-19 pandemic on tuberculosis management in India: A brief overview. https://core.ac.uk/download/579951024.pdf (accessed on 13th June 2025).

26. Chrisafis, G. C. (2017). Historical patterns of arboviral seroprevalence across Africa and Asia. https://core.ac.uk/download/84397690.pdf (accessed on 13th June 2025).

27. Clark, T. A., Cohn, A. C., Farley, M. M., Hall, A. J., et al. (2016). Meningococcal disease in patients with human immunodeficiency virus infection: A review of cases reported through active

surveillance in the United States, 2000–2008. https://core.ac.uk/download/323082103.pdf (accessed on 13th June 2025).

28. Coil, D. A., Dietz, L., Eisen, J. A., Fretz, M., et al. (2020). 2019 novel coronavirus (COVID-19) pandemic: Built environment considerations to reduce transmission. https://core.ac.uk/download/323069352.pdf (accessed on 13th June 2025).

29. Cookson, B., Kibbler, C., Kunori, T., Roberts, J., et al. (2002). Cost-effectiveness of different MRSA screening methods. *(Link not provided; no access date assigned).*

30. Cowden, J., Forbes, K. J., MacRae, M., Maiden, M. C. J., et al. (2013). Operationalizing factors that explain the emergence of infectious diseases: A case study of the human campylobacteriosis epidemic. https://core.ac.uk/download/18601300.pdf (accessed on 13th June 2025).

31. Cutler, S. J., Fooks, A. R., & van der Poel, W. H. M. (2010). Public health threat of new, reemerging, and neglected zoonoses in the industrialized world. https://core.ac.uk/download/pdf/29238214.pdf (accessed on 13th June 2025).

32. Djoko, C. F., Fair, J. N., Lebreton, M., Pike, B. L., et al. (2010). The origin and prevention of pandemics. https://core.ac.uk/download/323077529.pdf (accessed on 13th June 2025).

33. Gentile, G., & Micozzi, A. (2016). Speculations on the clinical significance of asymptomatic viral infections. https://core.ac.uk/download/98344656.pdf (accessed on 13th June 2025).

34. Grazzini, G., Liumbruno, G. M., Marano, G., Pupella, S., et al. (2016). Zika virus and the never-ending story of emerging pathogens and transfusion medicine. https://core.ac.uk/download/54532486.pdf (accessed on 13th June 2025).

35. Khalaf, N. F. (2022). Viral vaccine strategies. https://core.ac.uk/download/629276972.pdf (accessed on 13th June 2025).

36. Lewnard, J. A., & Reingold, A. L. (2019). Emerging challenges and opportunities in infectious disease epidemiology. https://core.ac.uk/download/323082106.pdf (accessed on 13th June 2025).

37. Pedersen, N. C. (2014). An update on feline infectious peritonitis: Diagnostics and therapeutics. https://core.ac.uk/download/323070220.pdf (accessed on 13th June 2025).

38. Todd, K. (2019). The promising viral threat to bacterial resistance: The uncertain patentability of phage therapeutics and the necessity of alternative incentives. https://core.ac.uk/download/213020895.pdf (accessed on 13th June 2025).

39. Wiethoelter, A. K., Bengis, R., Chardonnet, P., Beltrán-Alcrudo, D., Dehove, A., Kock, R., et al. (2015). Global trends in infectious diseases at the wildlife–livestock interface. https://core.ac.uk/download/36778662.pdf (accessed on 13th June 2025).

40. Zaragoza, G. (2019). Getting to zero HIV cases in San Francisco: Reconceptualizing housing as public health infrastructure in the framework of HIV prevention and treatment. https://core.ac.uk/download/287622090.pdf (accessed on 13th June 2025).

MEDICAL MYCOLOGY

5

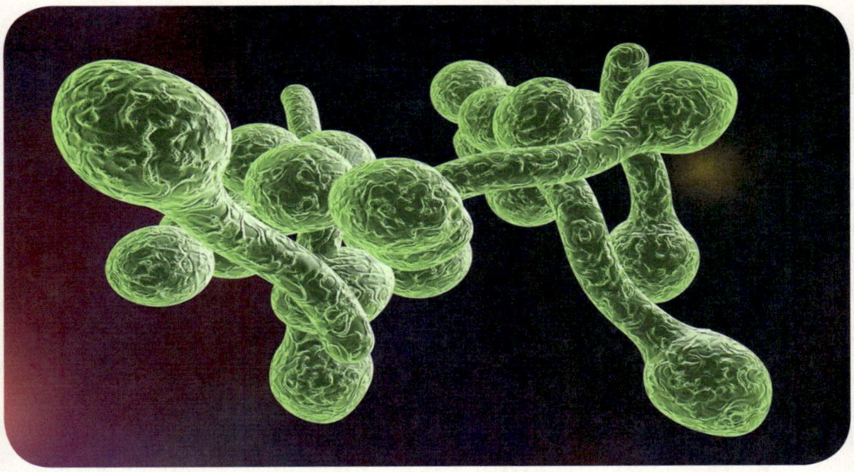

LEARNING OBJECTIVES

After studying this chapter, you will be able to:

1. Tell the basics of fungal biology;
2. Discuss usual fungal infections;
3. Seriously consider diagnosis of fungal infections;
4. Discuss treatment possibilities of fungal infections;
5. Learn epidemiology of fungal infections;
6. Address practical measures of prevention and control to reduce the burden of fungal pathogens.

Introduction

The medical mycology field has increased significance during the past decades because the role of fungal pathogens and their implications for human health have further evolved. Previously considered opportunistic pathogens, fungi of the kind that represent the Aspergillus genus have been associated primarily with immunocompromised patients. However, recent evidence highlights that invasive aspergillosis is also possible in non-neutropenic patients with pre-existing predisposing conditions, including corticosteroid treatment, chronic pulmonary disease, and solid tumor malignancies. Because of the growing incidence of fungal infections, particularly in intensive care units, healthcare workers must be aware of the possibility of identifying these pathogens and dealing with the risk in an efficient manner. This focus on epidemiology lays the foundation for the more in-depth investigation of diagnostic and therapeutic methods in medical mycology, so that it is a significant branch of medicine today. Diagnosis of fungal infections is exceptionally challenging, as the symptoms of such infections during clinical presentation are typically mimetic of bacterial or viral infection. Therefore, a higher clinical suspicion should be used in meeting critically ill patients with non-specific respiratory presentations. Methods , such as serum galactomannan assays, bronchoalveolar lavage, and some polymerase chain reaction (PCR) tests have developed to become critical tools in arriving at accurate diagnoses of illnesses , such as invasive aspergillosis. Care should, however, be taken when interpreting these diagnostic tests since false-positive and false-negative tests are also full of potential to mislead the management. Early initiation of antifungal therapy on suspicion, even when irrefutable evidence is not present, is critical in improving patient outcomes. Antifungal drug-based interventions using drugs , such as voriconazole and isavuconazole have shown promise in mortality reduction, highlighting the importance of accelerated diagnosis and treatment in the clinical setting (Bassetti & Bouza, 2017). Along with this, knowledge of the various risk factors associated with fungal infections and recognition of their courses clinically is important in clinical mycology. Mucormycosis, being rare, became a more prominent entity due to its presence in vulnerable populations, e.g., uncontrolled diabetes mellitus, open wounds, or immunocompromised status. Clinical presentations are marked by highly aggressive necrotizing lesions in vital anatomical locations, necessitating urgent medical care. Treatment interventions include not only immediate antifungal treatment, especially the administration of liposomal amphotericin B, but also radical surgical removal of infected tissue. In spite of improvements in diagnosis and treatment, mucormycosis mortality rates are still high, highlighting the necessity for continuous research and medical mycology education (Schauwvlieghe, 2020). In doing so, the medical fraternity can prepare to and combat the increasing threat of fungal infections.

Definition and Scope of Medical Mycology

Medical mycology is really all about studying and treating fungal infections that affect human health. As a branch of microbiology, it encompasses the identification, classification, and therapy of fungi that infect man, from superficial cutaneous infections to life-threatening systemic infections. Medical mycology also includes the epidemiology of these fungi, particularly in immunocompromised hosts, such as cancer patients or organ transplant recipients. The recent development of consensus definitions of invasive fungal diseases (IFDs) has played a crucial role in enhancing diagnostic and treatment strategies within the discipline. By standardizing proven, probable, and possible IFDs, such definitions enhance the precision of clinical trials and epidemiologic studies aimed at minimizing morbidity and mortality associated with these infections (Akan et al., 2019). One of the most important features of medical mycology is its interdisciplinary character, incorporating information from multiple disciplines , such as immunology, pharmacology, and public health. The cross-cutting nature enables a complete understanding of the interaction between fungal pathogens and the human host, where it commonly results in serious health complications. For example, the incidence of invasive fungal infections (IFIs) is not equally distributed globally; geographic and socioeconomic conditions play a major role in the incidence and handling of the diseases. The Netherlands and India, for example, demonstrate different backgrounds and policies regarding IFI management and uncover the necessity for customized strategies to achieve success in these different environments. Identification of unusual challenges and strategies in different healthcare systems is the foundation for proper planning of antifungal policies and awareness of fungal infections as a whole (Denning et al., 2025). Moreover, innovation of new antifungal drugs and diagnostic instruments has broadened the scope of medical mycology and posed new challenges to practicing it. Adaptive strategies are required because fungi keep evolving, with resistance to treatments that are already available. Medical mycology, on its part, must continually adapt and enhance its diagnostic criteria and prevention modalities, especially with the emergence of new fungal pathogens introduced by global change and internationalization. The present thrust of research activity in this field emphasizes the necessity for efficient surveillance and monitoring programs to identify and respond to outbreaks of fungal infections. With coordination among clinicians, scientists, and policymakers, medical mycology can be enhanced, ensuring improved patient outcomes and effective infection control, thus justifying its vital position in modern infectious disease management (Akan et al., 2019; Denning et al., 2025) (Figure 5.1).

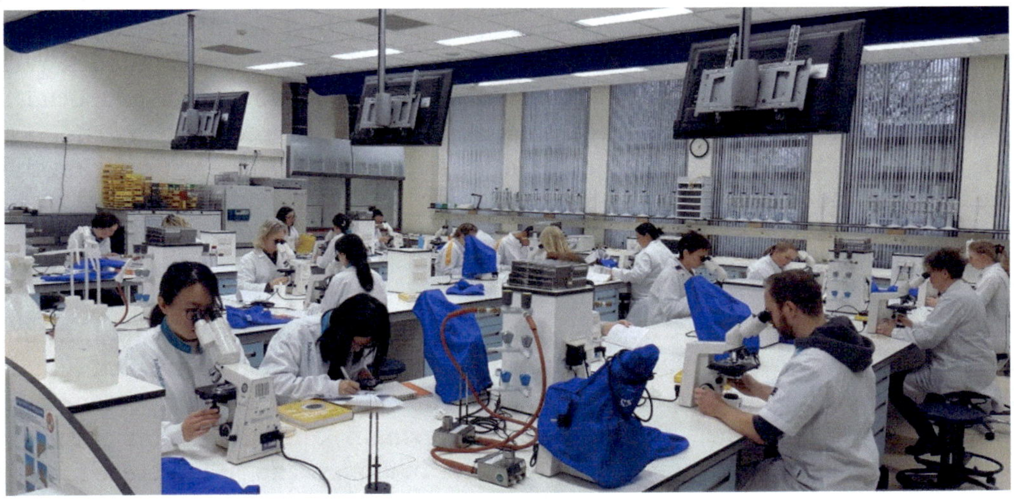

Figure 5.1. Medical mycology laboratory.

Source: https://www.atlasclinicalfungi.org/wp-content/uploads/Course.jpg.

Historical Background and Significance

The historical background to medical mycology is defined by significant events that reflect humanity's growing awareness of fungal pathogens and their impact on health. The realization that fungi are causative agents of disease began early in medicine, where disease and resulting morbidity were routinely attributed to miasma or the environment. At the close of the 19th century, advances in microbiology permitted the identification of single fungi as etiologic agents of disease in man, e.g., the Aspergillus species, marking the need for rigorous investigation into fungal participation in disease mechanisms. This foundation led to further research in the pathophysiology of mycotic infections, in clinical practice, and, as a consequence, the development of antifungal therapies, the dawn of medical mycology as a distinct field of medical science. Medical mycology has much broader significance than its clinical significance; it contains essential public health and bioethics concerns that have developed in the course of the last century. Since global growth in immunocompromised populations as a result of conditions like HIV/AIDS and more medical interventions, fungal infections have become major public health issues. The relationship between the emergent fungal diseases and ethics is gaining acknowledgment. For instance, as medical mycology has continued to progress, clinicians must consider the ethical limitations of research methodologies and treatment protocols. The call for a greater bioethical awareness among clinicians, as referenced in a study with postgraduate students of medical programs, points towards the integration of knowledge of ethical guidelines into medical programs regarding the progress of biomedical sciences (Bassetti & Bouza, 2017). This transition aligns with the broad discussion surrounding how pharmaceutical practices develop in response to evolving challenges in fungal pathogenicity. In the past decades, the establishment of international standards for the treatment of fungal infections has shed light on the previously significant role of the coordination of international health organizations. Following the Second World War, initiatives by the Food and Agriculture Organization (FAO) and the World Health Organization (WHO) have contributed significantly to the formulation of guidelines related to microbial safety, , such as fungi's role in food production and public health (Borowy et al., 2014). The controversies underlying the development of these standards mirror the need for a concerted and scientifically based approach to fungal pathogens, guiding the design of treatment regimens and prevention strategies across a broad variety of health environments. With ongoing advancement in medical mycology, ongoing interdisciplinary collaboration is crucial to provide for the strongest practices to be developed and implemented in reducing the impact of fungal infections on global health, and the establishment of appreciation for learning from the past that shapes contemporary medical practice.

Overview of Fungal Pathogens

Fungal pathogens are a significant threat to human health, particularly in immunocompromised individuals. Among the various groups of pathogenic fungi are yeasts, molds, and dimorphic fungi with varying mechanisms of pathogenicity and clinical manifestations. Important opportunistic pathogens include Candida species, Cryptococcus neoformans, and Aspergillus species, which are now being encountered with increasingly frequent rates in clinics. The rise in these fungal infections can be attributed to causes , such as increased use of immunosuppressive therapy, increased hospitalization stays, and advancements in medical equipment like catheters and ventilators. This has led to greater awareness regarding the need to create new therapeutic strategies and diagnostic methods to combat these pathogens effectively. It is critical to understand the epidemiology and biology of such fungi to formulate effective treatment regimens and minimize morbidity related to fungal infections. Fungal pathogens show wide diversity, which makes it very challenging to diagnose and treat them, particularly with the rising trend of antifungal resistance. Most fungi can change shape, making their identification more difficult for clinical diagnosis. Traditional approaches are based on culturing such organisms, which may consume a lot of time and slow down treatment. Next-generation sequencing and proteomics provide the field with exciting alternatives to rapid and precise identification of fungal pathogens. These technologies enable the identification of several species at once along with their drug susceptibility patterns and could transform clinical mycology. Even with such developments, moving these procedures from scientific research to clinical practice remains fraught with issues. Therefore, further work must continue to break the barriers that inhibit the general application of these new diagnostic tools (Consortium OPATHY, & Gabaldón, 2019). Recent work has only shown the potential of some fungal species not only as pathogens but also as causative agents for biological control of other fungal pathogens. For instance, Acremonium and Penicillium genera have been found to exhibit antagonistic activity against some pathogenic fungi, showing a dual role in disease and environment relations. It has been demonstrated that some isolates of Acremonium are able to suppress the growth of pathogenic fungi in co-culture, which can potentially result in the creation of biocontrol strategies in pharmacy and agriculture. These findings invite further investigation into the dynamics of fungal interactions and secondary metabolites produced under such interactions. Understanding these dynamics can lead to innovative therapeutics, not only to treat infection but also to combat agricultural attack from pathogenic fungi in the ecosystem (Felitti et al., 2017) (Figure 5.2).

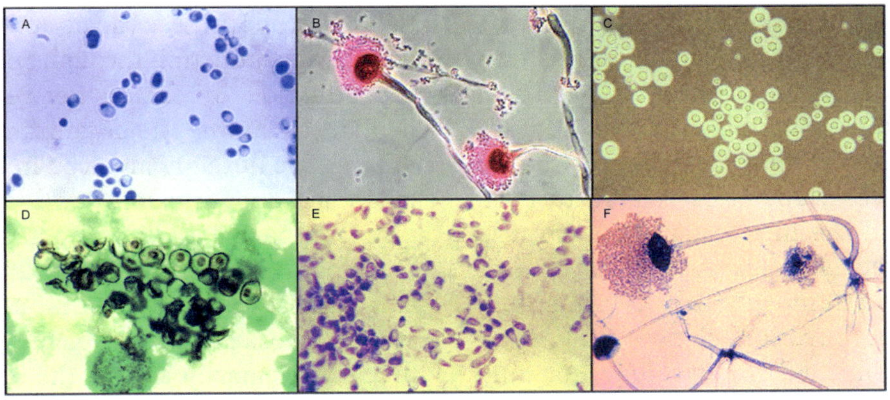

Figure 5.2. Photomicrographs of the most common fungal pathogens causing invasive diseases in humans. A: *Candida albicans* in its yeast phase; B: filamentous conidiophores of *Aspergillus fumigatus*; C: encapsulated yeasts of *Cryptococcus neoformans*; D: *Pneumocystis jirovecii* cysts; E: *Histoplasma capsulatum* in its yeast phase; F: reproductive sporangia of *Rhizopus oryzae*.

Source: https://www.researchgate.net/publication/345768329/figure/fig1/AS:957053673672704@1605190785007/Photomicrographs-of-the-most-common-fungal-pathogens-causing-invasive-diseases-in-humans.png.

5.1. Fungal Biology

Learning Outcome

1. Explain the structure and classification of fungi;
2. Explain the life cycles of pathogenic fungi;
3. Explain fungal growth and reproduction conditions.

Fungal biology is an integral part of medical mycology that tries to understand pathogenic fungi and their implications on human health. One prominent genus that has been in the spotlight is Candida, particularly *Candida auris*. Emerging in the last two decades, this opportunistic pathogen possesses a refined and evolving epidemiology. The ability of the yeast to rapidly develop resistance to multiple antifungal medications is a daunting obstacle to treatment and public health. It has been demonstrated that nearly 400 manuscripts have sought to clarify the various clades of *C. auris*, highlighting its conserved and unique pathogenic characteristics. The interrogation of these adaptive mechanisms is important for the identification of efficacious therapeutic interventions, as resistance patterns continue to evolve. Since *C. auris* and other fungi pose a growing threat to immunocompromised patients, and educational information about their biology is paramount when designing effective interventions and improving outcomes (Brown et al., 2020). The development of opportunistic infections by fungi underscores the imperative for medical mycology breakthroughs in diagnostic tools. Standard methods of fungal pathogen detection are conventional culturing procedures that are not only time-consuming but also risk patient management through delays in reporting. The increasingly diverse group of infectious yeast species poses a serious challenge to antifungal resistance that requires timely and efficient detection methods. New technologies in next-generation sequencing and proteomics have the promise of accelerating diagnostic speed and accuracy. These techniques provide windows for real-time identification of pathogenic fungi and their patterns of resistance, thus optimizing therapeutic strategies. Transfer of this research into practice has to meet several obstacles related to cost, accessibility, and the implementation of these sophisticated technologies in general clinical practice (Consortium OPATHY, & Gabaldón, 2019). The incorporation of new diagnostic techniques within medical mycology not only benefits patient outcomes but also aids the body of knowledge regarding fungal biology. The quick identification of the exact yeast pathogens causing infections by clinicians can then be used to customize antifungal therapy to successfully cover resistance patterns. Not only does this facilitate easier management of patients, but it also helps provide an enhanced understanding of the epidemiology of fungal infections. As our knowledge of fungal biology evolves, an in-depth examination of species-specific traits and mechanisms of resistance will guide future treatments and public health initiatives. Further, an understanding of the evolutionary dynamics of important pathogens like *C. auris* can be used to inform the creation of new therapeutic modalities, confirming the interconnectedness of fungal research and clinical application in the fight against mycological disease (Consortium OPATHY, & Gabaldón, 2019; Brown et al., 2020).

5.1.1. Structure and Classification of Fungi

The structure of fungi is very diverse, ranging from the unicellular yeasts to the multicellular complex organisms , such as mushrooms. At the cellular level, fungi are characterized by having cell walls that consist of chitin, marking them distinct from plants with cellulose walls. Fungal cells are usually made up of hyphae, which are filamentous and can develop into long, chain-like aggregates known as mycelium. This mycelial network is very important in nutrient uptake and interaction with the environment. Furthermore, fungi reproduce in a variety of ways, , such as asexual reproduction through spores and sexual reproduction by fusion between specialized hyphal structures. The organizational intricacies of fungi are not only involved in their ecological roles as decomposers and symbionts but also emphasize their importance in medical mycology, where pathogenic fungi morphology can affect identification and treatment strategies. Classification of fungi is a complex process, primarily due to the vast diversity of the kingdom as well as ongoing advances in genetic research. Historically, fungi were bound by morphology and reproductive structures, and hence the main divisions are Ascomycota and Basidiomycota. Due to recent advances in molecular techniques, most significantly DNA sequencing, it has been established that the majority of species bounded on morphology possess greater genetic diversity than was previously realized. This has thus resulted in the formulation of robust phylogenetic groupings among the fungal species. According to current research, the internal transcribed spacer of the nuclear ribosomal cistron region is of major importance for accurate species identification. Application of these molecular techniques ensures that fungal classification follows classical taxonomic systems, but, at the same time, takes into account genetic diversity as well, having an effect on our understanding regarding pathogenic fungi and their implications in human health (Schoch et al., 2014). Further, tools like MycoBank have an important role to play in the present trend towards unifying fungal nomenclature and taxonomy. By providing a comprehensive registration system for fungi, MycoBank is an important coordination hub that links various taxonomic databases. Formal registration of fungal names according to the

International Code of Nomenclature has significantly enhanced the quality and availability of fungal information. Recent additions to MycoBank have included advanced querying capabilities and the ability to record typification events, further automating classification. These developments better integrate DNA sequence information with taxonomic data and assist mycologists in finding fungi that are only known from genetic evidence. However, there are challenges with the precise associations between taxonomic names and DNA data, necessitating a continued advancement in the classification systems of fungi (Amor et al., 2013) (Figure 5.3).

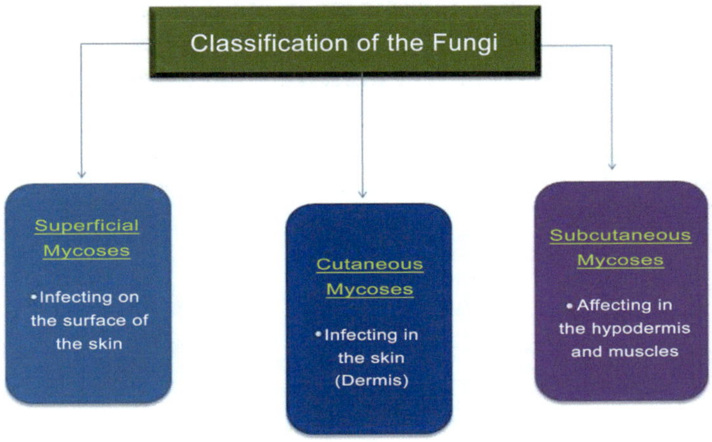

Figure 5.3. Classification of fungi.

Source: https://microbiologynotes.org/wp-content/uploads/2021/09/Classification-of-the-Fungal-Disease-on-the-basis-of-the-infection-site.jpg.

5.1.2. Life Cycles of Pathogenic Fungi

The pathogenic fungi life cycles consist of intricate processes that can play a great role in determining their pathogenicity and adapting capacity. These organisms usually possess two principal mechanisms of reproduction: sexual and asexual reproduction, both with significant ecological and evolutionary roles. Under asexual reproduction, structures , such as conidia or spores are formed and facilitate rapid colonization of new hosts and environments. Sexual reproduction, on the other hand, often entails the formation of specialized structures that allow for the recombination of genes, which can enhance pathogenic traits, e.g., drug resistance and virulence. The ability of fungi to switch between these two modes of reproduction in response to environmental stress underlies their evolutionary success across a variety of ecosystems. This adaptability is particularly evident in opportunistic pathogens capable of sustaining themselves in shifting host conditions, making effective clinical intervention and management of systemic infections difficult. Moreover, environmental stimuli triggering the pathogenic fungi's life cycles are of utmost significance to comprehend their behavior and interaction with hosts. Temperature, humidity, and nutrient levels rank among the significant factors that contribute powerfully to the growth and reproductive strategies of fungi. In particular, temperature fluctuations may trigger the shift from saprophytic forms to pathogenic forms, e.g., in fungi like *Candida* spp. Also, the development of mycelia can be stimulated in some conditions, while sporulation can be induced by stress or lack. The life cycle of fungi can impact their transmission behavior, particularly in how they enter the host, infect, and spread subsequently. The impact of these environmental parameters could vary among different fungal species to indicate the need for specific research in medical mycology to provide effective antifungal intervention. Pathogenic fungi's life cycles are not only critical in understanding their biology but also in designing diagnosis and treatment procedures in medical mycology. Molecular identification techniques have improved the earlier diagnosis of fungal infections, and thus, timely interventions are facilitated. For instance, quality-controlled ITS database production has provided medical practitioners with a reliable tool in species identification, thus making treatment procedures easier. However, since new fungal species are continually being discovered, there is an urgent need to carry out regular research and database analysis. New technology , such as genetic barcoding, boosts our capability for screening and identification of pathogenic fungi in real-time. This integrated approach underscores that a profound understanding of the life cycles of fungi is important in combating the risks associated with fungal infections and indirectly assists in gaining better patient outcomes in medical mycology (Alastruey-Izquierdo et al., 2015; Felitti et al., 2017) (Figure 5.4).

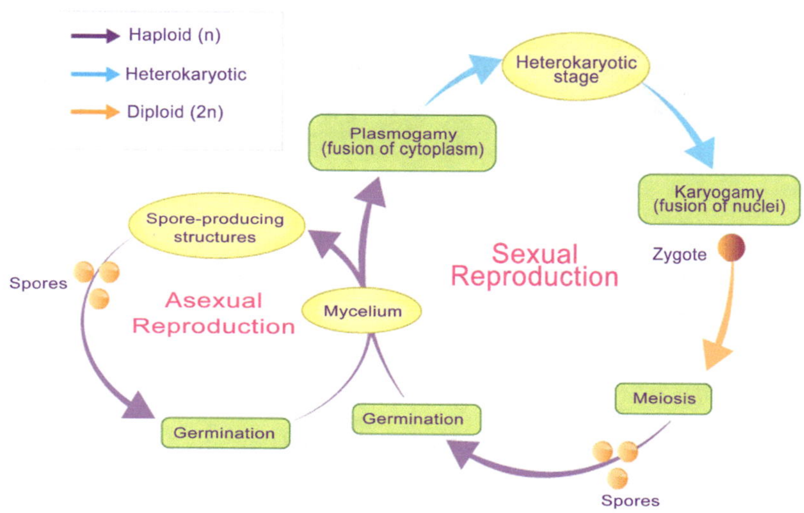

Figure 5.4. Life cycles of fungi.

Source: https://cdn1.byjus.com/wp-content/uploads/2022/08/Life-cycle-of-fungi.png.

5.1.3. Fungal Reproduction and Growth Conditions

The intricate processes of the reproduction of fungi are at the heart of their viability and dispersal, greatly determining their ecological and medical significance. Fungi predominantly reproduce through asexual and sexual reproduction. Asexual reproduction commonly occurs through the production of spores, which can be mass-produced and distributed by abiotic factors , such as wind and water. This kind of adaptability in reproduction enables fungi to spread to new environments efficiently. On the contrary, sexual reproduction forms the combination of compatible mating types, leading to genetic diversification necessary for survival under different conditions. This genetic diversification is also the cause of the development of antifungal resistance, which forms a critical issue in medical mycology (Rajendran et al., 2012). It is critical to be aware of such reproductive processes to develop effective treatments against fungal infections and manage their impact on the environment. The growth conditions that fungi require to live are also diverse and can vary significantly from species to species. Fungi are highly tolerant and will thrive in various environments, like soil, decaying organic matter, or as a parasite on living hosts. The ideal growth conditions typically require accurate temperature regulation, water content, and nutrient availability. Most pathogenic fungi have an affinity for warmer temperatures, usually 20 to 30 degrees Celsius, corresponding to human body temperature, thereby facilitating colonization of the host during infection (Joshaghani et al., 2013). Furthermore, a humid and nutrient-rich environment, e.g., rotting foods, promotes further fungal growth. These are conditions that necessitate controlling humidity and temperature in clinical settings to inhibit fungal growth and prevent opportunistic infections. Fungal biofilms also represent a key feature of fungal growth conditions, especially from a medical standpoint. Fungal biofilms are found as dense aggregates of fungal cells trapped in a self-secreted extracellular matrix, conferring structural stability and built-in resistance to antifungal compounds. One of the interesting facts about such organisms is that many of them tend to develop biofilms on implanted medical devices or tissues, resulting in long-term infections that are difficult to eliminate. The causes for the formation of biofilms are the availability of nutrients, surface characteristics, and microbe interactions that permit the stable coexistence of fungal colonies (Rajendran et al., 2012). Knowledge of the conditions that permit biofilm formation not only helps in preventive procedures but also enables a better understanding of how these hardy structures provide the potential for pathogenicity in immunocompromised hosts (Figure 5.5).

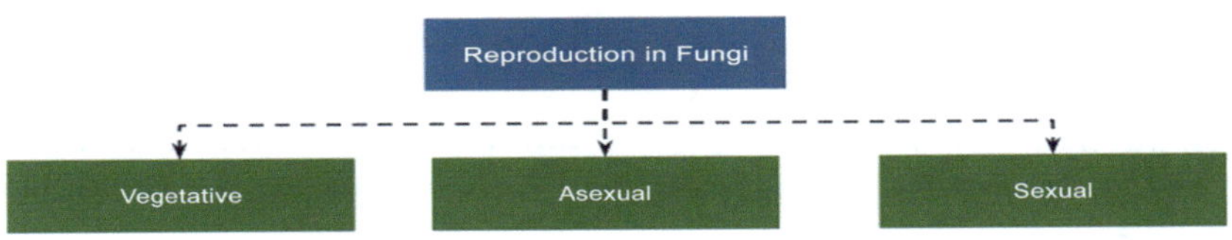

Figure 5.5. Reproduction in fungi.

Source: https://dcx0p3on5z8dw.cloudfront.net/Aakash/s3fs-public/inline-images/image9_23.png?7_d8iE3ytkEY4KJNKfeKSp_Ifqy2wzDJ.

Test Your Knowledge

1. What are the most crucial structural features that differentiate fungi from other microbes?
2. How and on what grounds do fungi become categorized into different groups based on their morphology and mode of reproduction?

5.2. Common Fungal Infections

Learning Outcome

1. Describe superficial mycoses;
2. Define systemic mycoses;
3. Describe opportunistic mycoses.

The landscape of common fungal infections is vast and varied, reflecting the broad spectrum of fungal pathogens. Candidiasis, aspergillosis, and cryptococcosis are among the most prevalent fungal infections and present varying difficulties in diagnosis and treatment. Candidiasis, primarily caused by various species of the genus Candida, is particularly concerning due to its being one of the most common reasons for nosocomial bloodstream infection worldwide. Invasive infections have the potential to result in severe morbidity and increased mortality, particularly in the context of immunocompromised hosts. The challenge lies in the early treatment and detection of such infections, highlighting the requirement for sophisticated diagnostic methods capable of minimizing morbidity associated with such pathogens. Aspergillosis is a very common infection caused primarily by Aspergillus species that are present ubiquitously in the environment. It predominantly affects immunocompromised hosts, , such as those undergoing chemotherapy or organ transplantation. Diagnosis is likely to rely on a blend of clinical presentation, imaging studies, and laboratory findings, with categories of proven, probable, and possible invasive fungal diseases (IFDs) acting as a guideline for the right assessment. The expansion of the probable category highlights the need for clinicians to utilize appropriate use of diagnostic criteria to optimize patient outcomes, given the fact that such infections are more prevalent in high-risk groups (Akan et al., 2019). Host-virulence interactions involving the fungal pathogens and host factors are complex, necessitating an understanding of aspergillosis epidemiology and pathophysiology. Cryptococcosis, often due to Cryptococcus neoformans, is another serious fungal infection of note due to its impact on public health, particularly among immunocompromised patients, e.g., HIV/AIDS patients. The pathogen is primarily acquired by inhalation of spores with the ability to develop life-threatening pneumonia or meningoencephalitis, leading to substantial morbidity and mortality among affected groups. Proactive detection of susceptible patients, along with the early provision of antifungal therapy, like the administration of drugs like fluconazole, is important. However, resistance profiles observed in some cases highlight continued follow-up and research into the causes of resistance (Wissing et al., 2013). Raising further awareness and understanding about these endemic fungal infections through rigorous research can be beneficial in improving prevention, diagnosis, and treatment procedures among medical professionals.

5.2.1. Superficial Mycoses

Superficial mycoses constitute a diverse group of fungal infections affecting the outermost layer of skin, hair, and nails. They result from a variety of fungal causes, with dermatophytes being some of the most frequent culprits. They thrive in warm, humid environments and, therefore, some groups of the population, for example, those with certain outdoor activities or unhygienic practices, become extremely susceptible. The clinical manifestations of superficial mycoses range from mild to severe, such as tinea pedis (athlete's foot) to onychomycosis, which impacts the health of the nails considerably. Discovery of the epidemiology and pathogenesis of superficial mycoses is important in the development of proper prevention and treatment plans (Figure 5.6).

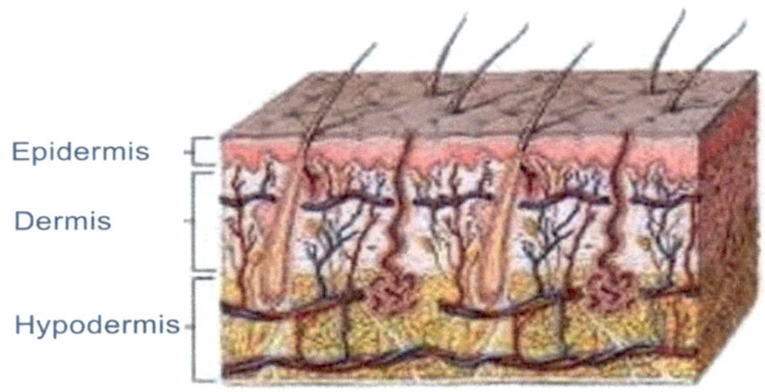

Figure 5.6. Superficial mycoses.

Source: https://cdn.slidesharecdn.com/ss_thumbnails/8-170821060809-thumbnail.jpg?width=640&height=640&fit=bounds.

Research indicates that individuals with poor socio-economic status are most vulnerable to the infection due to lack of access to healthcare facilities, poor hygiene, and more exposure to conditions favorable for the growth of fungi. Notably, a study at the Alupe Outpatient Clinic in Kenya established that superficial mycoses were prevalent among patients of undetermined HIV status, a result that confirms the coincidence between the two infections and immunocompromised conditions (Adungo et al., 2019). The coincidence determines that there should be particular interventions and education with an aim towards raising awareness and screening procedures among high-risk groups. *Scopulariopsis brevicaulis*, although less common, plays a serious part in the mycological scenario of superficial mycoses, particularly of onychomycosis. The organism has been isolated in clinical specimens of keratinized tissue infections in the context of toenail infections (Macura et al., 2015). It can be a minority of cases when contrasted with dermatophytes, but its occurrence confirms the need for accurate mycological analysis in nail infection diagnosis. Complications arising from undiagnosed superficial mycoses can manifest through secondary infections and extreme morbidity, hence necessitating early detection and treatment. Successful management relies on the identification of the causative organism as well as the selection of effective antifungal therapy, which can be tailored according to the inherent fungal species involved (Figure 5.7).

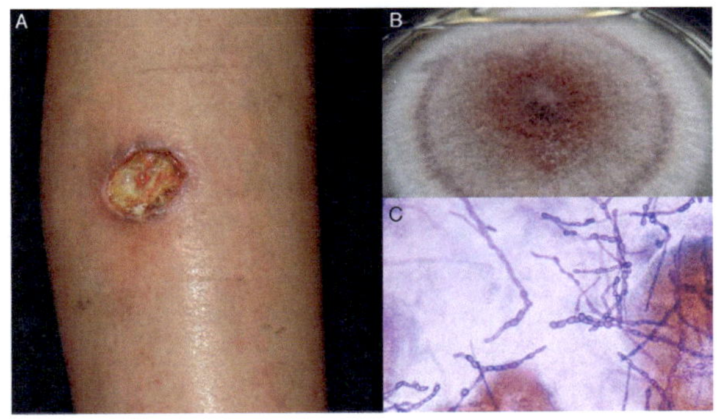

Figure 5.7. Cutaneous involvement in the deep mycoses.

Source: https://static.elsevier.es/multimedia/15782190/0000010700000010/v1_201611260103/S1578219016302402/v1_201611260103/en/main.assets/gr5.jpeg.

5.2.2. Systemic Mycoses

The pathogenesis of systemic mycoses has attracted increasing attention in the field of medical mycology due to the rising incidence of invasive fungal diseases (IFDs). Identified by their ability to spread through the body, systemic mycoses are capable of infecting more than one organ and system, particularly among immunocompromised individuals. Diabetes, HIV/AIDS, and certain malignancies predispose individuals to these infections and demand a thorough understanding of their pathogenesis and clinical presentation. Early diagnosis criteria have been streamlined and reevaluated to better encompass a larger population of high-risk patients beyond the groups undergoing oncology therapy, thus emphasizing the need for increased awareness on the part of medical professionals in the treatment of systemic mycotic infections (Akan et al., 2019). The need for effective and timely diagnosis cannot be overemphasized, as early intervention bears a significant effect on patient outcomes in this challenging area of infectious disease. Proper antifungal therapy is the main factor in systemic mycoses management, and proper selection is important in reducing morbidity and mortality of such infections as invasive aspergillosis (IA). Even though enhancement in prophylactic antifungal therapy has contributed to a decrease in IA infection cases among very susceptible populations, breakthrough infections are still a challenge to diagnose (Hoenigl & Jenks, 2018). These are due to the low sensitivities of conventional mycological tests, which could complicate making timely diagnoses. Therefore, guidelines now advocate for the use of mold-active agents, , such as voriconazole and isavuconazole, as first-line treatments. The ongoing revision of treatment guidelines attests to the evolving trends in the management of systemic mycoses, where targeted therapy remains essential for maximizing survival in susceptible patients. Lastly, the significance of continuous research and development in systemic mycoses cannot be overstated. As new diagnostic equipment and antifungal agents arrive, the therapeutic landscape of invasive fungal infections becomes more active by the hour. The emerging classifications and diagnostic guidelines issued by international groups reflect this change, allowing more astute clinical decision-making for a greater number of patients, including endemic mycoses (Akan et al., 2019). Further, studies on the alternative treatment options, , such as the use of echinocandins in salvage therapy, prove the need for adaptability in the case of chronic fungal infections , such as chronic pulmonary aspergillosis (CPA) (Hoenigl & Jenks, 2018). As new technologies and evidence-based strategies are revealed, the incorporation of the same will be the pivotal step toward successfully combating the threat posed by systemic mycoses (Figure 5.8).

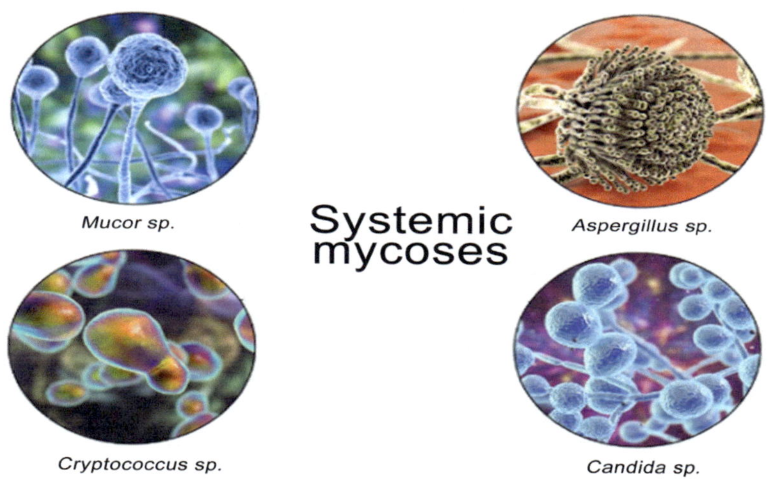

Figure 5.8. Systemic mycoses.

Source: https://microbialnotes.com/wp-content/uploads/2023/03/systemic-mycoses.webp.

5.2.3. Opportunistic Mycoses

Opportunistic mycoses are a significant issue in medical mycology, particularly in immunocompromised individuals, , such as cancer patients receiving treatment, organ transplant recipients, or HIV/AIDS patients. The infections usually take advantage of the weakened immune condition of the host and result in serious or life-threatening illnesses that may not be common in immunocompetent hosts. A broad spectrum of fungi, including Aspergillus, Candida, and Cryptococcus species, may manifest as opportunistic pathogens, underlining host defense-fungus virulence complex interactions. Because of ongoing improvements in medical treatment, improving survival rates for immunocompromised patients, the frequency of opportunistic infections has correspondingly increased in sympathy, making an urgent need to address successful preventive strategies and treatments. Recent studies have come to highlight the development of opportunistic mycoses in non-traditional settings, particularly with the onset of the COVID-19 pandemic. Critically ill patients with COVID-19 have been found to be at risk of invasive pulmonary aspergillosis despite the lack of traditional risk factors. For example, a case report of a patient aged 69 years who acquired this fungal infection two weeks after symptom onset shows how immunosuppression due to severe respiratory disease contributes to worsening fungal invasion (Prattes et al., 2021). This disturbing trend heralds a change in clinical practice and requires increased vigilance among medical care providers to identify and treat opportunistic fungal infections early in susceptible groups during and after pandemics. The historical context of opportunistic mycoses is observed to have been characterized by a dynamic influenced by social and medical advancements over the past two centuries. The evolution of medical treatments and increased reliance on immunosuppressive therapy have inadvertently created pathways for fungal infection to develop, particularly among chemotherapy or organ transplant recipients. Groundbreaking studies have blamed the causation of such diseases as candidiasis and aspergillosis on greater medical progress, i.e., the employment of antibiotics that disrupt normal flora and increase susceptibility to secondary infections (Homei & Worboys, 2020). Further, ecological shifts and demographic change—, such as population migrations and urbanization, have boosted the possibility of exposure to endemic fungi. This multifaceted interaction of factors needs an integrated approach to fight opportunistic mycoses by public health policy, enhanced diagnostic methods, and specific treatments that target both the fungal pathogens as well as host susceptibility in infected individuals (Figure 5.9).

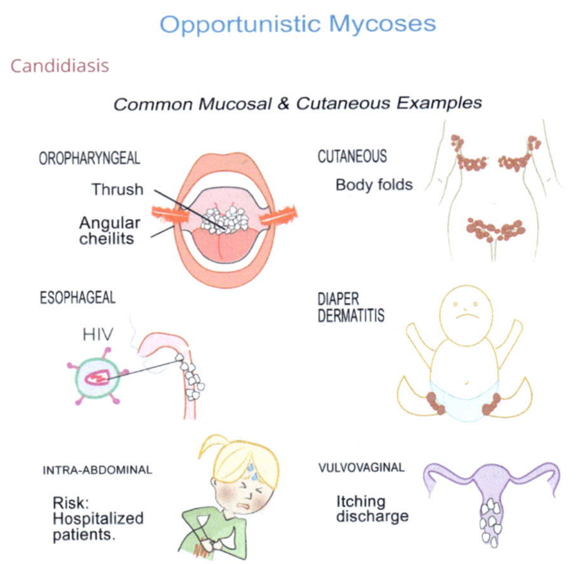

Figure 5.9. Opportunistic mycoses.

Source: https://d1j63owfs0b5j3.cloudfront.net/term/images/opportunistic-mycoses-candidiasis-yeast-infection-thrush-6326.png.

Test Your Knowledge

1. What are the key characteristics and examples of superficial mycoses?
2. How do systemic mycoses contrast with superficial fungal infections in terms of pathology and severity?

5.3. Diagnosis of Fungal Infections

Learning Outcome

1. Clinical symptoms in patients with fungal infection can be described;
2. New laboratory techniques for the correct identification of fungal pathogens can be explained;
3. The application of imaging in diagnosis can be described.

Correct diagnosis of fungal infections is a critical component of medical mycology, which has a significant impact on the treatment and survival rate in patients. Traditional diagnostic tests , such as culture techniques, have been a cornerstone for the identification of fungal pathogens for decades. However, these methods are cumbersome and not always capable of detecting rarer species of fungi. Newer advances in molecular diagnostics, including polymerase chain reaction (PCR) and next-generation sequencing, have facilitated the identification of fungi at a quick pace, allowing prompt intervention. Moreover, the prevalence of rarer molds like those of the *Fusarium* genus emphasizes the demand for enhanced diagnostic capability. Global collaboration has yielded guidelines to enhance diagnostic approaches, thereby seeking to address the challenge posed by such unusual but more familiar pathogens, as evidenced by efforts developed through the Global guideline for the diagnosis and management of rare mold infections (Hoenigl et al., 2021). In addition to traditional methods, serologic tests and imaging modalities have emerged as essential adjuncts to the diagnosis and evaluation of fungal infections. Serological tests that detect the levels of certain antibodies or antigens provide rapid insight into the reality of certain fungal infections, complementing the other diagnostic tools. Computed tomography (CT) and magnetic resonance imaging (MRI) are imaging technologies of further help in visualizing fungal lesions in infected tissues, providing clinicians with a sense of infection extent and severity. A significant area of concern is the increasing prevalence of invasive pulmonary aspergillosis (IPA) among critically ill patients, especially in the setting of COVID-19. Descriptions show that even patients without conventional risk factors may develop IPA, which calls for caution and an extended diagnostic workup in such high-risk groups (Prattes et al., 2021). This evolving scenario of diagnostic techniques is a reflection of the progression of fungal infections and the demands for ongoing research and adaptation. The nexus between diagnosis techniques and clinical results remains at the forefront in the realm of medical mycology. With fungal infections now being perceived as potential killers of immunocompromised patients, the demand for swift and accurate diagnosis grows stronger. New guidelines aim to encompass the concerns presented by rare molds in solving the prevalence of high levels of antifungal resistance increasingly reported in conjunction with these microorganisms. Through the incorporation of information from global specialists in the field, these guidelines aim to harmonize diagnostic and therapeutic methods worldwide, thus improving patient care. Prevalence and incidence of less common fungal infections will necessitate tailored interventions considering geographic variability in prevalence and local healthcare resources. In this regard, a sense of open collaborative culture among healthcare professionals is crucial to augment the quality of care and to ensure timely and suitable care for patients meeting their demands (Hoenigl et al., 2021).

5.3.1. Clinical Symptoms and Patient History

The clinical presentation is that of patients with fungal infections normally presenting in a broad range of presentation and therefore making diagnosis and management complicated. Presentations can be cough, fever, and skin lesions that can easily be mistaken for other conditions, thereby concealing the real mycological cause. For example, studies delineated the case of a 69-year-old patient who contracted invasive pulmonary aspergillosis (IPA) despite having no traditional risk factors, suggesting that even those without established immunocompromising disease can be at risk for potentially life-threatening fungal infections. This illustrates the point of the importance of careful clinical observation and history-taking, as atypical presentations will often lead to delays in proper management and poor patient outcomes, particularly in critically unwell groups like COVID-19 patients, in whom secondary fungal infection poses a concerning risk (Prattes et al., 2021). The patient's history also plays an equally important role in identifying the risk factors for fungal infections. Compilation of large histories allows clinicians to identify predispositions for specific mycoses effectively. For instance, a well-designed case-control study confirmed that foot dermatomycosis is closely linked with the development of acute bacterial cellulitis, and it provided a perspective into how the nature of fungal infection can predispose people to further complications (Sigurgeirsson et al., 2004). These associations demonstrate the importance of incorporating a thorough dermatological assessment in patient evaluations, particularly in those reporting recurring cellulitis. Through a review of the patient's history, including previous skin infections, chronic diseases, and even family histories of fungal infections, health care providers can better plan prevention and management techniques, ultimately leading to improved patient outcomes. Also, clinical sign patient history interaction is implicated in the identification of potential co-morbidities that will enhance the severity of fungal infections. For example, systemic diseases , such as diabetes or chronic pulmonary disease can be fundamental in dictating the progression of mycoses. Altered immunologic responses and excellent habitats for infection and colonization by fungi can ensue from these fundamental health issues. Hence, there is a need to value the complexity of each patient's medical history, including environmental and lifestyle exposures, that may guide a clinician's understanding of a patient's vulnerability to fungal infection. Thorough evaluation maximizes diagnostic precision in turn, enhancing appropriate treatment interventions and reducing medical mycology incidence burden among diverse populations of patients (Figure 5.10).

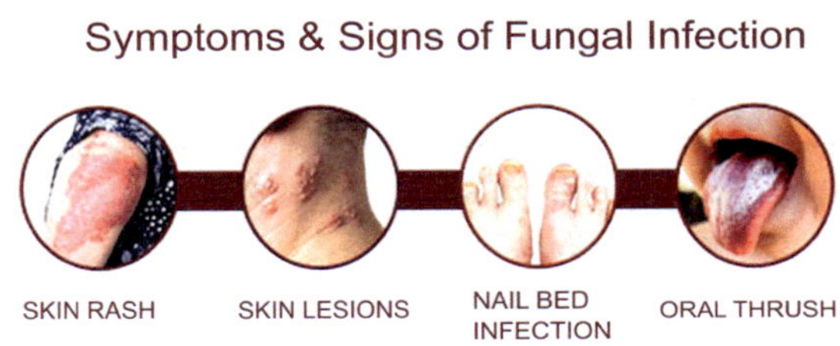

Figure 5.10. Symptoms and signs of fungal infection.

Source: https://images.medindia.net/patientinfo/450_237/symptoms-and-signs-of-fungal-infection.jpg.

5.3.2. Laboratory Techniques for Identification

Medical mycology relies to a large degree on novel laboratory techniques for accurate identification of fungal pathogens. Routine methods, such as the growth of microorganisms on differential media, have been the basis for the detection of mycotic infections but require lengthy incubation times and lack effectiveness against all fungal organisms. As such, molecular techniques have become essential tools of clinical mycology, particularly methods like the polymerase chain reaction (PCR). PCR facilitates rapid amplification and measurement of fungal DNA, hence making diagnosis quicker and more effective. For instance, in one study, endoscopically guided brush sampling of the middle meatus was done and fungal-specific quantitative PCR (QPCR) used to identify various species of fungi with a 45.9% rate of recovery from patients and control subjects with sinus disease, showing the applicability of the techniques in a clinical setting (Goldberg et al., 2006). In addition to PCR techniques, detection of fungi in the laboratory has also been upgraded with the use of imaging techniques and immunological tests. Imaging techniques, , such as computed tomography (CT) and magnetic resonance imaging (MRI), allow for visualization of the extent of the size of fungal infections within the body, thereby aiding in better clinical management. Complementing these imaging techniques are immunological tests, , such as enzyme-linked immunosorbent assays (ELISA). These tests detect specific fungal antigens or antibodies in patient specimens, providing rapid and specific confirmation of the presence of a fungal infection. Evolution of such laboratory tests has enabled clinicians to treat invasive fungal infection with increased specificity, leading to improved outcomes in patients. These advances are essential because invasive fungal disease is associated with high morbidity and mortality, particularly in high-risk groups (Akan et al., 2019). To further enhance the identification of fungi, the addition of next-generation sequencing (NGS) has become more relevant. With NGS technology, there is extensive examination of the fungal microbiome, allowing not only pathogenic but also non-pathogenic species of fungi within the clinical samples to be identified. Such knowledge is of greater significance for polymicrobial infection cases or immunocompromised patients. Also, the uniformity of laboratory techniques and definitions for the identification of invasive fungal infections has been emphasized by research organizations, which ensures consistency in clinical trials and in diagnostic assessment. With medical mycology moving forward, application of these advanced laboratory techniques will be critical to improve diagnostic accuracy and maximize therapeutic strategies for fungal infections (Akan et al., 2019).

5.3.3. Role of Imaging in Diagnosis

In clinical mycology, imaging plays a pivotal role in the diagnosis and management of invasive fungal infections (IFDs). Imaging techniques , such as computed tomography (CT) and magnetic resonance imaging (MRI) are essential to proving the dissemination of the fungal infection, particularly in organs , such as the lungs, brain, and sinuses. With such imaging modalities, clinicians can identify characteristic patterns associated with specific fungi, thus guiding appropriate treatment modalities. Distinguishing features of imaging, , such as ground-glass opacities or nodular consolidations, can unveil severe fungal infections like invasive aspergillosis, which warrants prompt intervention. As imaging technology continues to improve, it is easier to detect and monitor fungal infections, a control necessary for managing patient outcomes in high-risk populations, , such as those with compromised immune systems or underlying health conditions. The evolving IFD definitions, as highlighted by new guidelines, reinforce the relevance of integrating imaging into practice. According to recent consensus definitions by the Infectious Diseases Group of the European Organization for Research and Treatment of Cancer and the Mycoses Study Group, IFD classification has evolved to cover a broader spectrum of patients. This revision is intended to capture the awareness that optimized imaging can augment diagnosis, especially in patients who lack conventional risk factors for invasive fungal disease. Of note is the broadened definition of probable invasive fungal disease, which places greater emphasis upon imaging results combined with microbiological findings. This evolution in classification demonstrates the important role of imaging diagnostics in propagating the differentiated treatment of IFDs and encourages clinicians to employ these modalities for diagnosis and management. In addition, recent clinical series highlight imaging's key role in the diagnosis of atypical presentations of fungal infections in special patient populations, such as patients with COVID-19 infections. For example, a case report showed that a 69-year-old patient developed invasive pulmonary aspergillosis (IPA) two weeks following the presentation of COVID-19 symptoms, even though he did not have conventional risk factors for developing such fungal infections. Imaging findings were key to determining the development of IPA in this critically ill patient, highlighting the importance of increased awareness among practitioners. As challenges increase in differentiating viral from fungal etiology in the context of new emerging infectious diseases, the role of imaging in IFD diagnosis becomes increasingly relevant. This brings into focus the importance of continued innovation within imaging techniques in addition to clinical proficiency to diagnose and manage challenging cases of medical mycology effectively (Figure 5.11).

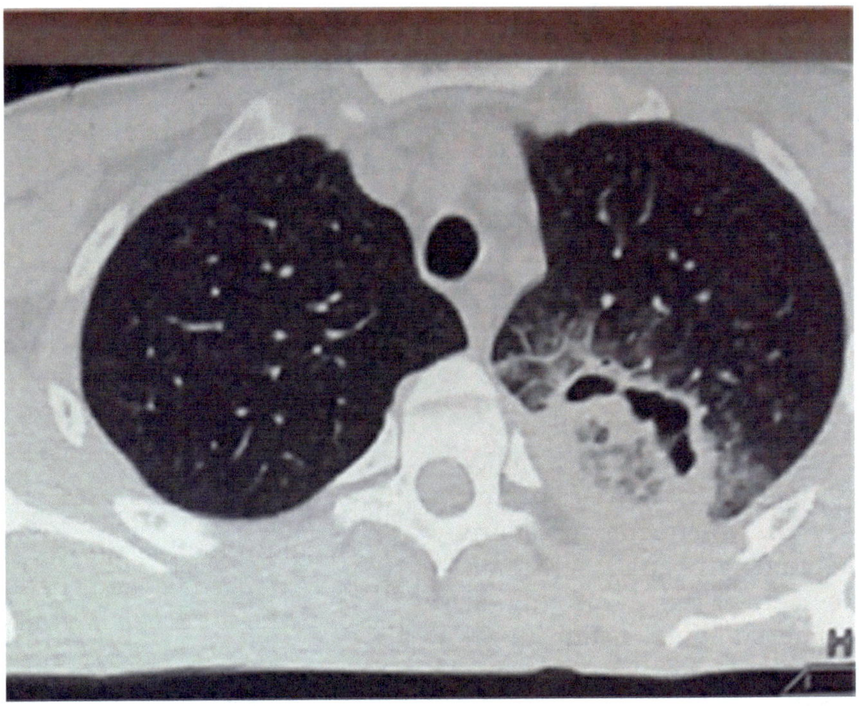

Figure 5.11. CT-scan of the chest in a patient with mucormycosis. Lung lesions with destruction. This Figure is reproduced in color in the online version of Medical Mycology.

Source: https://www.researchgate.net/publication/332121225/figure/fig1/AS:755111252983810@1557043960782/CT-scan-of-the-chest-in-patient-with-mucormycosis-Lung-lesions-with-destruction-This.jpg.

Test Your Knowledge

1. How can clinical signs and patient history guide initial suspicion of a fungal infection?
2. What are the most commonly used laboratory techniques for the detection of fungal pathogens and how are they different?

5.4. Treatment Options

Learning Outcome

1. Discuss antifungal drugs;
2. Elucidate the emergence of resistance to antifungal drugs;
3. Highlight alternative treatments and new therapy.

Treatment of fungal infections has evolved much in medical mycology, keeping pace with the diversity of various pathogens. Antifungals are the drug of choice, and such a class as azoles, echinocandins, and polyenes is optimally used. Azoles, , such as fluconazole and voriconazole, work by interfering with the formation of the fungal cell membrane, and this works in the treatment of a spectrum of fungi. Echinocandins, such as caspofungin, disrupt glucan formation in the fungal wall, thereby having particular effectiveness against Candida spp. The agents are often chosen according to the offending fungal species identified and their susceptibility patterns, highlighting the requirement for accurate diagnosis. The treatment procedure is intricate and challenging and relies on clinical expertise, knowledge of fungal biology, and an understanding of antifungal drug pharmacokinetics. The newly identified and rare fungal pathogens are increasingly being recognized to contribute significantly to morbidity and mortality, and tailor-made treatment approaches must be devised for them. The emergence of diseases caused by pathogens , such as *Fusarium*, *Lomentospora*, and *Scedosporium* species requires global management plans. These rare molds are known to have intrinsic resistance against commonly used antifungal agents, thereby complicating the management of the infections. In a way to combat this hindrance, the collaborative effort of international societies has culminated in the establishment of guidelines to improve diagnostic and management plans. As noted in recent literature, the Global guideline for diagnosis and treatment of rare mold infections provides clinicians with evidence-based recommendations to further enhance patient care of such infections (Hoenigl et al., 2021). Having additional therapeutic agents beyond the traditional therapies is a landmark step in the battle against such devious pathogens. In addition to drug therapy, adjunctive therapies form a critical part of the management of fungal infections. In severe cases, surgery must be undertaken to resect infected tissue to maximize clinical outcome. The pairing of antifungal therapy with supportive care, , such as resolution of immunosuppressive disease or optimization of patient nutrition, continues to maximize prospects for recovery. With every new antifungal drug that hits the market, either with an expanded range of activity or a novel mechanism of action, clinicians can modify treatment regimens on the fly. With the amount of antifungal research going on, the last word is really about being in favor of personalized medicine because its purpose is to deliver the best treatments to patients. Synergistic contributions and advances in medical mycology continually redefine the therapeutic horizon, strongly impacting the survival and quality of life of patients (Broenen et al., 2014).

5.4.1. Antifungal Medications

Fungal infections are managed to a large extent by antifungal agents, which are divided into several groups based on their mechanism of action, antimicrobial activity spectrum, and chemical nature. These comprise polyenes, azoles, allylamines, and echinocandins, each prescribed for specific therapeutic purposes. Polyenes, , such as amphotericin B, disrupt the fungal cell membrane by binding to ergosterol, leading to leakage and cell death. Azoles, however, inhibit the biosynthesis of ergosterol, a critical part of fungal membrane integrity, thereby being the most widely used antifungal drugs. The selection of the appropriate antifungal drug is significantly impacted by various factors, including the etiological fungal infection, patients' immune status, and drug-related adverse effects, proposing the use of individualized treatment strategies in medical mycology. Individualized treatment strategies are also required because of the complexity of the fungal infections, necessitating continuous evaluation of the safety and effectiveness of antifungal medications. One pressing issue is the growing rate of drug resistance among fungal pathogens, particularly Candida species. New resistance complicates treatment regimens, especially in immunocompromised patients, leading to poorer clinical outcomes. To find ways to overcome such issues, researchers are exploring novel antifungal drugs and other therapeutic alternatives to counteract resistance mechanisms. The new advances in molecular diagnostics also play a significant role in early diagnosis of fungal pathogens, with the prospect of more targeted treatment strategies. Integration of molecular methods with traditional culture techniques is a landmark development in the treatment of fungal infections, reflecting the interactive process between antifungal drug development and medical mycology. The effectiveness of the treatment with antifungal drugs is also influenced by the pharmacokinetic properties of the medications, their absorption, distribution, metabolic handling, and excretion in the organism. Oral formulations may be the treatment of choice for less serious infections in outpatient departments, while intravenous administration should be the first choice for more severe diseases needing hospital treatment. Furthermore, understanding the pharmacodynamics of antifungals can assist practitioners in maximizing dosage regimens for optimal therapeutic benefits and low toxicity. Such a recent study on the treatment of onychomycosis among elderly patients found alternative topical treatments like Mentholatum to be noteworthy, given the cost and health concerns of systemic antifungal therapy (Cappleman, 2003). Also, the need for ongoing surveillance of antifungal resistance is critical, particularly in Candida species, which continue to present diagnostic and therapeutic challenges in clinical practice (Al-Laaeiby et al., 2019). Hence, an evident understanding of antifungal drugs is crucial to address the developing scenario of fungal infections in medical mycology (Figure 5.12).

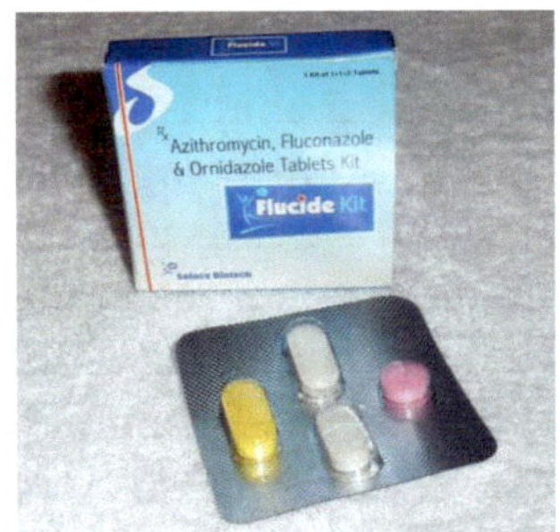

Figure 5.12. Antifungal medicine.

Source: https://img1.exportersindia.com/product_images/bc-full/dir_125/3737171/antifungal-medicine-2045195.jpg.

5.4.2. Resistance to Antifungal Agents

Development of drug resistance is one of the most severe issues confronting medical mycology and, consequently, impacts patient outcomes and the success of therapy. The opportunistic pathogen *Candida auris* serves best to perpetuate the growing issue as it possesses a remarkable potential for resistance to not only azoles, polyenes, and echinocandins but also to several classes of antifungal drugs in general. Uncovering mechanisms of resistance in *C. auris* is of critical concern to clinicians and scientists alike, considering how this drug-resistant yeast has rapidly disseminated across numerous health care institutions all over the world. With its clinical relevance, current studies have emphasized the need to identify the genetic and phenotypic mechanisms of resistance, and the role of environmental factors possibly facilitating the survival and adaptation of the yeasts to antifungal stresses (Kean et al., 2019). Biofilm formation is one of the important mechanisms of resistance that has been exhibited by most fungal species, particularly in the instance of chronic infections. Fungal biofilms form a complex environment that enhances the pathogen's resistance towards antifungal treatments. Particularly, Candida albicans is a model for resistance involving biofilm, and its processes of action involve the synthesis of an extracellular matrix (ECM) and increased efflux pump expression and the foundation of its survival. The ECM provides a protective layer, while efflux pumps actively transport antifungal compounds out of the cell, minimizing their drug effect. Moreover, the biofilm process of persisters also causes treatment failure because such persister cells become drug-resistant, typically leading to relapse or reinfection after treatment (Rajendran et al., 2012). In order to fight the issue of resistance to antifungals, it is not only important to adopt a multi-faceted approach but also to incorporate more effective diagnostic techniques, more therapy options, and strict infection control. With ongoing research, more and more efforts are being placed on developing new antifungal agents that have the capability to circumvent developed resistance mechanisms. Examination of combination therapy and the potential for adjunctive treatment further shows the resilience of medical mycology in overcoming the resistance problems. Training and awareness among the healthcare workforce about the risk of antifungal resistance are also crucial in ensuring successful treatment algorithms. Developing a complete understanding of resistance mechanisms, , such as those that have been described by *C. auris* and biofilm-forming fungi, will ultimately be essential to mitigating the emerging problem of antifungal drug resistance in the clinical environment (Rajendran et al., 2012; Kean et al., 2019) (Figure 5.13).

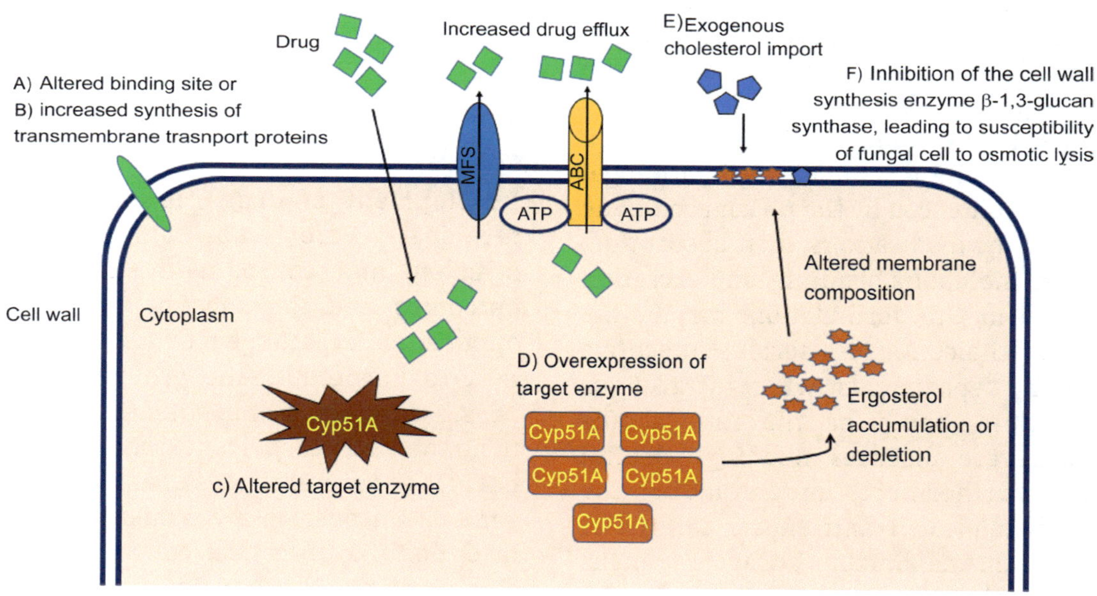

Figure 5.13. Graphical representation at the cellular level of the principal mechanisms of antifungal drug resistance relevant in the clinical practice.

Source: https://www.mdpi.com/biomedicines/biomedicines-11-01063/article_deploy/html/images/biomedicines-11-01063-g001.png.

5.4.3. Alternative Therapies and Emerging Treatments

The quest for new therapies and treatments is indispensable in dealing with the growing threats of drug-resistant fungal infections in medical mycology. Traditional antifungal monotherapies are ineffective against most filamentous fungi , such as Aspergillus fumigatus and various resistant strains, and this leads to high mortality rates (Vicente et al., 2016). As these infections continue to evolve and become resistant, synergistic antifungal combinations must be pursued as a possible solution. It has been observed through studies that effective combinations, , such as posaconazole combined with amphotericin B or anidulafungin, could potentially be more effective in treating refractory cases of aspergillosis than existing one-drug regimens. This investment in new therapeutic approaches not only holds out the potential for enhanced cure rates but also underscores the necessity of innovation in antifungal intervention as a metric of adaptation to increasingly resistant fungal pathogens. At the same time, advances in medical technology are paving the way for new diagnostic interventions and treatment options, further advancing outcomes in fungal infection in the patient. High-throughput screening and clinical big data analysis have emerged as powerful tools in the discovery of new pathogen profiles and potential targets for therapy (Jaiswal et al., 2023). Such techniques facilitate an improved comprehension of interactions between environmental drivers, fungal diversity, and host susceptibility, all necessary for personalizing interventions. For instance, the integration of molecular diagnostics, , such as Next Generation Sequencing and biosensor technology, enables quick and precise identification of fungal pathogens, thus accelerating effective therapy. Through integration into practice of advances in technology, medical providers can better navigate the complexities of fungal infections, ultimately reducing morbidity and mortality due to these diseases. Apart from this, alternative therapy, including herbal therapy and immunomodulatory drugs, is another new and exciting field of research for the management of fungal infections. Natural products with antifungal properties hold promise as adjuvants to conventional treatment protocols, particularly where antifungal resistance poses a significant clinical challenge. Further, therapeutic strategies to induce the host's response against fungal pathogens could prove beneficial, particularly in immunocompromised individuals (Jaiswal et al., 2023). With research continuing to unravel the complexities of the host-fungal interaction, the incorporation of these new therapies into patient treatment is set to provide enhanced management of fungal infection. These interdisciplinary approaches, in addition to augmenting the therapeutic arsenal available to the prescriber, will also drive responsible prescribing as antifungal resistance becomes an increasing problem.

Test Your Knowledge

1. What are the main categories of antifungal medications, and how do they function on fungal cells?
2. How does antifungal resistance arise, and what are the medical implications of resistant fungal infection?

5.5. Epidemiology of Fungal Infections

Learning Outcome

1. Explain about global incidence and prevalence rates of fungal infections;
2. Identify risk factors for infection in medical mycology;
3. Explain the impact of climate change on fungal diseases.

The epidemiology of fungal infection has also gained significance in the context of medical mycology, as it cause significant morbidity and mortality in patients. Invasive fungal infections (IFIs) target long-term in a surreptitious way, especially in immunocompromised hosts , such as cancer patients and transplant recipients. Recently available research describes at length the complex interaction between exposure, susceptibility, and baseline health status that produces these infections. Furthermore, antifungal drug resistance develops multiple levels of complexity for treatment and epidemiological assessment. The worldwide fungal disease burden is significant, with some Candida being identified as occurring commonly among nosocomial bloodstream infections. A solid grasp of these epidemiologic patterns is crucial for the establishment of effective prevention and therapeutic strategies in the clinical environment, having considerable influence on patient outcomes and health care resource planning. Surveillance data have shown that there has been a changing scene due to the epidemiology of fungal infections, indicating an imperative need for routine monitoring practice. For instance, Candida infections have also been reported to be prevalent in intensive care units, and patients there also present complicated cases of co-morbidities. The observed levels of resistance, particularly to medications like IV fluconazole, indicate the challenges faced in effective management. Of special significance, it has been seen through study that a large percentage of candida-infected patients carry strains that have demonstrated potential resistance, thereby complicating treatment models and further necessitating innovative therapeutic therapies. This epidemiologic shift calls for enhanced diagnostic guidelines as well as treatment methods, hence remaining in line with clinical study evidence and real-world patient outcomes that should be taken into account by medical practitioners. The revised clinical definitions of IFDs are an evolutionary response to increasing problems in fungal epidemiology. Not only are these changes more encompassing for a wider variety of affected groups, but they refine the classification system for IFDs as well. Proven, probable, and possible infections now encompass broader patient populations beyond those previously recognized to be immunocompromised. This transition is particularly relevant in the context of increased IFD rates among non-traditional patient groups. Given the changing global health landscape, effective epidemiological systems that account for these new categories will be instrumental in facilitating accurate diagnostic protocols, therapeutic initiatives, and eventually improved patient outcomes. Such research strategies will produce cogent information on the epidemiology of fungal infections and help come up with strategic interventions to control the public health implications of these diseases (Wissing et al., 2013; Akan et al., 2019).

5.5.1. Global Prevalence and Incidence Rates

The global picture of medical mycology witnesses a staggering prevalence of fungal infections that critically impact public health. More than 1.5 million deaths annually have been recently estimated to be caused by invasive fungal disease, primarily in immunocompromised hosts, , such as HIV/AIDS patients or those receiving immunosuppressive therapy. The epidemics of these infections are also complemented by the challenge of diagnosis, especially in regions where health infrastructures lack competency in fungal surveillance. With the current higher rates of fungal infections, particularly among non-neutropenic hosts, there is a critical need for better diagnostic agents and treatment modalities that are able to manage these infections and improve patient outcomes.

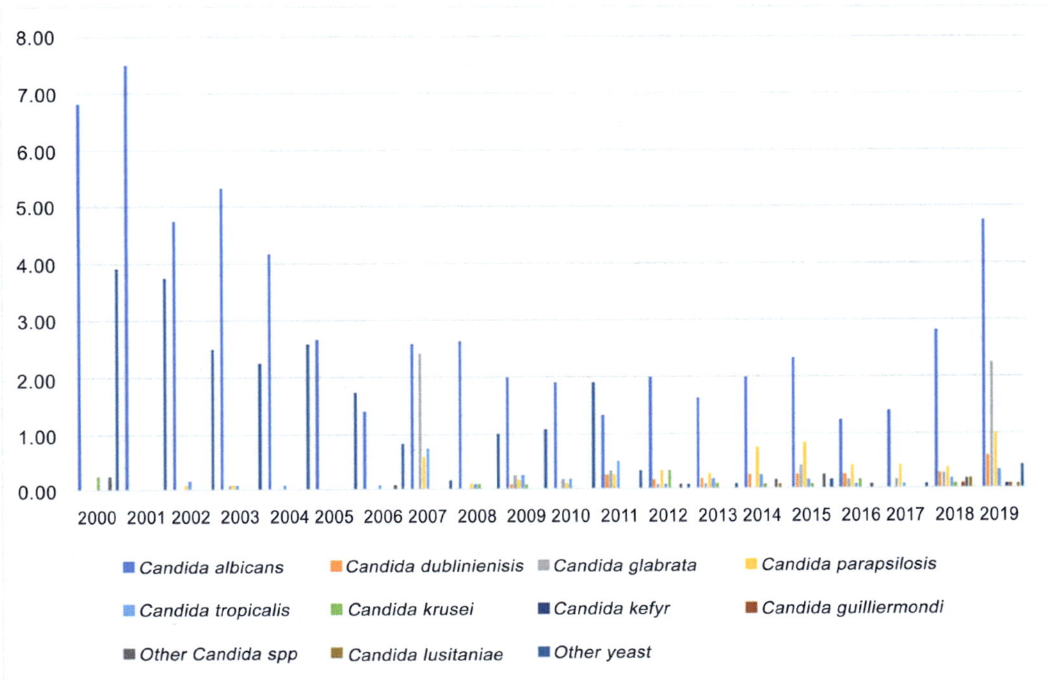

Figure 5.14. The year-wise prevalence of different fungal infections.

Source: https://www.researchgate.net/profile/Saad-Alhumaid/publication/356198074/figure/fig2/AS:1094561325678594@1637975164170/The-year-wise-prevalence-of-different-fungal-infection.jpg.

With the development of more global interdependence and travel, the spread of fungal pathogens across geographical boundaries has become apparent, and therefore, there is a requirement to come up with a concerted effort to tackle this public health challenge. Some fungi, , such as *Aspergillus* spp., are linked with undue morbidity and mortality. In the face of decreased incidence of invasive aspergillosis (IA) in populations at risk due to antifungal prophylaxis, breakthrough disease is still an ongoing characteristic that proves the need for timely and accurate diagnostic methods. Heterogeneous presentations in patient populations render clinical presentation complex and early diagnosis challenging. Current guideline recommendations advise the utilization of targeted systemic antifungal therapy, like voriconazole and isavuconazole, as first-line treatment for IA, an indication of patient-specific therapeutic planning. Moreover, the emergence of antifungal resistance has broken the continuity of current treatment protocols, emphasizing the necessity for healthcare systems across the world to invest in research, surveillance, and education regarding fungal infections (Hoenigl et al., 2018). In South and Central America, the lack of extensive epidemiological data on fungal infections exacerbates the problem. High prevalence rates for fungal diseases have been reported by research, with estimates for Pneumocystis pneumonia (PCP) ranging from 2.1 to 4.7 cases per 1,000 individuals, whereas Histoplasmosis prevalence ranges from 0.91 to 3.8 cases (Chaudhuri et al., 2022). Concerningly, the absence of mandatory reporting as well as national surveillance systems in these regions hinders an understanding of the true burden of fungal infections. The estimates that are provided are considered to be conservative, and the actual incidence is likely considerably higher. Prioritizing the implementation of nationally standardized surveillance strategies is critical in ensuring that these infections can be addressed appropriately and resources allocated to prevention and treatment programs. Closing gaps in surveillance of fungal diseases will not only enhance understanding of their epidemiologic trends but also inform public health policy worldwide (Figure 5.14).

5.5.2. Risk Factors for Infection

A multifaceted analysis of the risk factors for infection is paramount in the field of medical mycology, especially as fungal infections are on the rise in terms of prevalence and scope. A number of factors enhance the vulnerability of humans to fungal infections, including host immune status, the presence of underlying medical conditions, and certain therapeutic maneuvers. Severely ill patients, particularly those with associated comorbidities, such as diabetes mellitus or chronic pulmonary disorders, are at great risk for invasive fungal infections. In addition, with the immunocompromised state, the risk for opportunistic infections, such as invasive pulmonary aspergillosis (IPA) is amplified manifold. A clear example is given by Prattes et al. (2021), which demonstrates that even in otherwise healthy individuals, without standard risk factors , such as diabetes or prolonged antibiotic therapy, IPA can occur subsequent to a COVID-19 infection, indicating the unpredictable character of fungal infections in immunocompromised hosts. Aside from underlying medical diseases, hospitalization is a major risk factor for infection. Hospitals are a reservoir for various fungal pathogens, particularly in intensive care units (ICUs) where patients receive invasive devices and procedures. Evidence has demonstrated Candida spp., for instance, to be a frequent cause of nosocomial bloodstream infections that most often lead to serious complications or an increase in morbidity. Studies cited in Wissing et al. (2013) report ICU patients who received intravenous fluconazole and report dramatic resistance profiles of Candida infections that call for aggressive antifungal stewardship. With approximately 32% of patients revealing potentially fluconazole-resistant isolates, risk factors of hospitalization , such as antimicrobial therapy and repeated exposure to antibiotics, emerge as major concerns to enhance patient management and combat dangers posed by fungal infections. Besides, some medical treatments inadvertently augment the probability of fungal infections. Immunosuppressive therapy, commonly administered in the case of cancer patients receiving chemotherapy or in organ transplant recipients, compromises the body's resistance to opportunistic infections. This predisposition is further enhanced in settings where exposure to fungi is increased, e.g., hospital settings or with climatic/ecological changes that facilitate easy spread of fungi. The interaction between treatment protocols and increasing rates of fungal resistance requires vigilant monitoring and immediate intervention strategies. As argued in both Prattes et al. (2021) and Wissing et al. (2013), the emphasis on serious cases of COVID-19 patients developing infections and the high rate of fluconazole resistance is a red flag. Hence, an integrated effort in their identification and control is imperative to stem the flow and impact of infections in medical mycology.

5.5.3. Impact of Climate Change on Fungal Diseases

The intricate web of interdependence between climate change and the etiology of fungal diseases is a tremendous challenge to public health, particularly in the context of medical mycology. Increased temperatures and humidity fluctuations improve the viability and transmission of pathogenic fungi. For instance, the emergence of *Cryptococcus gattii* in the Pacific Northwest supports this ominous trend, having shifted from predominantly a tropical pathogen to a significant threat in temperate climates due to a change in climatic conditions. Studies show that such a fungus may have been unintentionally introduced by heightened human activity and shifting environmental patterns, thus altering its pathogenic pattern and geographical distribution (Wanke et al., 2018). As climate change continues to alter ecosystems, the range of infectious diseases transmitted by fungi is more than likely going to rise, making existing health systems more difficult to manage and overwhelming medical facilities.

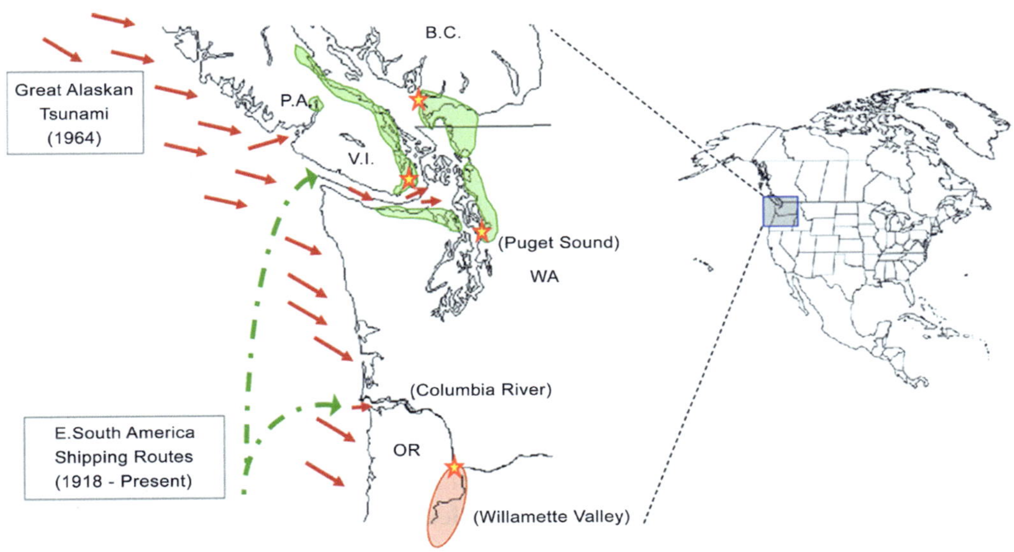

Figure 5.15. Map of the C. gattii Pacific Northwest dispersal hypothesis.

Source: https://www.researchgate.net/publication/336195991/figure/fig1/AS:809264146837505@1569955016734/Map-of-the-C-gattii-Pacific-Northwest-dispersal-hypothesis-Locales-of-VGIIa-endemicity.png.

Fungi thrive in various environmental conditions, and climate change offers the ideal conditions for their growth and dissemination. That fungi rely on some temperatures and humidity levels means that increasing temperatures on the globe can promote the growth of various fungal pathogens. Growth of fungi is boosted by high humidity, creating an ideal environment for diseases , such as blastomycosis and histoplasmosis to form in new regions. Such growth not only risks public health but also exacerbates existing vulnerabilities in immunocompromised individuals. As indicated in the ongoing debate among the experts, the overlap of fungal threats and climate change calls for a priority focus on developing effective mitigation measures, considering the need to undertake collaborative studies on the interaction of environmental conditions and fungal diseases (Berman et al., 2022). The socio-economic implications of climate-induced fungal infection are staggering, but just one of the many compounding factors in an already complex scenario. If fungal pathogens become all the more prevalent due to altered climatic patterns, healthcare systems can be anticipated to face escalating costs of treating such infections. Fungal disease-induced crop loss can become a food security threat in addition to the health risk generated by fungi in human populations. The race to harmonize ecological equilibrium with agricultural production becomes imperative as climate change continues to spur the adaptation and evolution of fungi. Overcoming these intricate problems will require cross-disciplinary skills combining medical mycology, environmental science, and public health programs to formulate and implement comprehensive strategies to guarantee resistance to the changing landscape of fungal infections (Berman et al., 2022) (Figure 5.15).

Test Your Knowledge

1. What are the rates of prevalence and incidence of prominent fungal infections globally, and where are they highest?
2. What are the primary risk factors for raising the risk of susceptibility to fungal infections?
3. How is climate change impacting the geographic spread and occurrence of fungal diseases?

5.6. Prevention and Control Measures

Learning Outcome

1. Understand public health interventions in controlling and reducing the impact of invasive fungal infections.
2. Discuss infection control in a health facility;
3. Describe educational and awareness programs for preventing invasive fungal infections (IFIs).

In medical mycology, effective prevention and control strategies are crucial in preventing the spread of fungal diseases, particularly within healthcare facilities. To combat the emerging threat of multidrug-resistant fungi, stringent infection controls must be applied. The outbreak of *Candida auris*, for example, underlines the need to have robust protocols in hospitals, where the pathogen has shown its capability to spread rapidly in vulnerable patient groups. A few of the main strategies include the early isolation of the infected patient and their contacts, frequent environmental cleaning, and the mandatory utilization of personal protective equipment by healthcare providers. These interventions not only stop outbreaks from spreading but also facilitate the identification of cases, emphasizing the need for early intervention to prevent nosocomial infection by fungal pathogens like *C. auris* (Abdolrasouli et al., 2016). Further strengthening infection control measures also involves ongoing education and surveillance within healthcare facilities. Informing staff on the identification of fungal infections, as well as understanding the value of rapid diagnostic equipment, ensures potential outbreaks can be rapidly contained before they become unmanageable. The application of advanced molecular techniques, , such as genotyping *C. auris*, enables efficient tracing of transmission routes and better insight into the behavior of the pathogens. Widespread screening of patients, particularly high-risk unit patients like intensive care, enhances the detection of asymptomatic carriers. In addition, decontamination interventions using efficient agents , such as chlorine-based cleaners and hydrogen peroxide vapors have been efficient in reducing environmental bioburden considerably, hence lessening infection risk (Wissing et al., 2013). Lastly, the implementation of antifungal stewardship programs within healthcare institutions is a key component of control and prevention measures. These programs are focused on judicious use of antifungal treatments, especially in the context of the high rates of resistance for fungal infections. As an illustration, the findings proving that a large proportion of Candida-infected patients are resistant to first-line treatment, , such as intravenous fluconazole, illustrate the necessity of customized therapeutic approaches. Through the creation of policies encouraging good prescribing practices and repeated susceptibility testing, hospitals will be able to improve the outcome in patients at the same time as minimizing potential increased resistance. Resolution of the problems through education, surveillance, and stewardship will be essential to the successful control of fungal pathogens within the clinical setting and for patient safety in the conduct of medical mycology.

5.6.1. Public Health Strategies

There is a need for good public health practice in the mitigation and management of invasive fungal infections, particularly since the burden of invasive infections is on the rise globally. Such practices entail an all-rounded effort that entails education, awareness, as well as policy mobilization targeting healthcare providers and the public at large. With the dissemination of awareness of invasive fungal diseases (IFDs), public health interventions can provide early diagnosis and best treatment, which are critical for better patient outcomes. By incorporating patient anecdotes, accounts of their passage through IFDs—the nonclinical outcomes of IFD infections , such as psychological distress and cost burden, are better appreciated. In addition, cooperative work between mycology experts and patient advocacy groups is emphasized as a key component of managing IFD strategically, as the success of the pan-fungal disease summit highlights (Castro et al., 2024). In addition to education, effective public health policies are also a key component of effective IFD management. A comparative analysis of antifungal policies in different countries lays bare dramatic gaps in identifying, prioritizing, and managing such infections. For instance, the majority of healthcare systems do not equip their healthcare workers with adequate training in the new diagnostic techniques and treatment regimens for IFDs. This deficiency is also supported by the failure to fully integrate fungal pathogens into all-inclusive antimicrobial resistance policies. These lacunas need to be bridged by widespread national, regional, and local policies centered on IFD management and instilling an antifungal stewardship culture. Not only do these policies increase awareness and education, but also ensure resources are utilized maximally to address the arising threat of invasive fungal infections, as revealed by detailed policy reviews (Denning et al., 2025). Ultimately, integrating patient-centered approaches into public policy will play a critical role in reshaping the face of medical mycology. Those programs that attempt to enhance patient involvement in research and clinical decision-making not only empower patients but also provide valuable insight into the challenges faced in the treatment of invasive fungal disease. With the active participation of caregivers and patients in policy-making for health, healthcare facilities are more capable of addressing the complex needs of IFDs and providing more integrated care. Such a partnership can lead to improved outcomes through tailored care education programs, enhanced peer networks, and targeted research programs. The recognition of patient experiences as pivotal in the development of public health strategies within medical mycology signifies a step towards a more efficient and equitable model of care, ultimately benefiting patients and clinicians alike (Castro et al., 2024) (Figure 5.16).

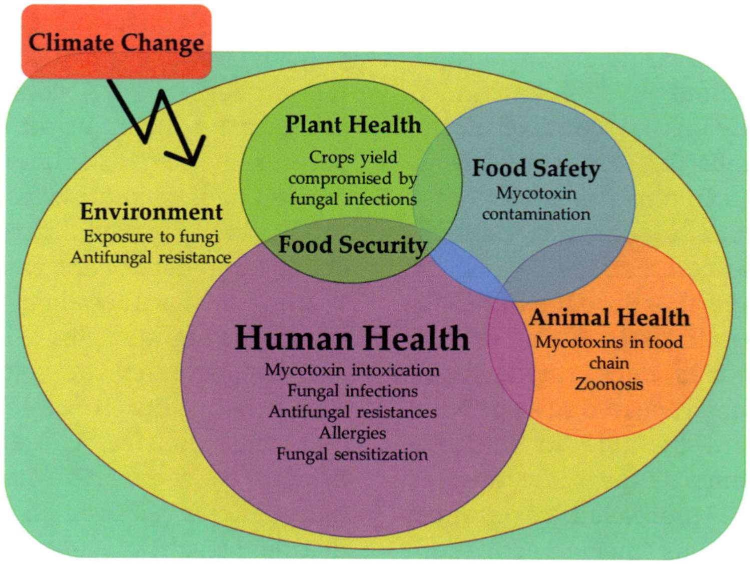

Figure 5.16. Fungal effects and interactions under the "One Health" perspective.

Source: https://www.mdpi.com/encyclopedia/encyclopedia-03-00064/article_deploy/html/images/encyclopedia-03-00064-g002.png.

5.6.2. Infection Control in Healthcare Settings

Infection prevention in a healthcare setting is very important in minimizing risk for fungal pathogens, particularly for multidrug-resistant organisms , such as *Candida auris*. The emergence of this yeast has brought about new challenges and emphasized the need for rigorous infection prevention practices. Procedures , such as extensive screening and isolation of affected patients are fundamental. Maintenance of environmental hygiene through effective cleaning procedures and regular monitoring of high-risk settings, particularly intensive care units, can be pivotal in slowing down the rates of transmission of *C. auris*. Observational studies highlight the importance of adherence to these procedures, with observations that even partial failure of infection control practices will trigger the onset of outbreaks, as evidenced in most health reports (Abdolrasouli et al., 2016). Therefore, it is critical to construct a robust system of infection control to protect vulnerable populations within the hospital setting. In addition to environmental control, compliance among hospital personnel with the use of personal protective equipment (PPE) is also critical in infection combat, specifically fungal infections like *C. auris*. Healthcare workers must be educated on the dangers of this organism and trained in the appropriate use of PPE, for instance, gloves and gowns. This is a critical training due to the reality that *C. auris* may be spread via dirty surfaces and healthcare providers. Infection control recommendations advocate for low-cost yet effective measures, including hand cleaning and skin disinfection by chlorhexidine, which are the first-line of defense against fungal spread (Abdolrasouli et al., 2016). Regular audits and inspections of PPE usage can promote a safety culture, where the health workers are ever vigilant against the nosocomial infection risk, finally resulting in better patient outcomes and reduced healthcare-associated infections. The central theme of infection control illustrates its place in the epidemiology of diseases, especially medical mycology. Outbreak response, especially with *C. auris*, requires a multidisciplinary response that combines epidemiological monitoring, laboratory experience, and timely clinical intervention. The

C. auris's specific genetic clades, through their resistance levels and particular pathobiological features, require ongoing research and surveillance. It is only through collaboration that healthcare facilities can devise the right interventions to contain this powerful threat. Continued education and communication among healthcare professionals, as well as investment in research on infection control practices, will enable institutions to more effectively combat fungal pathogens and ensure the health and safety of patients and healthcare providers.

5.6.3. Education and Awareness Programs

Awareness and education programs are progressively being recognized as being central to combating invasive fungal infections (IFIs) in the field of medical mycology. These programs serve a two-pronged purpose: they increase public awareness and inform medical personnel about rising rates of such infections. Public awareness programs can warn practitioners and patients alike about IFIs' signs, risk factors, and general treatment, which can result in earlier detection and treatment. The pressing need for enhanced education is identified by evidence showing an overall shortage of education and knowledge among healthcare personnel when it comes to IFI management, thereby increasing the burden of such conditions on patients and health systems. Closing these gaps via structured educational programs ensures that patients and healthcare professionals are both better informed and poised to manage more effectively the complex nature of fungal infections (Denning et al., 2025). Further, patient education and advocacy efforts have emerged as key measures in countering the burden of IFD. Fostering an interactive platform where caregivers, patients, and mycology experts converge can yield fruitful debates that unveil the real lives of people with such infections. The MYCology Advocacy, Research, & Education meeting is a case in point in the value of such interaction since it created a forum for different stakeholders to engage, put emphasis on education, and identify critical gaps in IFD knowledge. Members emphasized the nonclinical burdens of such infections, including psychological distress and economic burden, which further emphasizes the need for individualized educational programs that align with both the medical aspects as well as the individual aspects of life with IFD. These inter-professional efforts aim to normalize educational approaches to engage with patients' reality, in favor of improved outcomes in the area of medical mycology (Castro et al., 2024). In ensuring comprehensive education and information campaigns, inter-sectoral coordination of various sectors, the health sector, the research sector, and community activism, is required. Through this coming together of groups, education programs can be developed that are not merely informative but also culturally sensitive and accessible. In this manner, information provided will be relevant to a broad cross-section of people, responding to specific needs and concerns of the communities regarding IFIs. Also, through patient and healthcare provider feedback, the programs can be continuously updated and adapted to reflect the shifting landscape of fungal disease. Lastly, through the incorporation of robust education and awareness programs into the overall paradigm of medical mycology, clinical practices are not only enhanced but better-informed patients are empowered, enhancing their ability to successfully manage their healthcare experiences (Castro et al., 2024; Denning et al., 2025).

Test Your Knowledge

1. What are some effective public health practices to avoid the spread of fungal infections?
2. What role is played by education and awareness campaigns in lowering the rates of fungal infections?

SUMMARY

In outlining the comprehensive contributions of medical mycology, it is necessary to value the critical intersection of fungal biology and human health. Fungal pathophysiology has significant implications not only for the understanding of such illnesses as aspergillosis and candidiasis but for the overall practice of public health. The reported correlation of mycotoxin exposure, especially with staple food, raises food safety issues and its direct role in the occurrence of diseases. For example, high concentration of FB1 in rice and corn from high-risk areas, as evidenced in Golestan province, reflects the potential risk from infested foods. This critical connection indicates the imperative necessity for continued research and monitoring of fungal contaminants in our food supply as a preventive measure against adverse health consequences, including esophageal cancer (Aghasi et al., 2012). The exploration of mycological pathways not only expands the understanding of pathogenic fungi, but also the ecological relevance of these microorganisms is equally relevant. The example of the European Ash tree illustrates how invasive species bring with them fungi that are not known in advance, but will be catastrophic to native ecosystems if not addressed. The sudden and dramatic appearance in Europe of ash dieback caused by the pathogen *Chalara fraxinea* is a reminder of the ever-present nature of the threat posed by fungal disease. With the same processes presumably in action in new ecosystems, ongoing research into the fungi of invasive species is essential. Understanding of the natural and ecological background of fungi can guide conservation and prevention, explaining the symbiotic relationship between mycology and environmental medicine (Chen et al., 2012). Ultimately, the future of clinical mycology is best achieved by an interdisciplinary collaboration that brings researchers, clinicians, and public health workers together. Collaborative efforts must focus on utilizing advances in molecular methods to further define fungi and the role they play in human health. Also, public awareness campaigns can educate communities about food safety and the risks associated with mycotoxins, fostering a proactive stance toward prevention. As our knowledge of fungi expands, so too does our responsibility to address the complex challenges they present. By strengthening our understanding of both the health implications of fungal infection and fungi's ecological roles, we can make significant contributions to public health protection and ecosystem integrity.

Medical mycology has advanced significantly, particularly with increasing awareness that fungal infections are a major risk to human health. Understanding the taxonomy and diversity of fungi is instrumental in combating these pathogens. Advances in molecular techniques, especially DNA sequencing, have brought to prominence the limitations of traditional morphology-based species identification. Research has demonstrated that these techniques often fail to attain the achievement of perfecting fungal diversity, leading to false diagnoses and failure in treatment. As a countermeasure, constructing inclusive databases, which combine DNA sequence data with taxonomic data, has become the key to ensuring accurate recognition of species. These tools enhance our ability to accurately identify fungi, which is critical for proper and timely medical interventions, particularly in immunocompromised patients who are at higher risk of developing fungal infections (Schoch et al., 2014).

Further, the use of high-throughput sequencing technologies transformed our comprehension of fungal ecology and its role in human health. High-throughput studies based on microbiome analysis highlight the complex interaction between fungi and hosts, demonstrating that accurate species identification is essential to determining how these microbes impact health outcomes.

Accumulating molecular data necessitates standardized protocols for maximizing data quality to determine that new sequences are informative and reliable. By curation of reference sequences in public databases , such as the National Center for Biotechnology Information (NCBI), researchers are capable of facilitating effective species identification and contributions towards a growing reservoir of information needed to advance medical mycology (Schoch et al., 2014).

Furthermore, the clinical significance of knowing the diversity of fungi cannot be overestimated. Inaccurate identification of fungal pathogens can have a direct effect on therapeutic choices, with ensuing therapeutic failures or inappropriate use of antifungal medication. The pressure for re-annotation and type specimen sequence validation demonstrates the pressure to enhance our classification systems. Improved data quality in species identification is fundamental to limiting the misdiagnosis-related risks, as highlighted in recent research. Development of rigid protocols and use of strict standards in the practice will not only aid in clinical diagnosis but also aid in ongoing research into the evolving nature of fungal pathogens.

KEY TERMS FROM THIS CHAPTER

- Antifungal therapy
- Aspergillus species
- Chemotherapy
- Chronic pulmonary aspergillosis
- Cryptococcosis
- Echinocandins
- Extracellular matrix
- Fungal biology
- Fungal infections
- Immunocompetent hosts
- Aspergillus fumigatus
- Candidiasis
- Chlorine-based cleaners
- Comorbidities
- Diagnostic capability
- Environmental medicine
- Foot dermatomycosis
- Fungal epidemiolog
- Genetic diversification
- Immunosuppressive therapy

CRITICAL THINKING QUESTIONS

1. **Which of the following is a defining feature of fungal cell walls that differentiates them from bacterial cell walls?**
   a. Peptidoglycan
   b. Chitin
   c.
   d. Mycolic acid
2. **Which fungal organism is most frequently implicated in oral thrush in immunocompromised hosts?**
   a. *Cryptococcus neoformans*
   b. *Histoplasma capsulatum*
   c. *Candida albicans*
   d. *Aspergillus fumigatus*
3. **Which antifungal agent targets ergosterol and forms pores in the cell membrane of fungi?**
   a. Fluconazole
   b. Amphotericin B
   c. Terbinafine
   d. Caspofungin
4. **In which of the following groups are invasive fungal infections most typically seen?**
   a. Healthy children
   b. Diabetic elderly
   c. Immunocompromised (e.g., transplant recipients)
   d. Patients with viral upper respiratory tract infections
5. **What is the mechanism of action of Amphotericin B?**
   a. Inhibits DNA synthesis
   b. Inhibits protein synthesis
   c. Interferes with folate metabolism
   d. Interacts with ergosterol in fungal membranes

Short Answer Questions

1. Explain the primary structural differences between yeasts and molds. How do the differences influence their pathogenicity and mode of infection?
2. What are the most common opportunistic fungal diseases in immunocompromised individuals, and which fungi are most frequently involved?
3. Describe the clinical presentation and etiologic agents of superficial mycoses , such as dermatophytosis, candidiasis, and pityriasis versicolor.

4. What are the most common laboratory tests used to diagnose invasive mycoses? Describe direct and indirect techniques.
5. How do serologic testing and molecular testing increase the sensitivity and speed of diagnosing fungal infections?
6. Contrast mechanisms of action and clinical use of azoles, echinocandins, and polyenes in antifungal therapy.
7. What are the main challenges in the treatment of fungal infections, particularly antifungal resistance and host toxicity?
8. Explain the epidemiological trends in invasive fungal infections worldwide. Which environmental and health factors are accountable for their increasing occurrence?

Answer to Critical Thinking Questions

1. (b); 2. (c); 3. (b); 4. (c); 5. (d)

REFERENCES

1. Schoch, C. L., Robbertse, B., Robert, V., Vu, D., Cardinali, G., Irinyi, L., Meyer, W., Nilsson, R. H., Hughes, K., Miller, A. N., Kirk, P. M., Abarenkov, K., Aime, M. C., Ariyawansa, H. A., Bidartondo, M., Boekhout, T., Buyck, B., Cai, Q., Chen, J., Crespo, A., ... Federhen, S. (2014). Finding needles in haystacks: linking scientific names, reference specimens and molecular data for Fungi. *Database : the journal of biological databases and curation*, *2014*, bau061. https://doi.org/10.1093/database/bau061 (accessed on 13th June 2025).
2. Abdolrasouli, A., Armstrong-James, D. P. H., Chowdhary, A., Fisher, M. C., et al. (2016). First hospital outbreak of the globally emerging *Candida auris* in a European hospital. https://core.ac.uk/download/77018496.pdf (accessed on 13th June 2025).
3. Adungo, F., Bii, C., Makwaga, O., Matiru, V. N., et al. (2019). Factors associated with superficial mycoses in patients visiting Alupe Clinic and its environs in Busia, western Kenya. https://core.ac.uk/download/478368623.pdf (accessed on 13th June 2025).
4. Aghasi, M., Alizadeh, A. M., Ghiasian, S. A., Roshandel, G., et al. (2012). Fumonisin B1 contamination of cereals and risk of esophageal cancer in a high-risk area in Northeastern Iran. https://core.ac.uk/download/52204711.pdf (accessed on 13th June 2025).
5. Akan, H., Alexander, B. D., Andes, D., Azoulay, E., et al. (2019). Revision and update of the consensus definitions of invasive fungal disease from the European Organization for Research and Treatment of Cancer and the Mycoses Study Group Education and Research Consortium. https://core.ac.uk/download/287649722.pdf (accessed on 13th June 2025).
6. Al-Laaeiby, A., Al-Saadoon, A. H., & Ali, S. (2019). *Candida* species: The silent enemy. https://core.ac.uk/download/478291962.pdf (accessed on 13th June 2025).
7. Alastruey-Izquierdo, A., Giraldo, A., Alper, S., Altschul, E., Melo, A. S. A., Nishikaku, A. S., Normand, A. C., et al. (2015). International Society of Human and Animal Mycology (ISHAM)-ITS reference DNA barcoding database–the quality controlled standard tool for routine identification of human and animal pathogenic fungi. https://core.ac.uk/download/154274446.pdf (accessed on 13th June 2025).
8. Amor, A., Ben Daoud, S., Brouwer, C., Cardinali, G., et al. (2013). MycoBank gearing up for new horizons. https://core.ac.uk/download/323080827.pdf (accessed on 13th June 2025).
9. Consortium OPATHY, & Gabaldón, T. (2019). Recent trends in molecular diagnostics of yeast infections: from PCR to NGS. *FEMS microbiology reviews*, *43*(5), 517–547. https://doi.org/10.1093/femsre/fuz015(accessed on 13th June 2025).
10. Wissing, H., Ballus, J., Bingold, T. M., Nocea, G., Krobot, K. J., Kaskel, P., Kumar, R. N., & Mavros, P. (2013). Intensive care unit-related fluconazole use in Spain and Germany: patient characteristics and outcomes of a prospective multicenter longitudinal observational study. *Infection and drug resistance*, *6*, 15–25. https://doi.org/10.2147/IDR.S38945 (accessed on 13th June 2025).
11. Bassetti, M., & Bouza, E. (2017). Invasive mould infections in the ICU setting: complexities and solutions. *The Journal of antimicrobial chemotherapy*, *72*(suppl_1), i39–i47. https://doi.org/10.1093/jac/dkx032(accessed on 13th June 2025).
12. Berman, J., Blehert, D., Case, N., Cowen, L. E., et al. (2022). The future of fungi: Threats and opportunities. https://core.ac.uk/download/541700436.pdf (accessed on 13th June 2025).
13. Borowy, I., Codex Committee on Food Hygiene, Crane, P. H., Dahms, S., Edel, W., Food and

Agriculture Organization, et al. (2014). The emergence of international food safety standards and guidelines: Understanding the current landscape through a historical approach. https://core.ac.uk/download/42138184.pdf (accessed on 13th June 2025).

14. Broenen, E., Brüggemann, R., Kamphuis-van Ulzen, K., Mavinkurve-Groothuis, A. M. C., et al. (2014). Screening of the central nervous system in children with invasive pulmonary aspergillosis. https://core.ac.uk/download/131024764.pdf (accessed on 13th June 2025).
15. Brown, A. J. P., Brown, G. D., Gow, N. A. R., Netea, M. G., et al. (2014). Metabolism impacts upon *Candida* immunogenicity and pathogenicity at multiple levels. https://core.ac.uk/download/25497610.pdf (accessed on 13th June 2025).
16. Brown, J., Gulmez, D., Kean, R., Ramage, G., et al. (2020). *Candida auris*: A decade of understanding of an enigmatic pathogenic yeast. https://core.ac.uk/download/293868702.pdf (accessed on 13th June 2025).
17. Cappleman, S. (2003). Effects of Mentholatum on onychomycosis of the toenail. https://core.ac.uk/download/480740732.pdf (accessed on 13th June 2025).
18. Castro, G. K., Chiller, T. M., Davis, T., Ferretti, G., et al. (2024). Shared vision for improving outcomes for serious fungal diseases: Report of a patient, caregiver, and clinician summit. https://core.ac.uk/download/619402116.pdf (accessed on 13th June 2025).
19. Chaudhuri, U. (2022). Fungal burden of disease in Central and South America. https://core.ac.uk/download/621349787.pdf (accessed on 13th June 2025).
20. Chen, J. (2012). Fungal community survey of *Fraxinus excelsior* in New Zealand. https://core.ac.uk/download/11988644.pdf (accessed on 13th June 2025).
21. Hoenigl, M., Levitz, S. M., Schuetz, A. N., Zhang, S. X., & Cornely, O. A. (2021). All You Need to Know and More about the Diagnosis and Management of Rare Mold Infections. *mBio*, *12*(1), e02920-20. https://doi.org/10.1128/mBio.02920-20(accessed on 13th June 2025).
22. Prattes, J., Valentin, T., Hoenigl, M., Talakic, E., Reisinger, A. C., & Eller, P. (2021). Invasive pulmonary aspergillosis complicating COVID-19 in the ICU - A case report. *Medical mycology case reports*, *31*, 2–5. https://doi.org/10.1016/j.mmcr.2020.05.001(accessed on 13th June 2025).
23. Felitti, S. A., García Lemos, A., Gil Cardeza, M. L., Gomez, M., et al. (2017). Fungal endophytes in species of *Paspalum* and *Bromus*, occurrence and *in vitro* antagonistic activity assessment. https://core.ac.uk/download/224999098.pdf (accessed on 13th June 2025).
24. Goldberg, A. N., Murr, A. H., & Vesper, S. (2006). Fungal speciation using quantitative polymerase chain reaction (QPCR) in patients with and without chronic rhinosinusitis. https://core.ac.uk/download/323072535.pdf (accessed on 13th June 2025).
25. Denning, D. W., Perfect, J. R., Milevska-Kostova, N., Haderi, A., Armstrong, H., Hardenberg, M. C., Chavez, E., Altevogt, B., Holmes, P., & Aram, J. A. (2025). Antifungal Policy and Practice Across Five Countries: A Qualitative Review. *Journal of fungi (Basel, Switzerland)*, *11*(2), 162. https://doi.org/10.3390/jof11020162(accessed on 13th June 2025).
26. Hoenigl, M., & Jenks, J. D. (2018). Treatment of aspergillosis. https://core.ac.uk/download/323064842.pdf (accessed on 13th June 2025).
27. Homei, A., & Worboys, M. (2020). Chapter introduction. https://core.ac.uk/download/478128193.pdf (accessed on 13th June 2025).

28. Jaiswal, K. P., & Pandey, A. K. (2023). An update on medical mycology big data analytics and antifungal therapies. https://core.ac.uk/download/652722955.pdf (accessed on 13th June 2025).

29. Joshaghani, H., Kohsar, F., Namjoo, M., Niknejad, F., et al. (2013). Mycoflora of fungal contamination in wheat storage (silos) in Golestan Province, north of Iran. https://core.ac.uk/download/52204649.pdf (accessed on 13th June 2025).

30. Kean, R., & Ramage, G. (2019). Combined antifungal resistance and biofilm tolerance: The global threat of *Candida auris*. https://core.ac.uk/download/293867055.pdf (accessed on 13th June 2025).

31. Macura, A., & Skóra, M. (2015). 21-year retrospective study of the prevalence of *Scopulariopsis brevicaulis* in patients suspected of superficial mycoses. https://core.ac.uk/download/286324201.pdf (accessed on 13th June 2025).

32. Martín Vicente, A. (2016). Development of new strategies for the treatment of emerging opportunistic fungal infections. https://core.ac.uk/download/78460177.pdf (accessed on 13th June 2025).

33. Rajendran, R., Ramage, G., Sherry, L., Williams, C., et al. (2012). Fungal biofilm resistance. https://core.ac.uk/download/9650980.pdf (accessed on 13th June 2025).

34. Schauwvlieghe, A. F. A. D. (2020). *Risicofactoren, Diagnose En Behandeling Van (Azole-Resistente) Invasieve Aspergillose*. https://core.ac.uk/download/328852271.pdf (accessed on 13th June 2025).

35. Sigurgeirsson, B., Paul, C., Dupuy, A., Guberman, D., Korting, H. C., Kerl, H., Hull, P. R., et al. (2004). Chronic dermatomycoses of the foot as risk factors for acute bacterial cellulitis of the leg: A case-control study. https://core.ac.uk/download/16432790.pdf (accessed on 13th June 2025).

36. Wanke, B., Roe, C. C., Lysen, C., Hepp, C. M., Engelthaler, D. M., Overy, D. P., DeBess, E., et al. (2018). Dating the *Cryptococcus gattii* dispersal to the North American Pacific Northwest. https://core.ac.uk/download/323069956.pdf (accessed on 13th June 2025).

GENERAL PARASITOLOGY

6

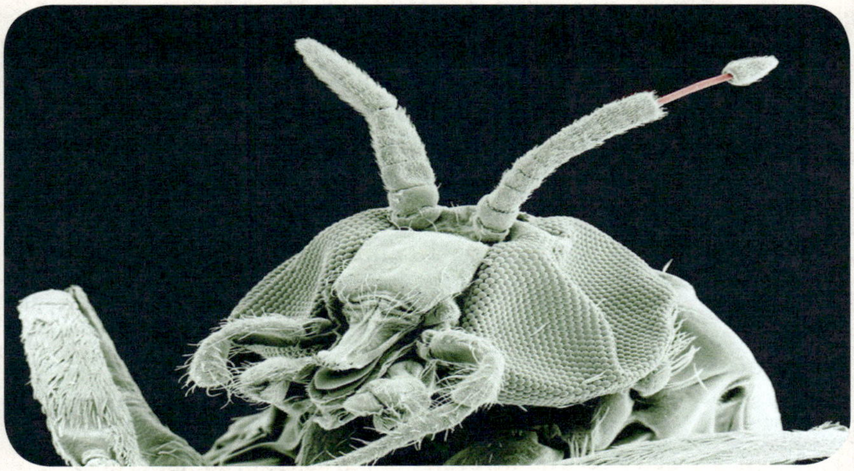

LEARNING OBJECTIVES

After studying this chapter, you will be able to:

1. Explain the types of parasites;
2. Discuss life cycles of parasites;
3. Appreciate the host-parasite relationship concept;
4. Define pathogenesis and disease;
5. Prepare to diagnose parasitic infections;
6. Zero in on the treatment and control of parasitic infections.

Introduction to Parasitology

In light of the intricacies in parasitology, consideration of the relationships underpinning parasitic interactions should be made. Parasitology examines how organisms establish symbiotic associations, one of which benefits at the cost of the other. The broad discipline examines a vast array of organisms, primarily eukaryotes, although work on bacterial and viral parasites remains significant. Parasitic organisms are stunningly varied in size, ranging from extremely diminutive protozoa to massive flowering plants , such as Rafflesia. Each parasitic species possesses its unique life cycles with mechanisms for survival in specific milieus and hosts. Through detailed examination of this array of parasites, scientists are able to better appreciate not just their complexity but also their ecological and medical significance, which goes beyond understanding disease in human beings, animals, and plants as well. This basic knowledge provides the foundation for subsequent interdisciplinary study in parasitology (Chalmers et al., 2016). The importance of parasitology becomes increasingly insistent when environmental sustainability and public health are considered. Complex conditions , such as climate change and globalization, in recent years, have multiplied the transmission of parasitic diseases. For instance, while some regions have shown decreasing incidence of malaria, access to potent treatment remains a priority. The development of drug resistance is a significant problem, particularly for *Plasmodium falciparum* malaria, which demands a requisite improvement in the availability of treatment and diagnosis initiatives. Initiatives like the Affordable Medicines Facility for Malaria have the potential to enhance the availability of effective drugs. The availability of health infrastructures of different countries poses a limitation to implementing such initiatives, particularly in rural areas (Marriot et al., 2011). This highlights the importance of uniting social, economic, and environmental elements in parasitic disease management and underscores the call for continued research and interdisciplinarity. Perhaps most importantly, however, the One Health idea has become an influential model for addressing the intersection of human, animal, and environmental health in the context of parasitology. By understanding the intricate relationships between these disciplines, researchers are better able to overcome the multi-faceted challenges faced by parasites. Interdisciplinary research promotes cooperation between biologists, physicians, environmental scientists, and policymakers upon a firm groundwork for reacting to the public health impact of parasites. The British Society for Parasitology's 2015 Autumn Symposium is one such effort promoting this expanded thinking regarding parasitology. By engaging early-career scientists and embracing diversified subject matter beyond mainstream parasitology, such programs can promote innovative science and leadership. Ultimately, embracing the One Health concept might lead to ground-breaking solutions to efficient and sustainable control of parasitic disease (Chalmers et al., 2016).

Definition of Parasitology

Parasitology, a discipline within the biological sciences, examines the intricate associations that exist between parasites and hosts. This field focuses on the complexities of parasitism, a form of symbiosis in which one organism—the parasite—advantages at the cost of a second organism, the host. Parasitology is comprehensive, covering various organisms from microscopic protozoa to large organisms , such as helminths and ectoparasites. An awareness of these associations is significant since parasites can significantly impact their hosts' health, ecology, and even general behavior. This interaction often leads to infectious diseases that affect not only individual hosts but also populations and ecosystems, and thus the study of parasitology is crucial in advancing medical research, veterinary health, and environmental science. The diversity of parasitic organisms also challenges the necessity of a comprehensive definition of parasitology. Defined in recent literature, the field traditionally focuses on eukaryotic life but also incorporates a wide variety of infectious agents, including bacteria and viruses; these are studied separately but provide an additional perspective on organism interaction. From obligate intracellular parasites to organisms with more complex life cycles, parasitology concerns a broad array of forms of life. The applicability of these studies extends beyond the biological sciences, increasingly transgressing into agriculture, wildlife conservation, and public health due to the significant role parasites play in ecosystems. This far-reaching strategy emphasizes the need for integrating knowledge from each field in order to meet the challenges posed by parasitic infections, thus emphasizing the necessity for a converging body of knowledge in the field. New paradigms like the One Health approach have thus been established to facilitate more cohesion of learning parasitology in terms of bridging human, animal, and environmental health. The philosophy recognizes that parasitic diseases tend to cross species barriers and thus points out the ecological dependencies involved. Zoonotic disease is a case in point, where there is transmission between humans and animals, highlighting the need for multi-disciplinary research methods and collaborative interventions in addressing parasitic threats. Symposia like the British Society for Parasitologys Autumn Symposium are promoting multi-disciplinary debate, leading a multi-disciplinary discourse involving individuals of different disciplines. While scientists further explore the interface between health and ecosystems, the discipline of parasitology will adapt to incorporate new findings from varied scientific research (Charlier et al., 2008; Chalmers et al., 2016) (Figure 6.1).

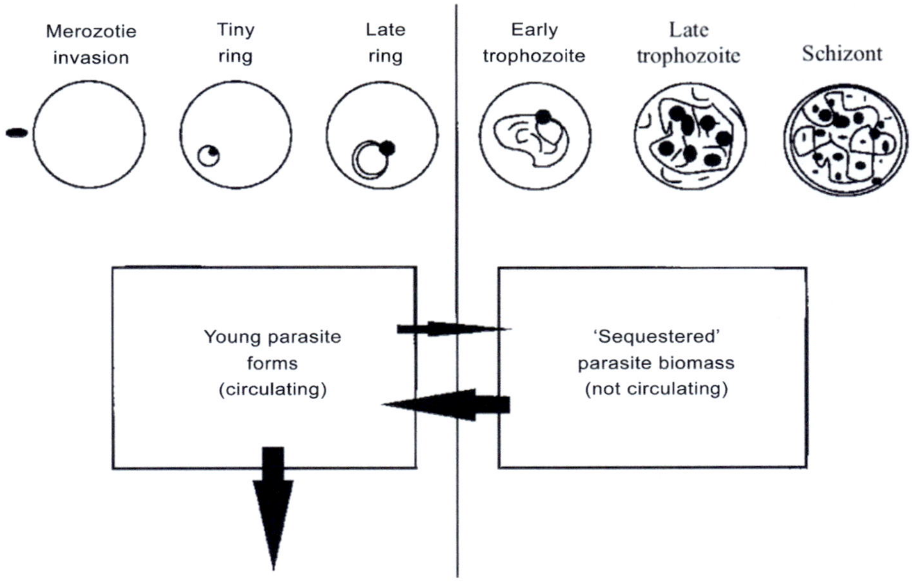

Figure 6.1. Schematic diagram showing broad stages of parasite development across the 48-h life cycle of *Plasmodium falciparum*.

Source: https://www.researchgate.net/profile/Timothy-Davis-25/publication/13932949/figure/fig1/AS:601743566065669@1520478254439/Schematic-diagram-showing-broad-stages-of-parasite-development-across-the-48-h-life-cycle.png.

Historical Background of Parasitology

The history of parasitology has deep origins entwined in the overall history of medicine and biology. As an emergent discipline in the 19th century, parasitology was first molded by early observational research on the varying life forms that live in other organisms. Pathfinding researchers , such as Antonie van Leeuwenhoek, who first delineated protozoa, and Rudolf Virchow, who developed the theory of cell theory, laid the groundwork for understanding coexistence among species. This new awareness of host-parasite relationship was fundamental in that it transformed our comprehension of causation of disease from a simplistic contagion to an understanding of sophisticated biological interaction. The earlier history of such advances is brought out by the evolving relationship between man and his parasitic opposite, which has continued to influence present research and public health practice in parasitology. With disciplinary maturity came the predominance of interdisciplinary approaches, which merged knowledge from zoology, microbiology, and veterinary medicine. The introduction of methods , such as microscopy and, later, molecular techniques facilitated groundbreaking discoveries in understanding parasitic life cycles and transmission modalities. During the late 19th and early 20th centuries, significant advancements were catalyzed by the identification of parasites responsible for diseases like malaria and Trichinosis. These discoveries not only propelled the field of parasitology forward but also spurred broader discussions on zoonotic diseases—those transmitted from animals to humans. The recognition of interdependence between human and animal health served as the foundation for what would eventually be the One Health movement, which is an all-encompassing approach to health that includes greater than one species and specialty, as captured in the historical narratives of contemporary medicine. , such as their interconnected relationships with veterinary medicine (Bresalier et al., 2017). The establishment of specialized organizations and professionalization of parasitology also advanced it. Research efforts flourished following World War II with the founding of institutions specialized in tropical diseases, which were predominantly found among poor communities. The period was characterized by the development of new therapeutic approaches and diagnostic techniques for addressing parasitic infections that had long plagued heavily populated humans. Laboratory procedures and historical collections also offered insights into how parasitological research methods change over time. Examination of historical documents, such as ancient books on medicine and conserved samples, lent substance to the scientific advancement in the past decades (Jardine et al., 2019). Such cumulative insight into the history of parasitology offers not only the host-parasite interaction intricacies but also the need for ongoing research amidst global health emergencies, like climate change and deterioration in biodiversity (Figure 6.2).

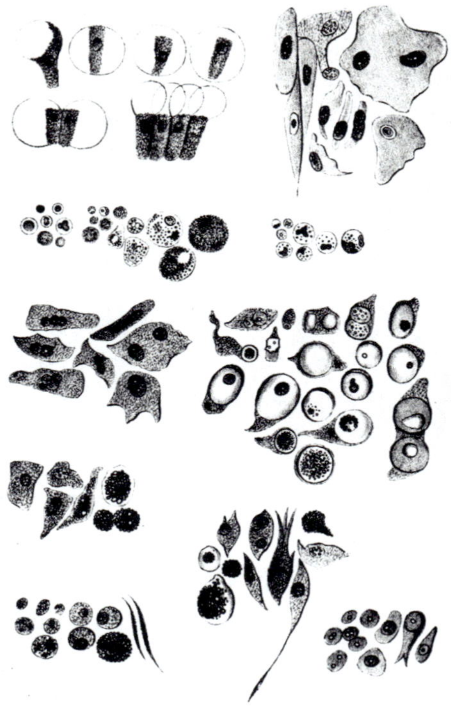

Figure 6.2. Illustration of Virchow's cell theory.

Source: https://upload.wikimedia.org/wikipedia/commons/thumb/7/7b/Virchow-cell.jpg/320px-Virchow-cell.jpg.

Importance of Studying Parasites

Parasite research is of utmost significance in an effort to comprehend the complex relationships of parasites with hosts, resulting in revolutionary advances in medical and environmental science. Parasites , such as protozoa, helminths, and ectoparasites possess intricate life cycles and evasive mechanisms that pose critical challenges to human and animal hosts alike. By the exploration of these organisms, researchers are able to gain information on host-pathogen interactions and immune evasion mechanisms. Methods like the DMU e-Parasitology e-learning package complement study activities by transferring artificial microscopes and vast databases of digitized tissue so that learners and practitioners can become familiarized with the morphology of various parasites (Acosta et al., 2019). These teaching efforts are significant in exposing the next generation of scientists and medical practitioners to the knowledge necessary in treating parasitic infections, their prevention, and their management of health impacts. Beyond the health aspect, parasites also play a significant role in the discipline of ecology in general, wherein these animals contribute heavily to determining biodiversity and ecosystem operations. Many parasites are host-specific in association with a complex life cycle that has implications for the host populations and communities. For example, the parasitization by a particular parasitic species can reduce host animal populations, which in turn reconstructs the predator-prey interaction and ecosystem function. These processes not only reveal information regarding the evolutionary pressures within biological communities but also regarding conservation strategies. The applications of parasitology extend beyond medicine because the effects of these organisms have the potential to echo across entire ecosystems. True comprehension of these interactions allows ecologists and conservationists to implement informed measures in managing wildlife populations and their habitats to most effective. Moreover, developments in technology and computer biology have broadened the scope for research on parasites, leading to path-breaking discoveries that enhance our understanding about various parasitic diseases. Antigenic variation in malaria, particularly in Plasmodium knowlesi and its interactions with the host in monkey hosts, illustrate the efficacy of high-resolution research in informing treatment protocols (Ay et al., 2018). Through an investigation of these factors using longitudinal analysis and multi-omic approaches, scientists can establish the molecular processes of disease process and resistance. The recent advances in parasites improve diagnostic and treatment facilities but also promote innovation in vaccine and epidemiological surveillance. Since globalization facilitates the spread of parasites, research becomes more urgent. Public health and safety worldwide are more required today, hence accentuating the significance of parasitological research today.

6.1. Types of Parasites

Learning Outcome

1. Describe ectoparasites;
2. Define endoparasites;
3. Differentiate between obligate and facultative parasites.

Taxonomy of parasites encompasses a broad range of organisms, which all collectively fall under the headings of protozoa, helminths, and ectoparasites. Protozoa are unicellular organisms capable of producing disease in a variety of hosts, including humans. Examples include Plasmodium spp., the pathogens of malaria, and *Giardia lamblia*, the cause of gastrointestinal infections. Gaining knowledge of their life cycles and mode of transmission is crucial in the development of effective treatment and prevention protocols. The dynamics of their interactions with hosts can best be explained through studies on antigenic variation, , such as the case of *Plasmodium knowlesi*, which indicated the adaptive mechanisms employed by such parasites to evade the immune response of their hosts (Rousing et al., 2011). These findings are exceedingly valuable to undertake research in protozoan pathogenesis and also essential for planning public health interventions. Helminths, however, are multicellular parasites that belong to three broad categories: cestodes or tapeworms, nematodes or roundworms, and trematodes or flukes. The parasites commonly infect the gastrointestinal tract but can also inhabit other systems in the host body. Their multicellular life cycles often involve intermediate hosts that not only serve as a source of nutrition for parasites but increase their transmission rate as well. Helminthology is vital, as helminthic infections can lead to a great amount of morbidity, influencing nutrition and overall well-being, particularly where they are endemic. Epidemiological studies on the helminth infection have initiated massive intervention programs, , such as mass school deworming, to reduce the population burden of helminthiasis (Rousing et al., 2011). The interventions underscore the importance of understanding the ecological habitats and life cycles of helminth parasites in public health. Ectoparasites, as opposed to their endoparasitic relatives, reside on the exterior of their hosts, deriving sustenance and protection at the cost of frequently terrible pain and illness. Ectoparasites consist of lice, fleas, and ticks, each having distinct biological and ecological characteristics. Each not only "borrows" the hosts blood but also serves as a vector for a range of infectious agents, complicating disease control even further. For instance, ticks also act as vectors of pathogens responsible for Lyme disease and other tick-borne diseases, which serves to emphasize the need for integrated vector management. Population control of ectoparasites typically involves environmental management practices and imposition of specific treatment strategies. The multi-factorial nature of ectoparasitism serves to emphasize the need to carry out more research into the understanding of their association with hosts and the impact thereof on health outcomes in affected groups (Ay et al., 2018).

6.1.1. Ectoparasites

Ectoparasites, which live on the external surfaces of their hosts, encompass a wide variety of organisms, e.g., fleas, ticks, lice, and mites. Ectoparasites exert significant influences on host survival and well-being and can inflict harmful physiological consequences. Infection by ectoparasites can result in skin irritation, nutrient loss, and vulnerability to secondary infections. For instance, infestations by the dinoflagellate *Amyloodinium ocellatum* in fish , such as gilthead sea bream induce severe gill damage and lead to anoxia and systemic infection as a consequence of compromised osmoregulatory function. Knowledge of ectoparasitic infection dynamics is central to enlightening the contribution of such infections to the health and mortality of host populations, with the importance highlighted by the call for expanded research into host responses to ectoparasitic infestations and their long-term consequences for various species (Moreira et al., 2017). The impact of ectoparasites also extends beyond individual hosts since they are known to act as vectors for diseases, amplifying their role in disease transmission dynamics. Larval ticks of the Ixodes scapularis, for example, have the capacity to transmit pathogens that lead to Lyme disease, anaplasmosis, and babesiosis and exert significant influence on wildlife populations and human health. Research on white-footed mice, the carriers of such pathogens, has shown that high tick burdens do not necessarily lead to decreased survival rates. In fact, higher tick burdens may enhance various ecological interactions, thus stabilizing both vector and host populations (Hersh et al., 2014). This complicated interaction underscores the ecological and epidemiological significance of ectoparasites, making their role as parasites and regulators in ecosystems a subject to be viewed more extensively. Ectoparasite infestations are extremely difficult to control in wildlife as well as in agricultural ecosystems due to the impact on the health of the host and ecosystem processes. Effective control measures should consider not only the immediate effects of these parasites on their hosts but also their roles within greater ecological contexts. Integrated pest management approaches incorporating the association of biological control, environmental monitoring, and the use of specific anthelmintics may offset the adverse effects of ectoparasites. Dynamic resistance of ectoparasites to treatment underscores the need for continuous research and the creation of novel management strategies. By refining our understanding of how ectoparasites operate in host populations and of their complex interactions with pathogens, we are better positioned to inform strategies for protecting the health of both humans and wildlife in a more globalized world (Figure 6.3).

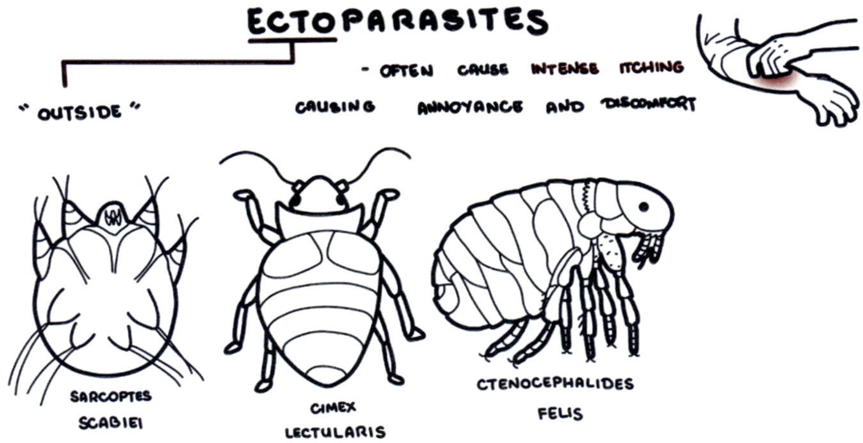

Figure 6.3. Ectoparasites.

Source: https://i.ytimg.com/vi/LSqiJozPpF0/maxresdefault.jpg.

6.1.2. Endoparasites

Endoparasites, living animals inside the hosts' bodies, pose serious health risks to humans as well as agricultural productivity. These parasites, represented by a diverse array of helminths and protozoa, possess complex life cycles with many hosts and different stages in contrasting environments. Understanding the ecology and biology of endoparasites is required for control measure planning. In addition, the economic effects are of global concern: infestations may lead to extensive losses in livestock production, which results in a setback to food security and economic stability. As highlighted in several studies, the endemicity of endoparasitic infection in livestock indicates the necessity of generating sustainable management practices that minimize chemical intervention but maintain animal welfare (Anonymous et al., 2025). The employment of anthelmintic drugs conventionally in the management of endoparasites is being challenged by resistance development and public health concerns of chemical residue in farm produce. This has prompted research into alternative control measures that emphasize integrated pest management (IPM) strategies. The non-chemical alternatives, , such as biological control, managing pasture properly, and the use of bioactive forages, are increasingly being emphasized as sustainable controls. For instance, better nutrition in animals can improve host immunity, thus reducing the susceptibility to infection. Furthermore, selective breeding for genetic parasite resistance has also proved lucrative in other animal species with the prospect of resulting in a more sustainable agriculture system (Rahmann et al., 2006). Scientific research into novel anthelmintic therapies, including phytotherapy, has also been recognized as an important area of study. Studies indicate that numerous plant chemicals exert anthelmintic properties, demonstrating one such avenue to reduce reliance on synthetic medicines. It is, however, important to subject these treatments to rigorous scientific trials to determine their safety and efficiency. With the market transitioning to organic farming and sustainability, such alternatives will definitely find greater demand. Current research on such alternative prospects highlights how innovation can be utilized to fight endoparasitic infection while achieving economic viability as well as ecological balance. Lastly, addressing the issue caused by endoparasites requires a multidisciplinary approach that involves both traditional and new approaches (Rahmann et al., 2006) (Figure 6.4).

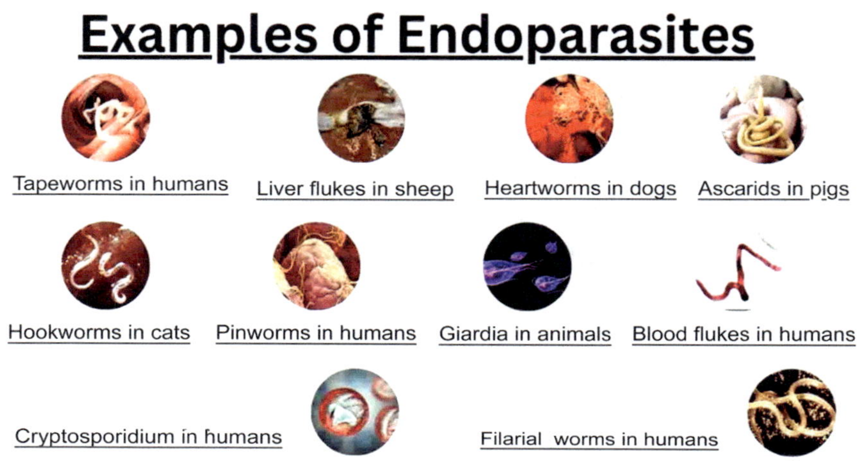

Figure 6.4. Examples of endoparasites.

Source: https://eduinput.com/wp-content/uploads/2023/05/Examples-of-Endoparasites-image-1024x555.jpg.webp.

6.1.3. Obligate Versus Facultative Parasites

Obligate and facultative parasites differ simply when considering the host-parasite relationship in the context of general parasitology. Obligate parasites are entirely dependent on their hosts for their existence, conducting essential life functions , such as reproduction and nutrition within the host environment. This strict dependence usually results in specialized adaptations for obligate parasites, which enable them to exist while also transforming the biological integrity of the host. For instance, certain obligate parasites can manipulate host immune mechanisms in order to support their existence, testament to the complex co-evolutionary dynamics between such organisms. Because obligate parasites are likely to find a high degree of specificity with a host species, their life cycles are functionally integrated and play a significant role in the dynamics of transmission and ecological balance in their habitats. Facultative parasites, on the other hand, follow a more flexible way of living and are capable of existing independently or as a commensal in addition to a host. This flexibility allows facultative parasites to exploit a greater range of environmental conditions and be more reliable in fluctuating ecosystems. Even though they are able to benefit from a host when found, facultative parasites are not host-dependent for the completion of their life cycle, which can influence their evolutionary strategies. Facultative parasites, for example, may have opportunistic behavior wherein they scavenge on weakened or moribund hosts, hence influencing the dynamics of the host populations. Further, such flexibility could increase gene flow and genetic diversity in facultative parasites to better suit them to exist in diverse environments. Their ecological roles may, therefore, strongly vary from those of obligate parasitic species, so much so that special difficulties arise in regulating their impacts. Such differences have significant implications in applied fields, , such as aquaculture and disease management. In aquaculture, for example, obligate parasites can wipe out fish stocks and cause severe economic losses due to their intricate life cycle and relationship with a specific host. Of particular concern is the development of drug resistance in obligate parasites, which creates formidable challenges for aquaculture businesses, as indicated by documented losses of up to 40% in fish output due to some diseases (Vaughan, 2018). Alternatively, facultative parasites may also present a distinct set of challenges as they can thrive in more than one environment, thereby complicating management practice. Successful control measures are highly dependent on an understanding of these differences. Through continuous research, incorporating new information on the life cycles and activity of both obligate and facultative parasites will guide a strategy that will minimize their impacts on hosts and the environment (Kasl, 2016) (Figure 6.5).

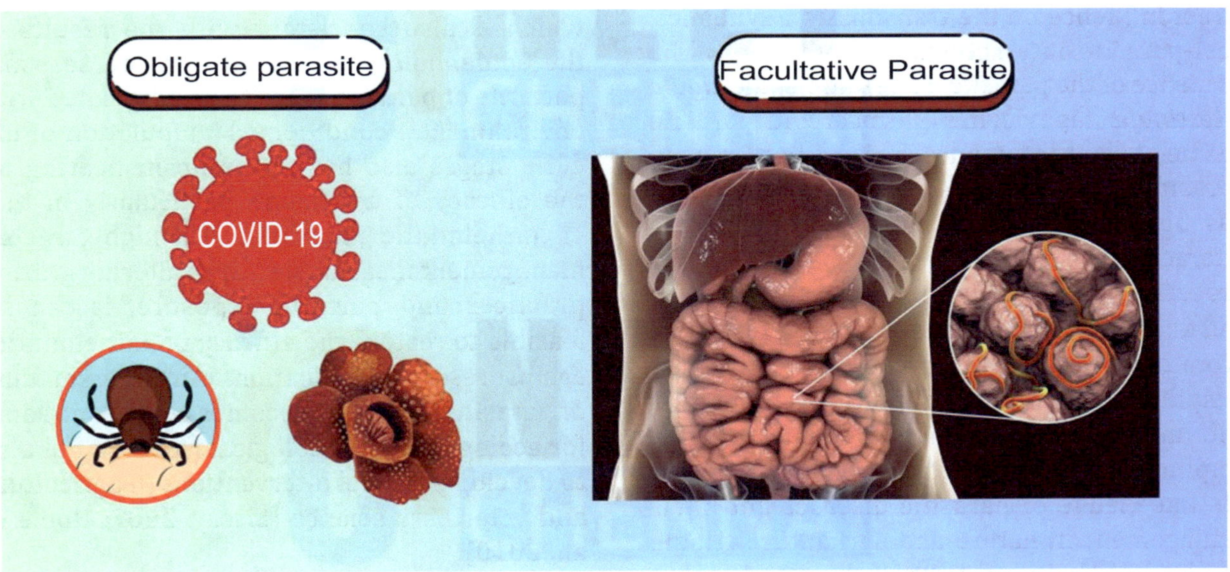

Figure 6.5. Obligate vs. facultative parasites.

Source: https://www.neetchennai.com/wp-content/uploads/2024/10/42.Difference-between-Obligate-Parasite-and-Facultative-Parasite-1024x576.jpeg.

Test Your Knowledge

1. What are the differences between ectoparasites and endoparasites in terms of where they live on or inside the host?
2. What specializations do obligate parasites have to make them dependent solely on their hosts?

6.2. Life Cycles of Parasites

Learning Outcome

1. Describe direct life cycles of parasites;
2. Describe the concept of indirect life cycles in parasitology;
3. Understand the concept of complex life cycles to understanding the evolutionary strategy and biology of most parasites.

Parasite life cycles are complex and can include over one host, thereby enabling the organism to exploit multiple ecological niches. Understanding such life cycles is significant in general parasitology because they have a direct influence on the transmission dynamics, host-parasite interactions, and ultimately the virulence of the parasite. For example, the *Ligula intestinalis* tapeworm's plerocercoid parasite has been used as a model to examine metazoan parasites. There is considerable research that has demonstrated that parasite-cyprinid fish interaction can offer insights into basic biological processes, , such as immunological responses and even environmental stressors like pollution. From these studies, researchers have obtained insight into parasite adaptations to persist and multiply within diverse environments, emphasizing the importance of life cycles in the knowledge of parasitic diseases and their management in nature and agriculture (Hoole et al., 2010). Epidemiological patterns that are evident in parasitic infections significantly enhance our knowledge of parasite life cycles, especially in livestock. In a comprehensive two-year field study in eastern Ethiopia, researchers collected parasitological information on goats and sheep to reveal helminth infection prevalence and distribution. Through the results, clear associations between fecal egg counts, packed cell volume, and indicators of animal health were apparent, thus reflecting the intricate associations between parasites and hosts. The nematode *Haemonchus contortus* was particularly widespread, affecting the productivity and health of small ruminants. This illustrates the influence of environmental drivers, for example, seasonal rain, on parasitic life cycles, which results in fluctuating infection rates and intensities. With the understanding of these trends, effective management strategies can be devised to mitigate the impact of parasites on livestock health and productivity (Sissay, 2007). In addition, parasite life cycles are tied to their evolutionary strategy, which yields several adaptations that ensure survival and transmission. For instance, there are some parasitic species that possess very good arrested development abilities, which allow them to adapt to adverse conditions. This was extremely observed in *H. contortus* during dry weather, which is also consistent with the results of the epidemiology studies that noted seasonal patterns of parasite loads to be associated with environmental conditions. Manipulation of life cycle stages also has a significant bearing on the efficacy of treatment, particularly in that of anthelmintic resistance. Through targeted management measures, such as altering grazing practices and parasite exposure, it can be feasible to restore the efficacy of anthelmintics against resistant populations. An understanding of parasite life cycles becomes central, not only for ecologizing and biological research but also to develop practical interventions in agriculture and veterinary science (Sissay, 2007; Hoole et al., 2010).

6.2.1. Direct Life Cycles

Direct life cycles constitute a basic aspect of parasitology, with the focus being on the interaction between hosts and parasites without intermediate hosts. In the case of direct life cycles, a single host species is both the definitive and intermediate host, which facilitates an efficient process of transmission. The simplicity of direct life cycles will predispose them to higher transmission rates as the parasite is able to grow and breed in a single host. This is not just augmenting the parasite's evolutionary fitness but also rendering host populations increasingly unable to handle infestations. Through research on the direct life cycle of various parasites, scientists have a deeper understanding of the mechanisms behind the parasitic persistence within ecosystems and host health and biodiversity implications.

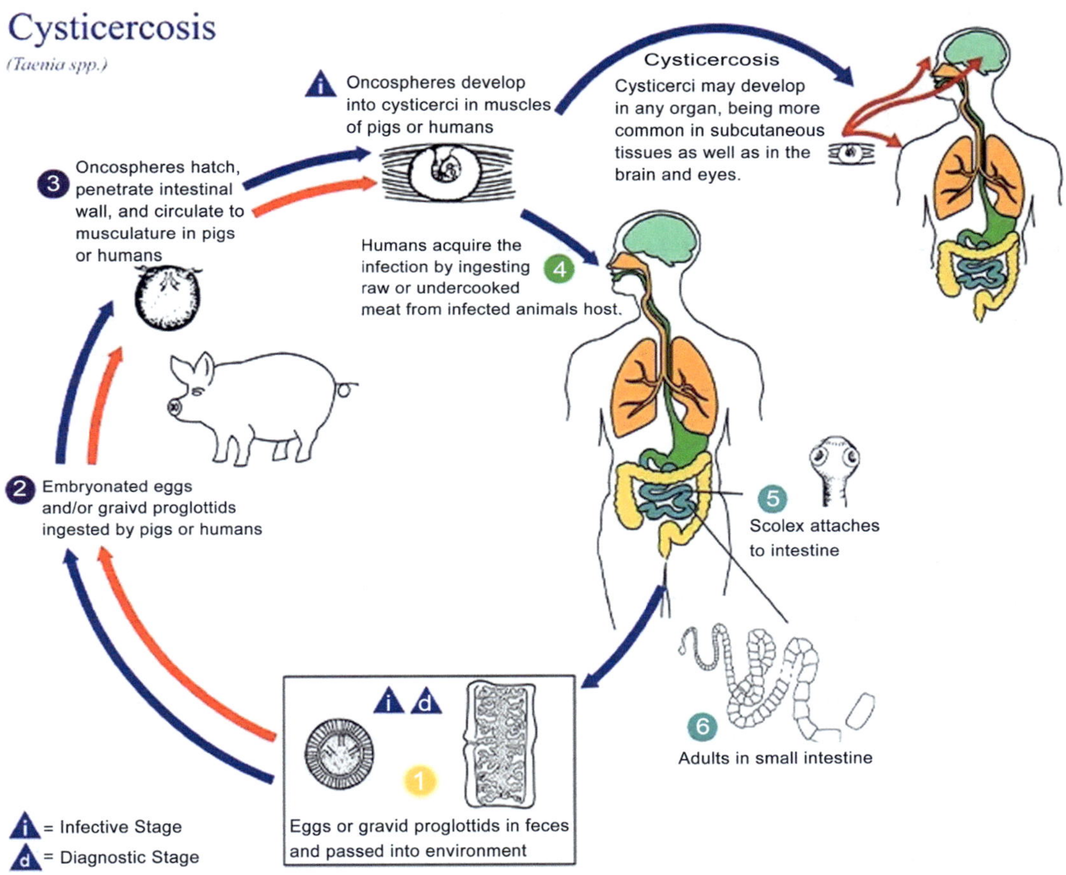

Figure 6.6. Tapeworm life cycle.

Source: https://media.geeksforgeeks.org/wp-content/uploads/20240602181708/Tapeworm-Life-Cycle.webp.

The tapeworm *Ligula intestinalis* plerocercoid is a perfect model to study direct life cycles and their impact on the host populations. Its life cycle consists of infection via feeding, with fish as the primary host to sustain the parasites' growth to their mature form. The association has been explored extensively, with considerable information given on host-parasite relationships and ecological interactions. Over six decades of research have highlighted the sophisticated biological forces involved, bordering on physical and ecological factors and molecular technology's function in decoding parasite diversity. Therefore, *Ligula intestinalis* has broadened our knowledge of direct life cycles and parasitology in general, and how environmental pressures , such as pollution and host immunology, are connected to parasite ecology and genetics (Hoole et al., 2010). Direct life cycles also emphasize the importance of genetic variation within pathogen populations. This genetic heterogeneity can influence virulence as well as adaptations to environmental change, making it more difficult to control disease. The application of the classic evolutionary models of hard and soft selection provides a model with which to predict how such forces affect pathogen life cycles. These models illustrate that the timing and form of control efforts can affect pathogen density and evolutionary directions, thereby affecting host susceptibility and disease processes. Scientists point towards future theoretical and experimental work to examine these relations in more detail since understanding them may yield better methods of control for infectious diseases involving direct life cycles (Alizon et al., 2013) (Figure 6.6).

6.2.2. Indirect Life Cycles

Parasitology is based on the indirect life cycle theory, which is central to understanding the complex relationships between the parasite and the host. Indirect life cycles involve a range of hosts, frequently definitive and intermediate hosts, which are involved in supporting the development and transmission of the parasite. Frequently involved are a series of developmental activities, where the parasite experiences drastic morphological and physiological changes. For example, the majority of helminth parasites , such as *Ascaris suum* and *Trichuris suis* have intricate indirect life cycles with intermediate hosts or environmental stages before they infest their definitive hosts. Intermediate hosts enhance parasite dispersal as well as utilizing multiple ecological niches, thus increasing the chances of infection of the definitive hosts. The knowledge of these life cycles is fundamental not only in the regulation of infections, but also in interpreting the ecological processes that affect parasitic populations in different habitats. Besides, indirect life cycles are central in establishing the epidemiological dynamics of parasitic infections. Furthermore, the dynamics between the environmental conditions, host populations, and the phases of the life cycle of the parasites have direct effects on prevalence and transmission. For instance, studies have shown that environmental conditions , such as the nature of the soil, level of humidity, and temperature, have a significant effect on determining the survival of parasite eggs and larvae in the environment. In the case of helminths, recent studies have shown that *A. suum* and *T. suis* eggs survive in pastures for weeks or even months, and this can pose a persistent threat to outdoor livestock production (Mejer et al., 2011). This persistence in the environment is an indicator of the importance of understanding ecological determinants of indirect life cycles. This information can be helpful in the development of sustainable control measures that mitigate the potential of zoonotic infections in animal and human populations. The influence of indirect life cycles is also seen with host immunity immunomodulation, as the interaction with various hosts can influence immune dynamics. The parasites, like *A. suum* and *T. suis*, have evolved immune evasion strategies against their definitive hosts through altering host immuneresponse and creating Th2-skewed environments (Mejer et al., 2011). This immunomodulation can result in increased susceptibility to secondary infection, thus making disease control more difficult. Moreover, alterations in intermediate host density and prevalence can significantly affect larval digenean transmission within specific environments. These linkages define the intricate association of ecological processes and host-parasite interaction, demanding that effective control of parasitic diseases depends on a fine appreciation of their indirect life cycles and the associated ecological processes (Figure 6.7).

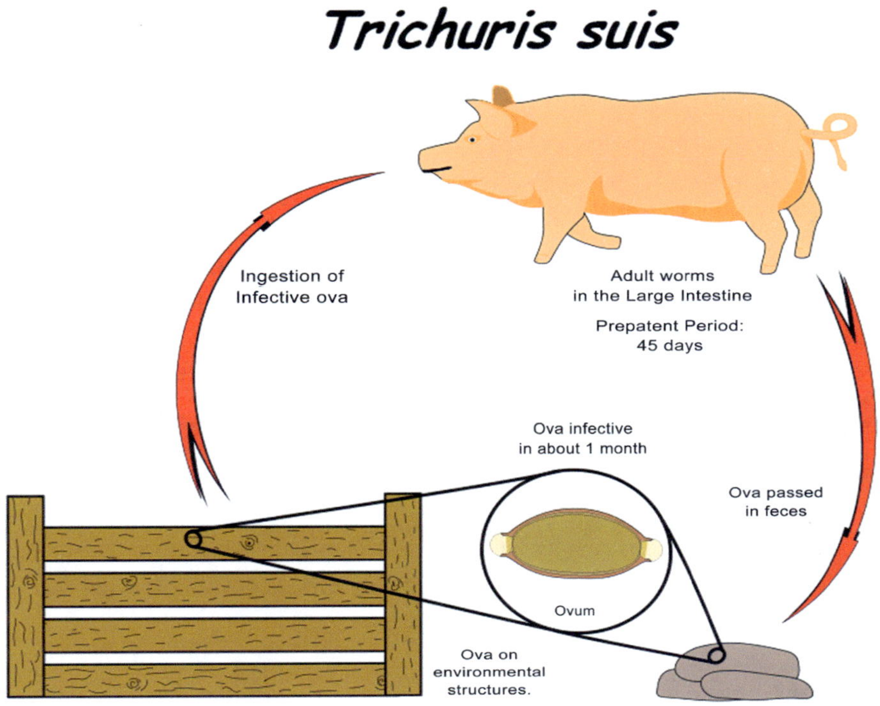

Figure 6.7. Trichuris suis life cycle.

Source: https://parasitology.cvm.ncsu.edu/life_cycles/nematodes/enoplids/graphics/trichuris_suis.png.

6.2.3. Complex Life Cycles

The concept of complex life cycles forms the core concept of understanding the biology and evolutionary strategy of most parasites. Such life cycles are multihost and multistage, allowing parasites to occupy rich ecological niches. The plerocercoid larva of *Ligula intestinalis*, for instance, has been taken as a paradigm for the study of host-parasite interaction in its fish intermediate host. In the past sixty years, there has been relatively extensive work that deconstructed the ecological significance of such interactions, showing how parasites can manipulate host numbers and alter community structure. The intricate life cycles of the organisms reflect the selective pressures underlying their adaptations and enabling them to utilize fluctuating environments. Comparing such life cycles with simpler ones provides significant information regarding selective advantages accrued from complexity and implications for ecosystem function and biodiversity (Hoole et al., 2010). Multistep life cycles present unique challenges and opportunities for parasitic disease management. The genetic variation shown by parasite populations is a significant part of their ability to adapt, particularly in response to changing environmental conditions. An understanding of the evolutionary process of these pathogens is essential to the application of effective control. The hard versus soft selection models idea further elucidates how parasite virulence and polymorphism are influenced by density-dependent forces. These models suggest that specific control interventions can affect not just the evolution of pathogenic traits but also stability in host populations. Thus, examining the complexity of complex life cycles justifies anticipating the evolutionary trajectory of parasites and, therefore, targeting future therapeutic and ecological interventions to reverse their impact

(Alizon et al., 2013). In addition, the significance of complicated life cycles goes beyond the mere comprehension of host-parasite dynamics; they also play a role in constructing larger narratives in ecology and conservation. Having multiple hosts allows for the transmission of disease across ecosystems, and it underscores the significance of interspecies relationships. Whereas scientists investigate the mechanism by which parasites adjust their life cycle as an adaptation to changing environments—pollution or global warming, for example—it is evident that complex life history can serve as a parasite bioindicator of ecosystem health. In this context, the research on parasites like *Ligula intestinalis* not only builds our theory of parasite biology but also advises ecological monitoring and conservation policy. By grasping the intricate interrelationships inherent within complex life cycles, we are in a better position to appreciate the intricate role performed by parasites within ecosystems and the consequences of their continued evolution (Hoole et al., 2010).

Test Your Knowledge

1. Define a direct life cycle in parasites and provide an example.
2. How are indirect life cycles different from direct life cycles, and what is the function of intermediate hosts?
3. What are the most significant features of complex parasite life cycles, and why are they favored by evolution?

6.3. Host-Parasite Interactions

Learning Outcome

1. Explain the types of hosts;
2. Recognize mechanisms of host manipulation;
3. Discuss co-evolution between hosts and parasites.

The intricate dynamics of host-parasite interactions are one of the most important areas of study in the science of parasitology. The dynamics can be explained by a sequence of evolutionary adaptations that impact both the parasite and the host. As an example, parasites can evolve mechanisms for manipulating host behavior or physiology to enhance their transmission and survival. The tapeworm *Ligula intestinalis* plerocercoid larva is a prime example. These investigations have demonstrated significant biological and ecological interactions between this parasite and cyprinid fish hosts. Over the decades, studies of such interactions have clarified essential aspects of immunology, parasite ecology, and evolutionary consequences of infection and host response and clarified general themes in parasite-host relationships (Hoole et al., 2010). Such observations underscore the need for continued research, particularly as ecological change introduces new variables to these age-old associations. Furthermore, understanding inter-individual variability in parasite assemblage and infection burdens in wild animal populations is critical for host-parasite dynamics. Interests are influenced by a range of factors, from the mechanisms of resistance among hosts to environmental factors that affect or impede parasite transfer. For example, a study involving spotted hyenas in Tanzania demonstrated that infection loads, in this instance, Ancylostoma and Cystoisospora infections, were set by the population density of members within a clan, reducing contact with infectious agents (Bush et al., 2019). Reducing encounter effect highlights how social structure serves to minimize parasite transmission. Further, the work discovered that juvenile survival rates were inversely impacted by high rates of infection, which further underscores both the role of individual health and social status within the broader ecological context.

These findings suggest interventions to examine host behavior and population dynamics to be very crucial in wildlife health management. Apart from ecological and social factors, age variation also plays a significant role in host-parasite dynamics. Young hosts, particularly juveniles, are more susceptible to infections due to immature immune systems and behaviors that increase exposure to parasites. Among the juvenile spotted hyenas, increased age was linked with reduced parasite loads and increased survival to adulthood, showing a key aspect of fitness in such interactions (Bush et al., 2019). This dynamic not only underscores the pivotal function of age as an infection risk factor but also suggests the potential physiological accommodations reached with maturity. Honoring these nuances in host development and parasite interactions can unleash targeted conservation measures and control methodologies that minimize the fitness burden of parasitic infection, generally favoring healthier wildlife populations within their respective ecosystems (Figure 6.8).

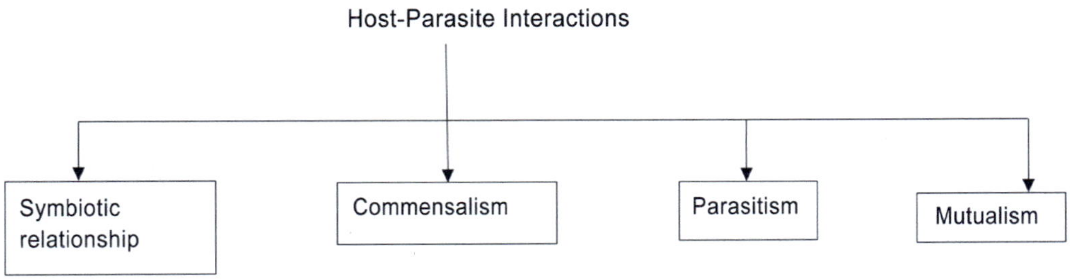

Figure 6.8. Host parasite interactions.

Source: https://microbenotes.com/wp-content/uploads/2024/12/Host-Parasite-Interactions.jpg.

6.3.1. Types of Hosts (Definitive, Intermediate, Reservoir)

In the study of parasitology, understanding the types of hosts is vital for grasping the complex interactions between parasites, their hosts, and the environments in which they exist. Definitive hosts are organisms in which parasites reach maturity and reproduce, playing a critical role in the life cycle of the parasite. For example, in the case of tapeworm *Echinococcus granulosus*, the final host is the canines, which allow the reproductive cycle of the parasites to be fulfilled. Definitive host determination is essential in creating effective control strategies for decreasing transmission. Without regulation of definitive host dynamics, parasitic infection will continue to be self-sustaining and will grow, thus posing serious public health problems and highlighting the importance of intervening within ecosystems. Intermediate hosts are the organisms that hold immature or larval stages of the parasite. Intermediate hosts are essential in the life cycle of the parasite since they typically serve as a link for parasites to reach their definitive host. For instance, in the life cycle of the trematode *Schistosoma* spp., the intermediate host is the freshwater snail, facilitating larval development, which subsequently infects the definitive host , such as the human. Understanding of the intermediate hosts' function enhances our understanding of transmission patterns, since intermediate hosts influence the prevalence of parasitic disease in populations of humans. The fact that there are a large number of intermediate hosts, particularly in peri-urban or rural communities, would exacerbate infection spread in most situations, and thus, ecological considerations become integral to disease prevention and control measures. Reservoir hosts, as opposed to definitive and intermediate hosts, are hosts where parasites are harbored without the host necessarily showing significant signs of disease. Reservoir hosts themselves are sources of infection for other potential hosts, including man, and therefore make control harder. The existence of animal reservoirs can significantly alter the epidemiology of zoonoses. For example, some of the strains of the etiologic agent of schistosomiasis, *Schistosoma* spp. have been identified in many wild and domesticated animals, which have caused great challenges to public health programs attempting to control the transmission. As highlighted by recent research, the relationship between reservoir species and human populations can lead to enhanced transmission dynamics, thus adding to the challenges of controlling it. Reservoir hosts knowledge is paramount in an integrated public health approach as it realizes the interconnection between animal, human, and environmental health, which demands multi-dimensional approach strategies as a response to the multi-dimensionality of parasite dynamics in contemporary dynamics (Webster et al., 2015; Borlase et al., 2017) (Figure 6.9).

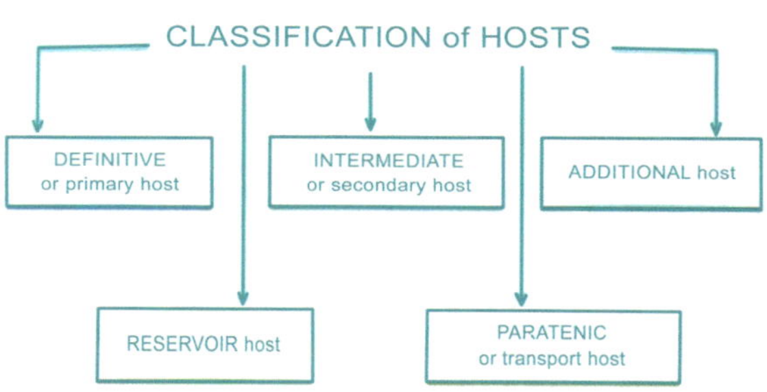

Figure 6.9. Classification of hosts.

Source: https://microbeonline.com/wp-content/uploads/2022/02/Classification-of-hosts.png.

6.3.2. Mechanisms of Host Manipulation

The intricate interaction between hosts and parasites often reveals profound mechanisms of manipulation that are beneficial to the parasite's survival and reproduction. Host manipulation refers to the various mechanisms by which parasites manipulate the behavior, physiology, or development of their hosts to enhance transmission possibility. For instance, the *Ligula intestinalis* plerocercoid shows how parasites can render their fish intermediate host more susceptible to predation by birds, the parasite's definitive hosts (Hoole et al., 2010). This is a demonstration of how parasites can exploit the behavioral ecology of the host, effectively using it as a transport host for themselves in order to finish their own life cycles. These interactions not only affect particular organisms but also have cascading effects on ecosystems via effects on species interactions and food web associations. Further, the temporality of the manipulation of the host is a critical consideration for understanding these interactions. Scientists have begun exploring the cycles of biological processes, noting that parasites, in most cases, synchronize their life cycles with host cycles, such as daily or seasonal activity (Helm et al., 2015). Synchronization often leads to more effective transmission strategies, as the parasites exploit periods of heightened host activity for optimal reproduction and spreading. For example, seasonal changes in immune responses can dictate infection timing to permit vulnerability exploitation by parasites. The interconnection of chronobiology and parasitism illuminates the adaptive significance of manipulation strategies and emphasizes the importance of taking temporal considerations into host-parasite research. Ultimately, understanding the mechanisms of host manipulation not only increases our knowledge of parasitology but also offers avenues for future research in ecological and evolutionary dynamics. By examining how various parasites manipulate their hosts, scientists can gain more universal implications for disease control and conservation policies. With such parasites as *Ligula intestinalis*, researchers are able to study the environmental and genetic reasons for host susceptibility and immunity to manipulation (Hoole et al., 2010). Further, looking at the temporal aspects of parasitic strategies can provide a view of co-evolutionary patterns in hosts and parasites, which suggest that the survival arms race is conducted in a high temporal context (Helm et al., 2015). These arguments ultimately emphasize the complex and dynamic nature of host-parasite interactions, offering critical information on ecological balance and biodiversity (Figure 6.10).

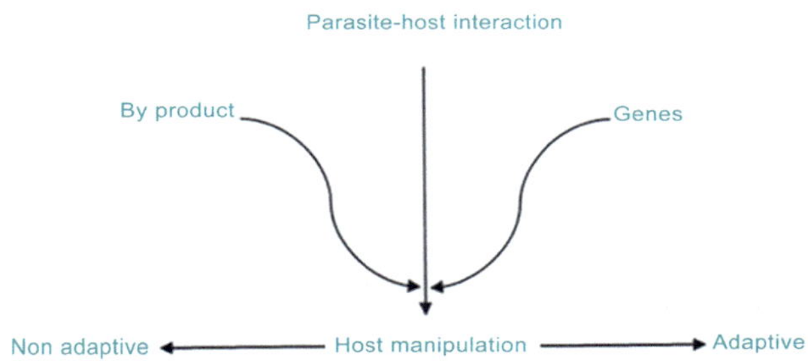

Figure 6.10. The schematics illustrate the modes of manipulation.

Source: https://www.intechopen.com/chapters/1204224.

6.3.3. Co-Evolution of Hosts and Parasites

Host-parasite co-evolution is a pivotal theme in the study of the dynamics of parasitic relationships. This is a process of adaptation wherein hosts evolve defense strategies against parasitic infection, and the parasites evolve countermeasures to circumvent such defenses. This evolutionary struggle leads to complex ecological and genetic interactions that can have long-lasting effects on both parasite and host populations. One of the most important aspects of this co-evolution is its influence on transmission dynamics; successful parasites that manipulate their hosts will enhance their own reproductive success. As hosts develop resistance traits, the continuous adaptation shown by parasites is characteristic of the continuous struggle for survival, exemplifying the intricacies of natural selection in practice. Therefore, observing the co-evolution between hosts and parasites enables scientists to observe the broader biological implications, , such as the potential for emergent infectious diseases that are caused by these interactions. Above all, host manipulation explains the strategies by which parasites enhance their fitness. For instance, some parasites manipulate the behavior of their hosts more efficiently to enhance transmission, as is observed in the cestode *Schistocephalus solidus*, which manipulates its copepod host in an attempt to reduce the threat of predation. This manipulation, while serving the parasite, could have deleterious effects on the host, creating an interesting paradox that leads to the hosts fitness being compromised for the parasites benefit. This mechanism puts evolutionary pressure on hosts, facilitating the evolution of resistance mechanisms that can effectively counter manipulative strategies. The host versus parasite fitness competition is a better example of the interplay between complex evolutionary strategies and adaptations that lead to rich ecological histories and knowledge development that guides existing research in general parasitology. Moreover, ecological history co-evolution knowledge is crucial in addressing NZD-related issues. Evolution of transmission patterns and host switching would dominate disease epidemiology among animal and human populations. There is a need to adopt an integrated, One Health approach that involves understanding ecological interactions and evolutionary dynamics in the management of NZDs. Parasite evolution and disease ecology are both relevant because they illuminate pathways through which diseases arise and spread. Effective control programs must thus be directed towards the complexity of host-parasite interactions and guided by the evolutionary history and ecological context of such interactions. By illuminating these connections, scientists can present meaningful evidence reinforcing prevention strategies for avoiding the public health impacts of neglected diseases (Webster et al., 2015; Hafer-Hahmann et al., 2019) (Figure 6.11).

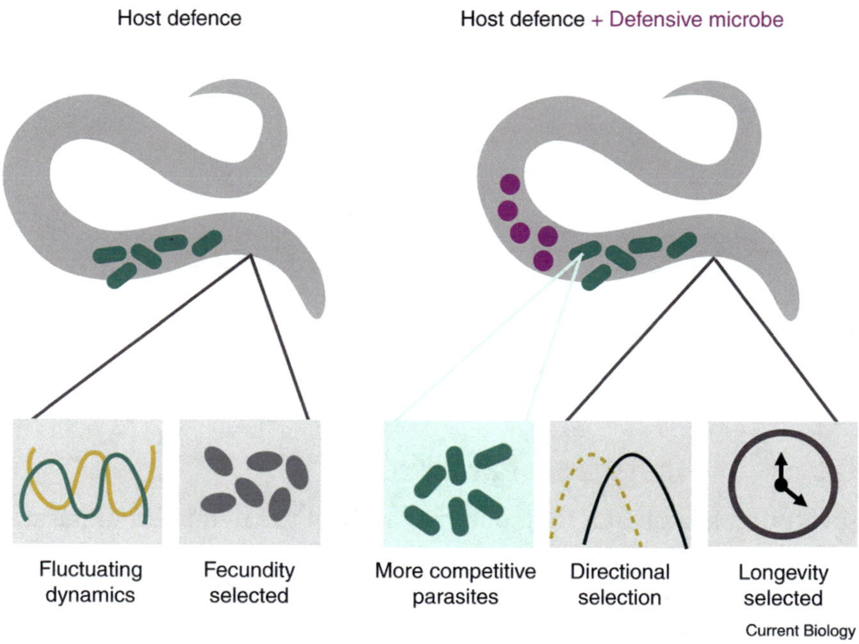

Figure 6.11. Worm hosts with defensive microbes show different coevolutionary dynamics with parasites and evolve different life-history responses to infection; meanwhile, parasites evolve to become more competitive against defensive microbes.

Source: https://ars.els-cdn.com/content/image/1-s2.0-S0960982222002470-gr1_lrg.jpg.

Test Your Knowledge

1. What are the differences between definitive, intermediate, and reservoir hosts in the parasite life cycle?
2. Provide examples of co-evolution of parasites and hosts and how this affects their interaction.

6.4. Pathogenesis and Disease

Learning Outcome

1. To comprehend common diseases caused by parasites;
2. To describe the disease development process;
3. To discuss the role of parasitology in public health.

The mechanism of pathogenesis of parasitic infections is defined by a complex interplay between host and parasite, particularly in relation to mechanisms involved in the causation of disease by parasites. Parasitic cells can play tricks on host cell functions in a manner that supports their survival by various mechanisms, , such as immunomodulation or evasion. As a model example, host cell-released extracellular vesicles (EVs) play a pivotal role in such interactions since they are capable of carrying molecules that modulate immune responses and can act as mediators in communication between pathogens and host cells. As per recent research findings, EV release rises when cells are under infection-induced stress, influencing the host's metabolic equilibrium and potentially leading to further pathological effects. Clarification of these interactions is crucial for the development of targeted therapeutic and diagnostic approaches in parasitology, highlighting the significance of EVs here (Gavinho et al., 2019). Pathogenesis of parasitic disease is often exacerbated by the interaction between the vector and the parasite. Consider, for example, the interaction of filarial nematode *Brugia malayi* with its endosymbiotic partner, Wolbachia. The infection of Wolbachia is essential for the growth and development of *B. malayi* since it provides metabolites that are critical for survival in the nematodes. This symbiosis points to the complexities in parasitic pathogenesis as well as how parasites manage to use symbiotic associations to enhance their survivability within hosts. The genome of Wolbachia demonstrates uniform degradation compared to other bacteria and raises concerns regarding evolution and adaptation under parasitic lifestyles. Additionally, the study of these genomic features may provide insight into novel targets for treatment of associated diseases, explain host-parasite relationships and filarial disease pathogenesis. Lastly, the pathogenesis of parasitic infections is a multifaceted process that is affected by evolutionary adaptations and intricate host-parasite interactions. The dynamic extracellular vesicle release during infection highlights the capacity of the parasites to manipulate host biology, justifying the need for new research approaches to further explore these interactions. Research in symbiotic associations, such as *B. malayi* and Wolbachia, is relevant in the context of understanding parasitism evolution as well as potential avenues of intervention. This intricate web of interactions emphasizes the fact that parasitic disease knowledge requires an integrated strategy that encompasses molecular biology, immunology, and evolutionary theory. Ultimately, additional research on pathogenesis in parasitology will contribute to effective therapeutic strategies, improving public health status in parasitologically impacted populations.

6.4.1. Common Diseases Caused by Parasites

There are a great number of diseases caused by parasites, which impact humans and animals quite significantly. One of the most prevalent is infection with gastrointestinal nematodes, particularly in small ruminants , such as sheep and goats. The nematode *Haemonchus contortus* is an important pathogen with high levels of morbidity and mortality in infected animals. A study conducted in eastern Ethiopia compared the infection levels of various helminths among sheep and goats, and *H. contortus* had a high prevalence of 65-80% during wet seasons, where there was a correlation with greater fecal egg counts as well as lower packed cell volume in the host animals. This reaffirms the significant interrelation between environmental factors and parasitic infection level, calling for the understanding of local epidemiology in controlling disease in veterinary parasitology (Sissay, 2007). Zoonotic parasites create serious public health issues, contributing to a range of diseases in humans, frequently compounded by an incomplete understanding of transmission dynamics. Neglected Zoonotic Diseases (NZDs) are a group of such infections that are especially neglected, impacting the poorest in developing world regions. The population biology of such multihost parasites makes control more challenging, especially since ecological and evolutionary interactions can lead to drug resistance. The NZD study indicates that insights into host interactions and transmission routes are imperative to informing effective intervention strategies. Without a coordinated One Health approach, which brings together human, animal, and environmental health, traditional control measures like preventive chemotherapy are likely to fall short in the battle against these endemic infections (Webster et al., 2015). Prevalence of parasitic diseases highlights starkly the necessity for innovative host-directed and parasite-directed control measures. The propagation of drug resistance, particularly among helminths like *H. contortus*, requires a redevelopment of the treatment practices in veterinary clinics. Based on research, the imposition of a new management system, which includes the elimination of existing parasite infestations and alteration in grazing practices, will improve the effectiveness of commonly used anthelmintics. Through exploitation of refugia and integrated parasitic management practices, a delay in the establishment of resistance to anthelmintics is possible. This approach not only ensures the safety of animal health but also assures the sustainability of agricultural practices, hence marking the significant intersection between animal health and food security under the umbrella of general parasitology (Sissay, 2007; Webster et al., 2015) (Figure 6.12).

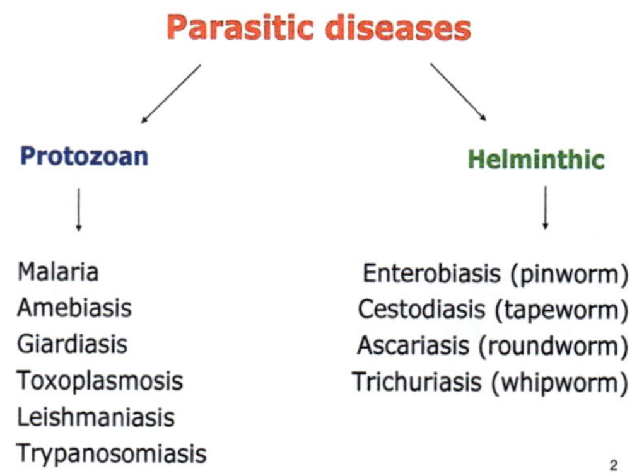

Figure 6.12. Parasitic diseases.

Source: https://slideplayer.com/slide/13260459/79/images/2/Parasitic+diseases+Protozoan+Helminthic.jpg.

6.4.2. Mechanisms of Disease Development

Disease development mechanisms in parasitic infections generally consist of complex interactions between parasite and host. One of the most important features is the ability of parasites to reorganize their life cycles in response to environmental pressures in the host. *Toxoplasma gondii*, for instance, demonstrates this adaptability through the ability to change from tachyzoite, the agent of acute infection, to bradyzoite, latent in tissue cysts. This stage transition not only protects the parasite from the host's immune response but also allows long-term transmission and survival. These stage switching mechanisms allow one to comprehend how *T. gondii* can survive and proliferate and infect a wide range of hosts, hence having a significant impact on human health and ecology (Jeffers et al., 2018). Another mechanism of disease development exists in the genetic and molecular complexity of parasites like *Trypanosoma cruzi*, the causative agent of Chagas disease. The unconventional genetic and biological features of *T. cruzi* complicate the development of effective treatments, particularly when the disease has entered its chronic phase. Genomic sequencing has identified numerous new mechanisms the parasite employs to overcome host protective mechanisms as well as adapt to the variability of different environments. This data is significant in the production of novel therapeutic solutions, especially since existing antiparasitic treatments are not particularly successful. The simple fact that *T. cruzi* has a life cycle complicated by the parasite's ability to manipulate immune responses within host organisms makes it obvious to see the need for novel solutions to address the long-standing issue this parasite poses (Vazquez, 2007). Understanding the disease processes in parasitic infections also involves an investigation of the immune response of the hosts. In the majority of cases, the immune response of the host and the interaction of the parasite determine the course of the disease. For example, in *Toxoplasma gondii* infection, the host's immune response can be effective in initially controlling the acute infection; however, poor activation of the immune system can allow the parasite to develop into the bradyzoite form, leading to chronic infection. Similarly, in Chagas' disease, *T. cruzi* can evade and hide from detection and killing by the immune system through many mechanisms , such as antigenic variation and manipulation of host cell metabolism. This intricate interaction of host and parasite discloses the dynamic nature of disease and points out where intervention could be therapeutic. Clarifying these processes is key to planning future approaches in the prevention and therapy of disease in general parasitology.

6.4.3. Impact on Public Health

The link between public health and parasitology is profound and complicated. Parasites have a significant impact on the health of humans and impose a heavy disease burden globally. In the majority of the world, particularly low- and middle-income countries, parasitic infections like malaria and schistosomiasis are among the primary concerns that lead to morbidity and mortality that strain the healthcare system and affects socioeconomic advancement. Malaria, which is due to Plasmodium spp., is a global public health issue that imposes enormous economic loss and disrupts community development. Additionally, the populations affected by such infections have demographic properties that reveal vulnerabilities, i.e., marginal and poor groups, meaning that effective public health measures will require equity as a first concern. Therapy for these infections requires an in-depth understanding of lifecycle phases and transmission routes, illustrating the necessity of interdisciplinary collaboration to devise effective control strategies that will eliminate this public health threat and promote overall societal well-being (Chalmers et al., 2016). Moreover, One Health has been an integral paradigm in addressing the public health aspects of parasitism. The philosophy embraces the interconnectedness of animal, human, and environmental health, necessitating disease prevention and control through a multidisciplinary approach. Having an understanding that parasites can shift between animals and humans underscores the necessity for surveillance and intervention efforts that go beyond classical paradigms of human health. For instance, zoonotic parasites , such as toxoplasmosis or *Leishmania*sis need collaborative efforts from veterinary and medical professionals in order to properly contain outbreaks. As the 2015 Autumn Symposium of the British Society for Parasitology stipulated, cross-disciplinary communication could usher in new avenues that enhance comprehension and management of parasitic infections (Bouwknegt et al., 2017). The successful implementation of the One Health strategy not only addresses current health issues but also prepares public health infrastructure for proactive response to future infectious hazards. Finally, education and public engagement cannot be overemphasized in the prevention and control of parasitic infections. Public health interventions should include sensitization campaigns that educate communities on transmission routes, preventive measures, and why symptoms of parasitic infection cases should be treated. These educational efforts are important for building community resilience against parasitic infection, especially in communities with limited access to health services. Empowerment with knowledge among communities promotes self-motivated health-seeking behavior and allows participatory strategies for surveillance and control measures. Furthermore, interventions done at the community level may enhance trust and collaboration among residents and health authorities and, consequently, increase the effectiveness of public health interventions. With the progress of the discipline of parasitology, it will be essential to integrate public health with education and community participation in addressing the burden that parasites present to global health (Chalmers et al., 2016).

Test Your Knowledge

1. What are some common diseases caused by parasitic infections?
2. What are the primary methods by which parasites get past the host's immune system during infection?

6.5. Diagnosis of Parasitic Infections

Learning Outcome

1. Be capable of describing laboratory techniques for the diagnosis of parasitic infections;
2. Discuss clinical signs and symptoms;
3. Highlight challenges in the diagnosis of parasitic infections.

Diagnosis of parasitic infections is a critical step in the effective control of parasitic diseases in human and veterinary medicine. Accurate diagnosis entails a combination of clinical assessments, laboratory investigations, and an understanding of epidemiological factors. Diagnosis depends on major techniques like microscopic analysis of fecal samples for helminth eggs or larvae, serological tests for antigen, and molecular tests , such as polymerase chain reaction (PCR) for the identification of specific parasites. Since parasitic infections vary geographically, the diagnostic approach may have to be tailored based on local epidemiology. The need for sensitivity and specificity of diagnosis is essential, as misdiagnosis or delayed diagnosis could enhance morbidity and economic loss, particularly in livestock within food production systems. In the past, GIN epidemiology has revealed their prevalence and economic losses on livestock that could have a direct impact on agricultural productivity. Recent studies, , such as those on small ruminants in eastern Ethiopia, have emphasized the need for detailed parasitological tests. Various parameters , such as eggs per gram of faeces (EPG), packed cell volume (PCV), and faecal culture larvae counts were utilized to assess infection burden in such studies. The findings revealed a high correlation of EPG with other parameters of health, , such as PCV and FAMACHA scores, which also reflected an integrated approach to evaluating parasite burden and animal health. An integrated diagnostic strategy is critical since it informs targeted treatments and highlights the value of ongoing health evaluations in infected herds (Sissay, 2007). In addition, the emergence of anthelmintic resistance has underscored the importance of effective diagnostic protocols, all the more in controlling and managing parasitic infestations. Studies have revealed that indiscriminate use of anthelmintics has resulted in the establishment of resistant populations, which complicates treatment and necessitates new methodologies for efficient worm control (Borges et al., 2011). Selective targeted treatment, for instance, aims to identify and treat only the animals carrying a significant parasitic load so that the efficacy of available anthelmintics is not compromised. Application of such selective measures requires accurate and prompt diagnosis so as to effectively limit the spread of resistance, thereby highlighting the widespread impact that an effective diagnostic strategy can have on both veterinary medicine and public health. Lastly, coping with the challenge of parasitic infections demands a dedicated effort to formulate diagnostic techniques that not only detect infections in time but also inform effective management protocols (Figure 6.13).

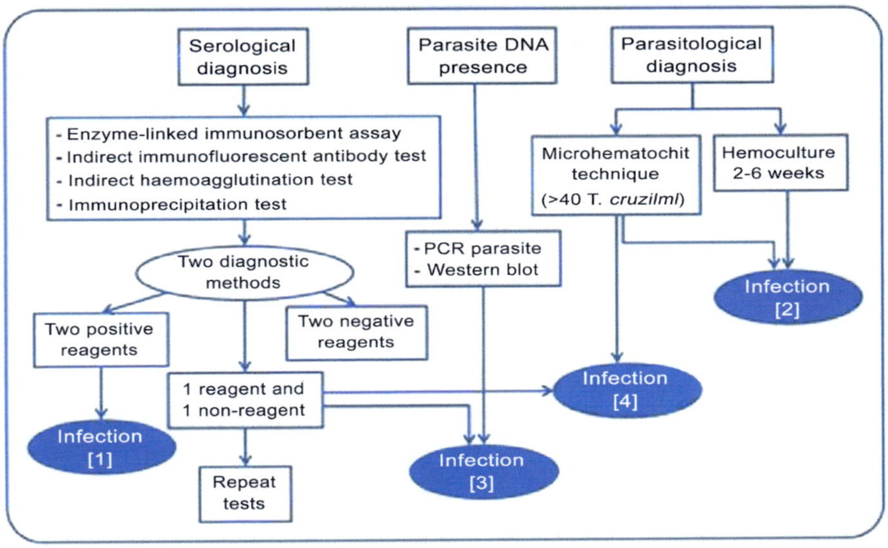

Figure 6.13. Diagnosis of Chagas disease through serology, parasite or parasite DNA detection.

Source: https://www.researchgate.net/profile/Faustino-Perez-Lopez/publication/44684316/figure/fig1/AS:601623822872589@1520449705704/Diagnosis-of-Chagas-disease-through-serology-parasite-or-parasite-DNA-detection-Two.png.

6.5.1. Laboratory Techniques for Diagnosis

Diagnosis of parasitic infections draws heavily on various laboratory methods that enable the detection and measurement of parasites in host organisms. Traditional methods , such as microscopy, remain central to the diagnostic process. The technique is direct observation of parasites in fecal samples, where eggs or larvae indicate gastrointestinal nematode infestation. In small ruminants, for instance, examination of fecal samples revealed the presence of a number of nematodes, *Haemonchus contortus* being most prevalent (Sissay, 2007). In addition to microscopic examination, nematode egg count per gram of feces (EPG) is valuable information in determining the infection level and informing treatment. It is critical to properly count EPG in that it allows veterinarians to ascertain the efficacy of anthelmintic medication as well as monitor resistance in parasitic populations. Laboratory developments have also included molecular methods, and these have immensely enhanced the diagnostic facilities in parasitology. The use of polymerase chain reaction (PCR) techniques can duplicate the target DNA sequences of parasites to ascertain their correct identification even in light infections. This is particularly valuable in the case of gastrointestinal nematodes, where infection is normally mixed and deceptive by conventional methods. In ruminant studies, molecular diagnosis has also been applied in the identification of drug resistance genes in nematodes to understand anthelmintic treatment efficacy (Borges et al., 2011). Molecular monitoring is vital in regions that are developing growing drug resistance-related issues because it facilitates early and efficient responses to risks. Through the integration of molecular techniques with traditional ones, researchers can produce an enhanced perspective of the parasite's dynamics in host populations.

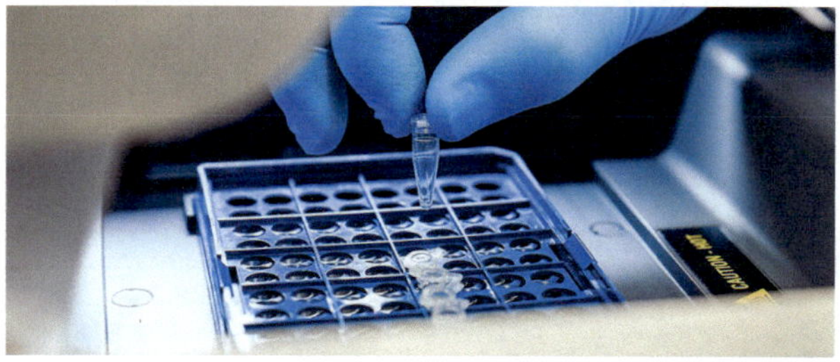

Figure 6.14. Molecular testing for parasite detection and disease diagnosis.

Source: https://todaysveterinarypractice.com/wp-content/uploads/sites/4/2021/02/TVP_MarApr21_ParasitologyPCR_MainImage.jpg.

Furthermore, through the integration of serological and haematological analyses, the diagnostic case for parasitic infection is widened. Serological analysis, which detects specific antibodies or antigens in the host, can provide insight into the host's immune response to parasitic infestation as well as systemic parasitic infection diagnosis. Concurrently, measurement of packed cell volume (PCV) can offer a secondary, indirect evaluation of parasitic infections' impact on host health, typically simultaneous with the intestinal nematode load (Sissay, 2007). Such approaches, particularly when done in tandem, can create a multifaceted view of the health and infection status of an animal. In addition, the use of specialized treatment protocols with thorough diagnostic testing can truly maximize the results in parasitology care, emphasizing the role of integrating varied laboratory procedures to better address the issue of parasitic infection management (Figure 6.14).

6.5.2. Clinical Symptoms and Signs

In parasitology, signs and symptoms are significant markers for infection, which will dictate diagnosis and treatment strategies. Parasitic infections show a range of symptoms that will be acute or chronic, based on the parasite and host immune response. Nematode infections, for instance, by *Angiostrongylus vasorum*, will present with respiratory issues, neurological abnormalities, and coagulopathy. Anorexia and gastrointestinal dysfunction are also frequently seen in infected can ids, necessitating meticulous clinical examination. Identification of specific clinical symptoms, i.e., respiratory distress and weight loss, is most important in directing further diagnostic procedures like imaging or laboratory tests towards successful parasitic disease control (Binst et al., 2011). Trichinellosis is another good example in which clinical features determine the course and severity of the infection. The zoonotic infection is caused by a rapid appearance of symptoms following the intake of infected pork, which typically leads to gastrointestinal and systemic symptoms. Clinically, the patients could have diarrhea, abdominal pain, and myalgia in the course of an average incubation period of only 9.5 days. The presence of fever and edema is a marker of a high inflammatory response to the larvae, which can indicate a high larval burden. As some outbreaks have caused hospitalization and death, it is important to understand these clinical manifestations to intervene early and respond to public health. The evidence of historical outbreaks in Vietnam supports the endemicity of this infection, which supports the importance of symptom identification to prevent recurrence (De et al., 2015). The polygenic character of clinical manifestations associated with parasitic infections highlights the quality of their impact on host health. Clinicians would be best advised to approach these cases with attention to the coalescing character of symptoms due to the fact that a majority of parasitic infections have a convergent host response. For instance, both *Trichinella spiralis* and *Angiostrongylus vasorum* infection can produce gastrointestinal and systemic manifestations, which require specific but not exclusive diagnostic criteria. The differential diagnosis requires most frequently the correlation of clinical presentation with epidemiological data, , such as feeding habits or environmental exposure. Against this background, it makes only practical sense to comprehend the clinical symptoms and signs of various parasites since, apart from being an academic exercise, it is an operational necessity that informs treatment regimens and prevention, thereby constraining the greater public health impacts of parasitic infections.

6.5.3. Challenges in Diagnosis

Parasitic infections are diagnosed with numerous challenges, which may make effective treatment and control efforts complicated. A significant one is the different life cycles of parasites, leading to fluctuating parasite loads at different seasons and developmental stages. For example, gastrointestinal nematodes can have bimodal infection patterns synchronized with environmental cues, , such as rain, so that the most suitable time for determining the status of infection cannot be ascertained for diagnostic purposes. This variability makes the establishment of an accurate notion regarding the status of infection of populations of livestock, particularly in regions afflicted by ineffectual veterinary services, challenging. Lastly, the complexity of parasite biology, as well as the effect of the environment, renders simple diagnostic processes less feasible, requiring more thoughtful and sophisticated techniques overall parasitology. Another challenge is the development of resistance to drugs within populations of parasites that complicates infection diagnosis and control of livestock. Over time, the continued use of anthelmintics has forced the evolution of resistant nematode populations, which have raised serious issues regarding the efficacy of conventional treatment protocols. Various studies have characterized how populations in Latin America, for instance, have characterized declining drug efficacy, leading to elevated mortality rates even following treatment (Borges et al., 2011).

Such resistance not only creates diagnostic challenges due to the persistence of infections but also raises ethical concerns regarding animal welfare and agricultural sustainability. Thus, researchers advocate improving diagnostic techniques and anthelmintic strategies to provide effective as well as responsible targeted therapies. The excessive reliance on traditional diagnostic methods, , such as fecal egg counts, also presents a significant challenge in accurately quantifying the impact of parasitic infections. Although these methods provide valuable data on infection levels, they may not adequately inform us regarding the dynamic nature of parasitic loads or host reactions. For instance, a detailed epidemiological study in sheep and goats from different geographic locations revealed considerable variation in the burden of gastrointestinal nematodes, which demonstrated how conditions in a given location can be very influential upon infection prevalence (Sissay, 2007). These observations underscore the necessity of inclusive diagnostic approaches that encompass both molecular and phenotypic markers. By casting a coherent image of infection patterns and synthesizing heterogeneous diagnostic approaches, researchers would be better able to address the challenges posed by parasitism in agriculture.

Test Your Knowledge

1. What are the most common laboratory techniques used to diagnose parasitic infections, and how do their sensitivity and specificity differ?
2. How can clinical symptomatology and patient history assist in initial suspicion of a parasitic infection?

6.6. Treatment and Control of Parasitic Infections

Learning Outcome

1. Acknowledge the role of antiparasitic drugs in controlling parasitic infections;
2. Discuss public health interventions and preventive measures;
3. Explain the role of vaccines in parasitology.

Effective treatment and control of parasitic infections are important to minimize their impact on animal health and productivity. Parasitic infestations, as expressed by gastrointestinal nematodes and liver fluke, have the capability to result in significant economic losses in agricultural production regions through compromising animal growth, milk production, and body condition. Approximately 70% of dairy herds reported high exposure to gastrointestinal nematodes, and consistent prevalence of liver fluke at approximately 30% from a 2009–2011 Belgian longitudinal survey (Charlier et al., 2013). These data mirror the endemicity of such infections and therefore the relevance of evidence-based intervention policies. Control strategies that account for geographical disparities in parasite exposure will maximize the efficacy of treatment models. Therefore, the organization of such programs should revolve around accurate monitoring and timely delivery of effective anthelmintics, as well as management strategies aimed at the environmental determinants facilitating parasite transmission. Anthelmintic treatment remains the cornerstone of parasitic infection management in livestock, but resistance against these drugs has emerged as a serious issue. Misuse or excessive use of anthelmintics leads to the emergence of resistance, which ultimately results in the failure of treatment and carries-over parasite populations. A study conducted at Götala Beef and Lamb Research Centre illustrated the stark differences in health performance between treated and untreated steers, a factor which indicated that the latter realized significantly higher weight gains while grazing compared to their infected counterparts (Johansson, 2017). Therefore, measures for preventing resistance, for instance, rotation among distinct classes of anthelmintics and including non-chemical control strategies, should be prioritized in treatment regimens. These approaches ensure anthelmintic effectiveness is not impaired but also provide sustainable parasite control in animal populations. Apart from pharmacological practices, behavioral and environmental factors need to be included in the treatment and parasitic infection control. Host behavior changes in the infected animals can provide input towards understanding the effectiveness of the treatment strategy. Observations have indicated that parasitized steers exhibit changes in activity level and social interaction, potentially changing overall herd dynamics and productivity (Johansson,

2017). These behavioral characteristics can indicate rising parasitic burdens that, if left uncontrolled, have the potential to exacerbate health deteriorations in herds. Behavioral data inclusion within monitoring schemes can offer enhanced insights into infestation dynamics and enhance management practices. In addition, integration of overall pasture management, e.g., rotational grazing and proper fecal management, can alleviate parasite loads and interrupt life cycles. Thus, promotion of an integrated approach that synthesizes pharmacological therapies with environmental and behavioral controls is critical for effective parasitic disease control in livestock.

6.6.1. Antiparasitic Medications

The role of antiparasitic drugs is central to the control of parasitic infections, which are of enormous health importance globally. These medications are employed either to kill parasites within the host or inhibit parasite development, and they are applied based on the parasite targeted. Antiparasitic drugs, for example, can be applied prophylactically, as a preventive measure against infections among risk populations, or therapeutically, as therapy for existing infections. A study in Paraguay testified to the extremely prevalent presence of "parasites" among patients, since 46% of patients diagnosed with these were prescribed antiparasitic medication. Interestingly, 78% of those who underwent screening for prophylactic application failed to be administered the medications they required, testifying to systemic barriers in health delivery. This difference highlights the necessity for a holistic approach that reconciles the benefits of preventive as well as curative antiparasitic practices to meet the omnipresent challenge of parasitic infection among vulnerable populations (Eick et al., 2013). Understanding the proper use of antiparasitic medications is a mandatory aspect of public health interventions among parasitologically high-risk populations. A Mexican study revealed that preventive knowledge was present in 72% of infected homes but with great lack of awareness in the use of proper treatments. The findings show a huge educational gap in health-seeking behavior, where infected individuals tend to accept parasitism as something part of life which cannot be avoided but only accepted. This emphasizes the necessity to create education campaigns that sensitize populations to the therapeutic benefits of antiparasitic medications, not only their potential in curative treatment of infections, but also in disease prevention. Increased awareness has the potential to be translated into increased compliance and improved levels of health among populations where parasitic infection is a concern (Faulkner et al., 1998). In addition, the effectiveness of antiparasitic medication relies considerably on health care access and socio-economic status. For instance, delivery of antiparasitic medicines can often be hindered by such logistical aspects as shortages of materials, erratic healthcare facilities, and absence of skilled medical personnel. The results of the Paraguay research clarify that treatment was provided to only half of those who were recommended, and it questions the systemic factors in effect more generally. Future efforts need to focus on building up local medical facilities as well as making sure there are sufficient supplies of antiparasitic drugs available to serve at-risk groups. Furthermore, implementing antiparasitic therapy regimens in conjunction with improved sanitation measures and community participation will most likely offer more efficient prevention, treatment, and eventually eradication of intestinal parasites (Eick et al., 2013) (Figure 6.15).

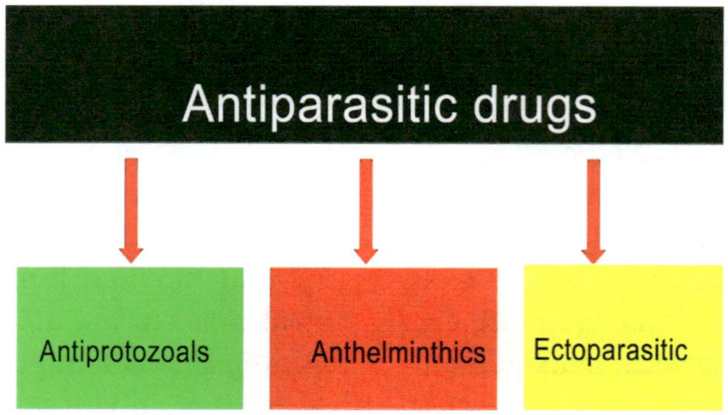

Figure 6.15. Antiparasitic drug.

Source: https://5.imimg.com/data5/SELLER/Default/2024/2/393950115/SW/II/UB/33400885/antiparasitic-drug.jpg.

6.6.2. Preventive Measures and Public Health Strategies

In general parasitology, preventive measures and public health interventions are critical in containing and controlling the impact of parasitic infestations on animal and human populations. Effective prevention tactics rely on a complete understanding of parasite life cycles and transmission patterns. For instance, utilizing stringent biosecurity practices in fields can reduce parasite transmission rates in livestock in an effective manner. These controls include proper sanitation, limited access to grazing areas, and regular health inspection of animals. These measures not only safeguard the well-being of individual animals but also safeguard the broader ecosystem by minimizing the risk of zoonotic disease spillovers affecting human populations. Other control measures have been increasingly popular in recent years, particularly in response to concerns regarding chemical treatments and their long-term effectiveness. Research has revealed the value of non-chemical solutions , such as biological control and pasture management, as hopeful avenues for sustainable parasitic control. Research into phytotherapy and the integration of bioactive forages presents a modern solution that could hold great potential for the therapy of resistant parasites. As per the literature, these emerging treatments hold promise but simultaneously reinforce the necessity of rigorous scientific confirmation to gauge their efficacy and viability across various farming systems (Rahmann et al., 2006). Second, the concept of a One Health approach is imperative in dealing with the interlinked relations among human, animal, and environmental well-being. Understanding the population biology of multihost parasites is critical in planning targeted public health interventions, particularly in nations burdened by neglected zoonotic diseases (NZDs). Coordination of veterinary and medical interventions can streamline our intervention for such diseases, particularly in developing countries where resource constraints always hamper effective control strategies. Through the understanding of complex interactions between human and animal reservoirs, public health can design more holistic responses with regard to ecological drivers of disease spread. As noted, NZD prevention depends on accurate study of transmission dynamics for modifying interventions accordingly, thereby improving health outcomes across and among species and habitats (Webster et al., 2015).

6.6.3. Role of Vaccines in Parasitology

Vaccination becomes more and more a central aspect of parasitology, especially since other traditional control methods, i.e., antiparasitic drugs, are faced with problems , such as drug resistance. For most parasites, especially helminths and protozoa, the development of good vaccines can become an important alternative for chemical therapy and foster sustainable control measures. Recently, the efficacy of vaccines has been demonstrated to manage parasitic disease that not only infects livestock but also significantly influences agricultural production on a huge economic scale. These diseases generally comprise complex life cycles and host-parasite relationships and hence, the development of vaccines is of concern to researchers working in this area. By helping to alleviate the load of such parasites, vaccines can thus improve the health and productivity of animals, with cascading effects on food security and economic stability in nation-states that depend considerably on livestock production. Vaccine development against specific parasitic infections has been suggested in a number of animal model systems, as in research involving organisms like *Neospora caninum*. This intracellular protozoan has been known to trigger substantial reproductive issues in some cattle herds, leading to enormous economic losses. Efforts to construct a recombinant subunit vaccine using the N. caninum antigen NcSRS2 reflect the potential of well-designed vaccines to induce appropriate immune responses against parasitic infection. Laboratory results revealed that such vaccines had the potential to significantly reduce parasitic DNA levels in infected animals to make them feasible. Besides, the ability of the vaccine to induce humoral and cellular immune responses suggests a multi-sided strategy that can confer stronger defense against such a complex parasite, paving the way for potential application in bovine health control (Pinitkiatisakul, 2007). In referring to the cumulative impact of vaccines, consideration must be given to their use in comprehensive disease control measures, especially as regards the issue of anthelmintic resistance in parasites. In Malaysia, for example, studies have found the emergence of resistance to commonly used anthelmintics in small ruminants to be a cause of significant concern, hence the implication of introducing new control measures. Methods that combine biological controls, , such as the use of nematophagous fungi like *Duddingtonia flagrans*, with vaccination methods can offer a sustainable exit. Taking the strengths of both biological and vaccine-based methods, farmers would be able to successfully reduce reliance on chemical controls. Hence, vaccines are not isolated products but a core component of an overall strategy against parasitic disease to achieve animal welfare and agricultural resilience in the face of progressing threats (Panchadcharam, 2004).

Test Your Knowledge

1. What are the major categories of antiparasitic drugs, and how do they act against different types of parasites?
2. What are the preventative measures that can be undertaken to restrict the transmission of parasitic diseases in endemic areas?

SUMMARY

In summarizing the general parasitology overview, it is imperative to note the significance of host-parasite interactions in determining ecological and health factors. This interactivity impacts the immediate hosts themselves but also has broader implications for agricultural productivity and economic sustainability. For instance, research indicates that immune reactions can significantly reduce the migratory larvae's population in hosts , such as pigs, affirming the delicate interaction between defense systems and parasitic infestations. Such findings suggest that the understanding of such interactions is crucial for the development of efficient management programs for lowering both health risks and financial losses incurred due to parasitic infestations, particularly in livestock populations (Chiers et al., 2013). In addition, the urgent need for sustainable solutions to parasite control should not be overstated, especially in light of mounting resistance to the conventional anthelmintics. The change towards non-chemical methods of control, including biological control and prudent management of pastures, offers potential for reducing dependence on drugs without compromising animal and environmental ill health. With the focus on alternative therapy , such as phytotherapy, researchers have established the promising potential of natural products to combat endoparasites in small ruminants. This novel shift provokes researchers to go further with the use of sustainable products that are harmonious with modern agricultural systems and tackle public concerns about chemical residue contamination and parasite resistance (Rahmann et al., 2006). Lastly, the incorporation of present research puts forth a demand for continuous research within the subject of parasitology, particularly host immunity and non-conventional methods of treatment. In reconciling findings of fragmented studies, it is understood that a general multi-dimensional approach must be taken to deal with the complexity of parasite control. Subsequent research needs to concentrate not only on validation of other interventions but also on building increased understanding around host defense, for example, as demonstrated through eosinophilic responses to infection (Chiers et al., 2013). Ultimately, gaining a better understanding of these interconnected themes will help stakeholders utilize more optimal solutions to ensure not only the health of livestock but also the long-term sustainability of agricultural practice as we move forward in addressing parasitic infection issues.

When approaching the complexities of parasitology, one should recognize the multifaceted interactions present between hosts and their parasitic counterparts. One of the topics of greatest concern is gastrointestinal nematode-livestock interaction, and this has been addressed traditionally through the utilization of anthelmintic drugs. Drug resistance renders it imperative to develop novel management plans. Scientists are investigating new alternatives , such as vaccination, supplementation, and selective breeding, aimed at enhancing the immunological response of the host. The application of fecal egg counts (FEC) to determine the intensity of infection is limited by inaccuracies, and it calls for novel markers that will provide more reliable measures of resistance by the host against parasites, in view of current studies (Mair et al., 2014). The ecology of host-parasite interactions extends beyond resistance and incorporates resource allocation and optimal parasite burdens in communities. A great deal of the significant research focuses on the host-parasite trade-off between investment in growth and immunity. Evidence suggests that there is a parasite burden at which hosts gain by allowing certain infections while they preserve overall health and reproductive return. For example, increased resource acquisition tends to give hosts the ability to spend more on immunity, giving rise to a cryptic interaction in which increased pathogenicity leads to lower optimum parasite loads and heightened exposure raises the acceptable infection level (Medley, 2002). This kind of paradigm underscores the necessity of model integration to be able to understand these dynamics. Furthermore, the meanings of these findings have broad implications for future research directions in general parasitology. An understanding of host condition-parasite burden relationship reveals a complexity of epidemiological patterns that are not reducible to unidimensional accounts. To present an example, it is anticipated that there is increased heterogeneity of parasite burdens among populations due to differential resource acquisition and exposure. This highlights the complicated and usually confusing interactions that demand robust analytical approaches. Generally, learning in this field not only enriches scholarship but also offers pragmatic information to improve livestock better and fight parasitic infections more effectively by sound planning and specific interventions (Medley, 2002; Mair et al., 2014).

KEY TERMS FROM THIS CHAPTER

- Anthelmintics
- Bioactive forages
- Density-dependent forces
- Diverse environments
- General parasitology
- Helminth infection
- Host-parasite relationships
- Immunity immunomodulation
- Neglected zoonotic diseases
- Osmoregulatory function
- Antiparasitic drugs
- Biological control
- Disease transmission dynamics
- Ectoparasites
- Global health emergencies
- Helminthology
- Immune system
- Microscopic protozoa
- NZD-related issues
- Parasite-host relationships

CRITICAL THINKING QUESTIONS

1. **What one of the following is an example of an ectoparasite?**
   a. *Plasmodium falciparum*
   b. *Giardia lamblia*
   c. *Pediculus humanus capitis*
   d. *Taenia solium*
2. **What term is used to describe a parasite that requires two or more hosts to finish its life cycle?**
   a. Facultative parasite
   b. Obligate parasite
   c. Direct life cycle parasite
   d. Indirect life cycle parasite
3. **Which host is usually responsible for sexual reproduction of parasites , such as Plasmodium?**
   a. Intermediate host
   b. Definitive host
   c. Paratenic host
   d. Accidental host
4. **A key mechanism through which parasites avoid host immunity is:**
   a. Inducing host fever
   b. Mimicking host antigens
   c. Increasing host RBC count
   d. Releasing digestive enzymes
5. **What is the definitive host in a parasite's life cycle?**
   a. A host where sexual reproduction occurs
   b. A host that harbors the larval stage
   c. A host where asexual reproduction occurs
   d. A host temporarily used for transport

Short Answer Questions

1. Differentiate between obligate parasites and facultative parasites, and give a single example for each.
2. Define the life cycle of *Plasmodium falciparum* in both its human and mosquito hosts.
3. Define the role of the intermediate host and definitive host in parasitic life cycles. Provide an example of each for *Taenia solium*.
4. What are the diagnostic tests most commonly utilized to detect *Giardia lamblia* infection? List at least two methods and how they work.

5. Establish three public health actions to control soil-transmitted helminth transmission.
6. Describe how travel across the world and climate change may influence the epidemiology of parasitic infections.

Answer to Critical Thinking Questions

1. (c); 2. (d); 3. (b); 4. (b); 5. (a)

REFERENCES

1. Moreira, M., Schrama, D., Soares, F., Wulff, T., Pousão-Ferreira, P., & Rodrigues, P. (2017). Physiological responses of reared sea bream (Sparus aurata Linnaeus, 1758) to an Amyloodinium ocellatum outbreak. *Journal of fish diseases, 40*(11), 1545–1560. https://doi.org/10.1111/jfd.12623 (accessed on 13th June 2025).
2. Acosta, L., Evans, M. D., Izquierdo, F., Magnet, A., et al. (2019). *Virtual Libraries of Tissue and Clinical Samples: Potential Role of a 3-D Microscope.* https://core.ac.uk/download/228195067.pdf (accessed on 13th June 2025).
3. Webster, J. P., Gower, C. M., Knowles, S. C., Molyneux, D. H., & Fenton, A. (2016). One health - an ecological and evolutionary framework for tackling Neglected Zoonotic Diseases. *Evolutionary applications, 9*(2), 313–333. https://doi.org/10.1111/eva.12341(accessed on 13th June 2025).
4. Akman, M., Lapidus, A., Altschul, S., Altschul, S., Amiri, M., Bhattacharyya, A., et al. (2005). *The Wolbachia Genome of Brugia malayi: Endosymbiont Evolution within a Human Pathogenic Nematode.* https://core.ac.uk/download/pdf/3629105.pdf (accessed on 13th June 2025).
5. Alizon, S., Barclay, V., Bell, A., Berngruber, T., Blanquart, F., Buckling, A., Bull, J., et al. (2013). *Killing Them Softly: Managing Pathogen Polymorphism and Virulence in Spatially Variable Environments.* https://core.ac.uk/download/28972996.pdf (accessed on 13th June 2025).
6. Anonymous, Baker, R. L., & Gray, G. D. (2025). *Worm Control for Small Ruminants in Tropical Asia.* https://core.ac.uk/download/pdf/6698925.pdf (accessed on 13th June 2025).
7. Ay, F., Fonseca, L. L., Galinski, M. R., Joyner, C., et al. (2018). *Plasmodium Knowlesi: A Superb In Vivo Nonhuman Primate Model of Antigenic Variation in Malaria.* https://core.ac.uk/download/323067423.pdf (accessed on 13th June 2025).
8. Binst, D., Claerebout, E., Daminet, S., Moeremans, B., et al. (2011). *Canine Angiostrongylus vasorum.* https://core.ac.uk/download/55801348.pdf (accessed on 13th June 2025).
9. Borges, F. de A., Chagas, A. C. de S., Fortes, F. S., Geldhof, P., et al. (2011). *Challenges of Nematode Control in Ruminants: Focus on Latin America.* https://core.ac.uk/download/55744143.pdf (accessed on 13th June 2025).
10. Borlase, A., Rudge, J. W., & Webster, J. P. (2017). *Opportunities and Challenges for Modelling Epidemiological and Evolutionary Dynamics in A Multihost, Multiparasite System: Zoonotic Hybrid Schistosomiasis in West Africa.* https://core.ac.uk/download/143477770.pdf (accessed on 13th June 2025).
11. Bouwknegt, M., Devleesschauwer, B., Dorny, P., Gabriël, S., et al. (2017). *Risk Ranking of Foodborne Parasites: State of the Art.* https://core.ac.uk/download/147046450.pdf (accessed on 13th June 2025).
12. Bresalier, M., Cassidy, A., Mason Dentinger, R., Woods, A., et al. (2017). *Animals and the Shaping of Modern Medicine: One Health and its Histories.* https://core.ac.uk/download/151259491.pdf (accessed on 13th June 2025).
13. Bush, A. O., Ferreira, S. C. M., Foreyt, W. J., Hofer, H., Kruuk, H., R Core Team, Roff, D., et al. (2019). *Parasite Infections in A Social Carnivore: Evidence of Their Fitness Consequences and Factors Modulating Infection Load.* https://core.ac.uk/download/225124809.pdf (accessed on 13th June 2025).

14. Hoole, D., Carter, V., & Dufour, S. (2010). Ligula intestinalis (Cestoda: Pseudophyllidea): an ideal fish-metazoan parasite model?. *Parasitology, 137*(3), 425–438. https://doi.org/10.1017/S0031182010000107 (accessed on 13th June 2025).

15. Chalmers, D., Blake, D. P., Fernandez Martin, A., Holland, C., Hosein, A., Johansen, M. V., Jones, B., et al. (2016). *One Health: Parasites and beyond.* https://core.ac.uk/download/76980844.pdf (accessed on 13th June 2025).

16. Charlier, J., Forbes, A. B., & Vercruysse, J. (2008). *A Survey of The Exposure to Ostertagia ostertagi in Dairy Cow Herds in Europe Through the Measurement of Antibodies in Milk Samples from The Bulk Tank.* https://core.ac.uk/download/55781452.pdf (accessed on 13th June 2025).

17. Charlier, J., Meyns, T., Soenen, K., Vercruysse, J., et al. (2013). *Monitoring Gastrointestinal Nematode and Liver Fluke Infections in Belgium by Bulk Tank Milk ELISA: Are We Making Progress in Parasite Control?* https://core.ac.uk/download/55844341.pdf (accessed on 13th June 2025).

18. Chiers, K., Geldhof, P., Masure, D., Van Den Broeck, W., et al. (2013). *A Role for Eosinophils in The Intestinal Immunity Against Infective Ascaris suum Larvae.* https://core.ac.uk/download/55807127.pdf (accessed on 13th June 2025).

19. De, N. V., Dorny, P., Dung, D. T., Minh, N. T., et al. (2015). *Trichinellosis in Vietnam.* https://core.ac.uk/download/55846724.pdf (accessed on 13th June 2025).

20. Eick, R. A. (2013). *Parasites in Paraguay: An Analysis of The Presentation and Management of Intestinal Parasites by Short-Term Medical Mission Volunteers in Paraguay.* https://core.ac.uk/download/36744120.pdf (accessed on 13th June 2025).

21. Etchegoin, J. A., Merlo, M. J., & Parietti, M. (2013). *Can the Studies at A Spatial Scale of 100s Meters Detect the Spatiotemporal Fluctuations of a Parasite Assemblage?* https://core.ac.uk/download/159284655.pdf (accessed on 13th June 2025).

22. Faulkner, C. T. (1998). *Household Management of Endo Parasitic Infection in A Border Community in Tamaulipas, Mexico.* https://core.ac.uk/download/268790840.pdf (accessed on 13th June 2025).

23. Gavinho, B., Combes, V., Dlugonska, H., Hart, E., Evans-Osses, I., Rossi, I. V., Inal, J., et al. (2019). *A New Landscape of Host–Protozoa Interactions Involving the Extracellular Vesicles World.* https://core.ac.uk/download/287580982.pdf (accessed on 13th June 2025).

24. Hafer-Hahmann, N. (2019). *Behavior Out of Control: Experimental evolution of Resistance to Host Manipulation.* https://core.ac.uk/download/231718168.pdf (accessed on 13th June 2025).

25. Helm, B., & Martinez-Bakker, M. (2015). *The Influence of Biological Rhythms on Host–Parasite Interactions.* https://core.ac.uk/download/42361213.pdf (accessed on 13th June 2025).

26. Hersh, M. H., LaDeau, S. L., Ostfeld, R. S., Previtali, M. A., et al. (2014). *When is a Parasite Not a Parasite? Effects of Larval Tick Burdens on White-Footed Mouse Survival.* https://core.ac.uk/download/159286852.pdf (accessed on 13th June 2025).

27. Jardine, B. (2019). *The Museum in The Lab: Historical Practice in The Experimental Sciences at Cambridge, 1874–1936.* https://core.ac.uk/download/334601514.pdf (accessed on 13th June 2025).

28. Jeffers, V., Kim, K., Sullivan, W. J., Jr., et al. (2018). *A Latent Ability to Persist: Differentiation in Toxoplasma gondii.* https://core.ac.uk/download/228066154.pdf (accessed on 13th June 2025).
29. Johansson, L. (2017). *The Impact of Gastrointestinal Parasites on Weight Gain, Activity Patterns and Behaviors in Cattle on Pasture.* https://core.ac.uk/download/161988609.pdf (accessed on 13th June 2025).
30. Kasl, E. L. (2016). *Phylogenetic Relationships in The Genus Alloglossidium (Digenea: Plagiorchioidea): Evolutionary Origins and Implications of Changes in Life Cycle Complexity.* https://core.ac.uk/download/79653939.pdf (accessed on 13th June 2025).
31. Mair, C., Marion, G., Matthews, L., Prada Jimenez de Cisneros, J., et al. (2014). *An Explicit Immunogenetic Model of Gastrointestinal Nematode Infection in Sheep.* https://core.ac.uk/download/42354689.pdf (accessed on 13th June 2025).
32. Marriot, A., Talisuna, A., Dondorp, A. M., Whitty, C., Cambodia National Institute of Public Health, Cambodia National Institute of Public Health, Cambodia National Institute of Public Health, & Malaria Consortium, et al. (2011). *Socially-Marketed Rapid Diagnostic Tests and ACT in the Private Sector: Ten Years of Experience in Cambodia.* https://core.ac.uk/download/2732099.pdf (accessed on 13th June 2025).
33. Medley, G. (2002). *The Epidemiological Consequences of Optimization of The Individual Host Immune Response.* https://core.ac.uk/download/48712.pdf (accessed on 13th June 2025).
34. Mejer, H., Nejsum, P., Roepstorff, A., Thamsborg, S. M., et al. (2011). *Helminth Parasites in Pigs: New Challenges in Pig Production and Current Research Highlights.* https://core.ac.uk/download/10931740.pdf (accessed on 13th June 2025).
35. Panchadcharam, C. (2004). *Problems in The Control of Nematode Parasites of Small Ruminants in Malaysia.* https://core.ac.uk/download/11694711.pdf (accessed on 13th June 2025).
36. Pinitkiatisakul, S. (2007). *Recombinant Subunit Vaccines Against Neospora caninum.* https://core.ac.uk/download/11695141.pdf (accessed on 13th June 2025).
37. Rahmann, G., & Seip, H. (2006). *Alternative Strategies to Prevent and Control Endoparasite Diseases in Organic Sheep and Goat Farming Systems–A Review of Current Scientific Knowledge.* https://core.ac.uk/download/10925183.pdf (accessed on 13th June 2025).
38. Rousing, T. (2011). *Final Report for Project no. 1904. Prevention of Selected Diseases and Parasites in Organic Pig Herds–By Means of HACCP Based Management and Surveillance Programmed (CorePig).* https://core.ac.uk/download/10932162.pdf (accessed on 13th June 2025).
39. Sissay, M. M. (2007). *Helminth Parasites of Sheep and Goats in Eastern Ethiopia.* https://core.ac.uk/download/11695158.pdf (accessed on 13th June 2025).
40. Vaughan, D. B. (2018). *Cleaner Shrimp as Biocontrol's in Aquaculture.* https://core.ac.uk/download/303788585.pdf (accessed on 13th June 2025).
41. Vazquez, M. P. (2007). *The Genetics and Genomics of Trypanosoma cruzi.* https://core.ac.uk/download/224998273.pdf (accessed on 13th June 2025).

PROTOZOAN INFECTIONS

7

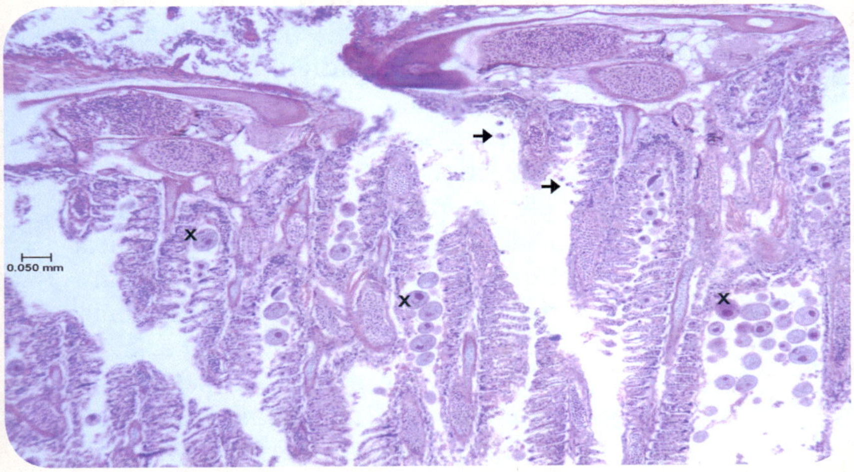

LEARNING OBJECTIVES

After studying this chapter, you will be able to:

1. Explain types of protozoan infections;
2. Explain transmission of protozoan infections;
3. Name symptoms of protozoan infections;
4. Explain the treatment of protozoan infections;
5. Prevent protozoan infections;
6. Give special consideration to the impact of protozoan infections on global health.

Introduction

Protozoan infections are a serious global health concern, infecting millions of individuals, particularly in tropical and subtropical regions. They are caused by unicellular organisms, specifically members of the *Trypanosoma* genus, *Plasmodium*, and *Leishmania*, among others. Some of the protozoan diseases have been classified as neglected tropical diseases because of the insufficient research and funding for their prevention and cure by the World Health Organization, for instance, malaria and Chagas disease. The epidemiology of such infections—ranging from diversity of life cycle to modes of transmission—coupled with the socio-economic characterization of the affected areas, magnifies their impact. The aim of this chapter is to explore the multi-dimensionality of protozoan infections, discuss transmission vectors, and identify challenges in their epidemiology and control, highlighting the compelling need for continuous research and public health interventions. These findings highlight the critical interaction between socio-environmental circumstances and protozoan infection transmission. For instance, vector-borne diseases caused by protozoan parasites have increasingly been observed in areas where ecological disturbance has occurred and, consequently, human exposure to infected vectors becomes elevated. A case in point is Chagas disease, in which the *Trypanosoma cruzi* parasite is transmitted primarily through feces of the triatomine bugs and infects millions in Latin America. In spite of remarkable progress in understanding its epidemiology, gaps in treatment continue to exist, exposing millions of people to the risk of acquiring serious health complications. The ongoing research to characterize the disease transmission dynamics provides useful information to design focused interventions and manage outbreaks effectively, identifying the contribution of interdisciplinary approaches to controlling protozoan infections (Sherman, 2019). The use of state-of-the-art diagnostic equipment and techniques has the ability to revolutionize the diagnosis and management of protozoan infections. A case in point is the utilization of high-throughput microfluidic real-time PCR technology that has been able to successfully describe tick-borne pathogen diversity in places like the Caribbean. This progress enables extensive epidemiological studies, offering rapid and reliable information needed to assess the risk of disease emergence and inform public health response. Perhaps most significantly, the ability to identify not only familiar pathogens but also novel microorganisms can significantly enhance our understanding of the ever-changing world of protozoan threats and their vectors. By integrating these advanced methodologies into surveillance programs, researchers can better forecast patterns of infection and develop timely interventions to reverse the impact of protozoan infections (Albina et al., 2020).

Definition of Protozoan Infections

Protozoan infections are caused by a single-celled eukaryotic parasite known as protozoa, which exist in numerous habitats, soil, water, and living hosts. These infectious agents may be classified into various groups based on their modes of locomotion , such as amoebae, flagellates, ciliates, and sporozoans. Protozoan infections are largely caused by food and water contamination with feces or by vectors like mosquitoes and ticks. These infective agents may utilize human hosts, particularly among immunocompromised individuals, to cause illness ranging from mild gastrointestinal upsets to severe systemic infections. Therefore, protozoan infections' public health significance is very important, particularly in regions of poor sanitation and health care accessibility. Clinical presentations of protozoan infections are highly varied and affect various organ systems. Diarrhea, abdominal pain, fever, and weakness are typical presenting symptoms, which are always related to such infections as amoebic dysentery and *Giardia*sis. Diarrhea, which is the result of some protozoan infections, is hazardous, especially in susceptible individuals, and contributes to high mortality and morbidity rates among children. In fact, diarrheal disease resulting from protozoa is a major cause of death in children throughout the world, hence the importance of knowing the causative pathogens. Against these infections, timely and appropriate interventions , such as rehydration therapy and antimicrobial medication are crucial in symptom management and prevention of further complications resulting from protracted illness (Caramia et al., 2015). Further, the ecological context of protozoan infections directs towards an intricate relationship among environmental determinants, host susceptibility, and successful transmission dynamics. For example, soil environments harbor diverse protozoa, which also find themselves as opportunistic pathogens when humans are exposed from infested materials. Soil's role in hosting such pathogenic organisms indicates the interrelation between the health of the environment and the health of human beings, necessitating prevention measures that are holistic in nature. In addition, community-level public health interventions aimed at increased sanitation, improved supply of safe water, and community education can regulate the prevalence of protozoan infections. As newer research uncovers the complexity of protozoan biology and transmission, it is important to develop targeted methods and interventions in a bid to combat these infections effectively, ultimately reducing their count and impact on world health (LEE et al., 2011) (Figure 7.1).

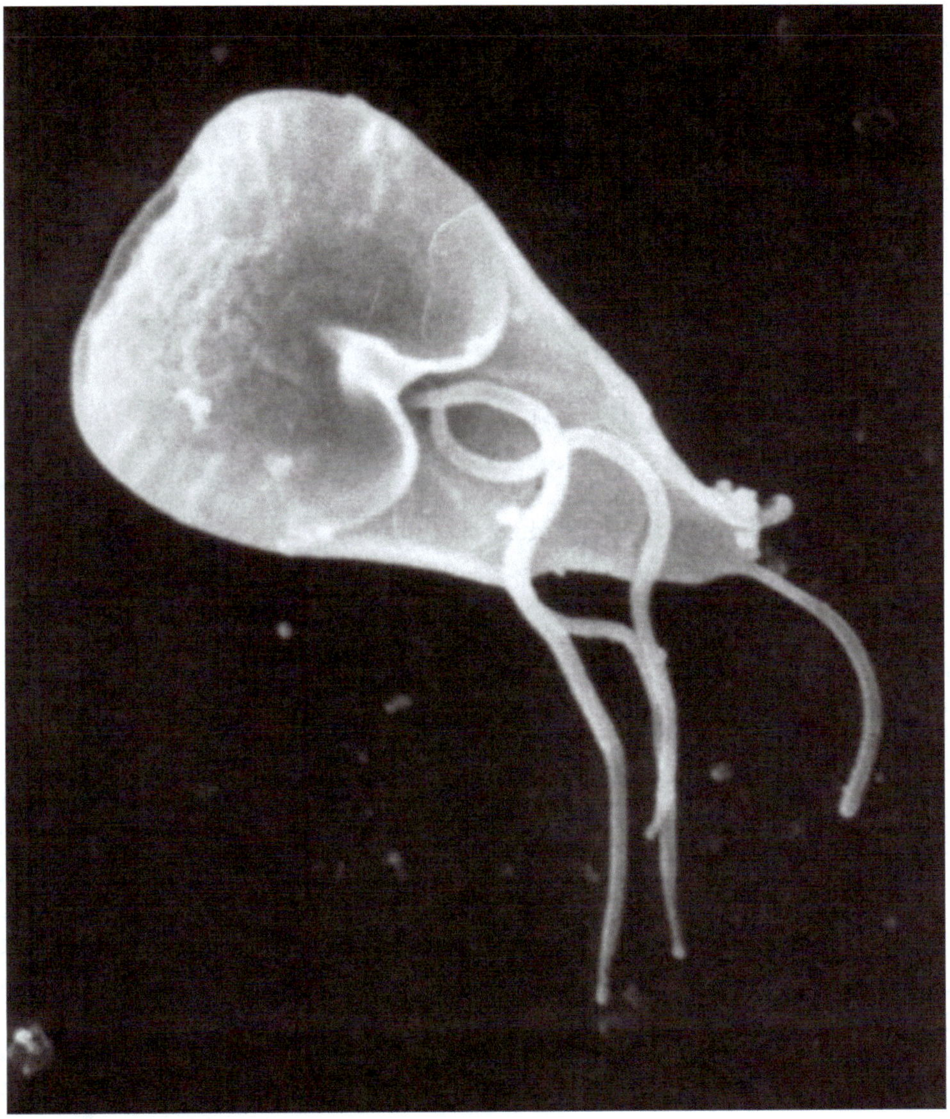

Figure 7.1. *Giardia lamblia*, an infectious protozoan.

Source: https://upload.wikimedia.org/wikipedia/commons/0/08/*Giardia*_lamblia_SEM_8698_lores.jpg.

Importance of Studying Protozoan Infections

The research into protozoan diseases is of extreme importance to both public health and epidemiology due to their pervasive impact on human health. Protozoans , such as *Toxoplasma gondii* and other malaria-causing species have implications that reach far beyond the health of the individual. As evidenced by the varying prevalence trends of *Schistosoma* spp. and intestinal protozoan infections, the prevalence of these infections is highly variable according to geographic and socioeconomic situations, emphasizing the necessity for target public health interventions (Coulibaly et al., 2012). Understanding how these pathogens are distributed among different groups will enable health workers to formulate effective prevention and control measures. Besides, the study of protozoan infections also helps in the understanding of vector dynamics and host-parasite interactions within ecosystems, which can inform environmental health programs and highlight the interlinkages among human, animal, and environmental health. Further significance in learning about protozoan infections is brought by the fact that these infections are able to cause morbidity and mortality not only in humans but in domestic and wild populations as well (Bahia-Oliveira et al., 2019). The zoonotic character of protozoan diseases demands a multidisciplinary approach to research and control involving veterinary sciences, environmental science, and human health perspectives. Because some protozoan infections have the capability of surviving within multiple environments—, such as the capability of surviving in several foods and environments by *T. gondiis* transmission dynamics need to be interpreted (Bahia-Oliveira et al., 2019). By describing transmission routes, researchers can identify intervention hotspots, preventing outbreaks in the process. The intricate dynamics between the settings and transmission vectors also attest to the need for extensive research in this field. Lastly, protozoan infection is a major public health problem that is being compounded by globalization, urbanization, and dynamic environmental changes. Knowing these infections enables the health authorities to predict and respond to new threats posed by protozoan diseases, which may mutate to take on new hosts or environments as global conditions are altered. The observed trends of compound infections, particularly in rural areas, show the complexity of managing these diseases and the necessity for ongoing surveillance programs that account for geographic variation in infection rates (Coulibaly et al., 2012). This alertness is essential to ensuring the health and welfare of risk groups. The value of studying protozoan infections thus cannot be overstated, for it gives us the ability and tools required to cope with an ever-evolving world of contagious disease.

7.1. Types of Protozoan Infections

Learning Outcome

1. Define amoebic infections;
2. Describe flagellate infections;
3. Describe ciliate infections.

The types of protozoan infections can be classified into different distinct types, predominantly separated based on their methods of transmission and body systems affected. Among the common ones is the flagellates, which are characterized by their whip-like appendages to enable movement. The prototype is that of *Trypanosoma cruzi*, the causative agent of Chagas disease, passed by the feces of triatomine bugs. The infection follows a sequence of acute and chronic stages to affect various body systems, primarily the cardiovascular, digestive, and nervous systems, with the principal health impact of this neglected tropical disease. The World Health Organization and the Centers for Disease Control emphasize the importance of Chagas disease, infecting millions and highlighting shortcomings in its research and epidemiological follow-up (Sherman, 2019). There is another very significant group of protozoan diseases that includes the amoebae, particularly *Entamoeba histolytica*, which cause amoebic dysentery. This parasite infects primarily through fecal-oral transmission, and most frequently through food or water contaminated with amoebae, resulting in severe gastrointestinal disturbances. Patients infected with *Entamoeba histolytica* may have mild diarrhea to fulminant dysentery, which is liable to be fatal if left untreated. The complicated life cycle and pathogenicity of amoebae create difficulties in public health, particularly in areas with inadequate sanitation and medical facilities. Knowledge of the epidemiology of amoebic infections is required to plan effective intervention measures, so much so that better personal hygiene measures and sensitization among risk groups are necessitated. Ciliates, although less frequent in the causation of human disease, are also causative agents in protozoan infections. A good example is *Balantidium coli*, most commonly found in swine and communicable to man, which causes balantidiasis. This infection is usually acquired in regions where human contact with contaminated food or water occurs, particularly where pigs are raised close to humans. Clinical presentation may range from asymptomatic infection to colitis, and, therefore, prevention efforts directed towards control of livestock and access to clean water sources are essential. The life cycle of *Balantidium coli*, which relies on both animal and human hosts, is tricky to control and poses the need for further exploration of its pathogenicity mechanisms and environmental reservoirs (Sherman, 2019). Hence, awareness about the different types of protozoan infections is crucial in planning targeted public health interventions.

7.1.1. Amoebic Infections

Amoebic infections, particularly those caused by the protozoan parasites *Entamoeba histolytica* and *Acanthamoeba* spp., are major public health issues globally. *Entamoeba histolytica*, the causative agent of amoebic dysentery, infects millions of people annually, predominantly in developing countries where there are poor sanitation facilities.

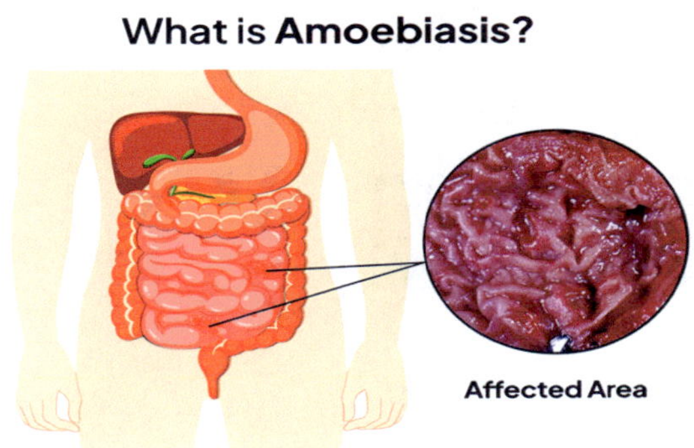

Figure 7.2. Amoebiasis.

Source: https://assets.truemeds.in/tm-cms-prod/what_is_amoebiasis_3d0467de23.jpg.

The life cycle of this protozoan includes transmission by fecal-oral contamination, leading to gastrointestinal disorder expressed as copious diarrhea and colicky pain. Vulnerable populations, especially children below the age of five, also show heightened risk of these infections due to factors like poor hygiene, environmental sanitation, and high population density (Unasho, 2013). These infections not only affect individual health but also carry economic burdens on healthcare systems and necessitate heightened scrutiny to guide communities on prevention. *Acanthamoeba* infection, while less frequent, carries special risk, particularly among contact lens wearers. The pathognomonic disorder is *Acanthamoeba keratitis*, which emphasizes the risk of insufficient lens hygiene and contact with contaminated environments. *Acanthamoeba* can lead to serious systemic infection in patients with compromised immune systems, further emphasizing the necessity to appreciate the virulence determinants and modes of transmission of the pathogens. Pathogens like *Acanthamoeba* thrive in various biotopes, including freshwaters and soil, leading to issues with restraining spread (Khan et al., 2004) (Figure 7.2).

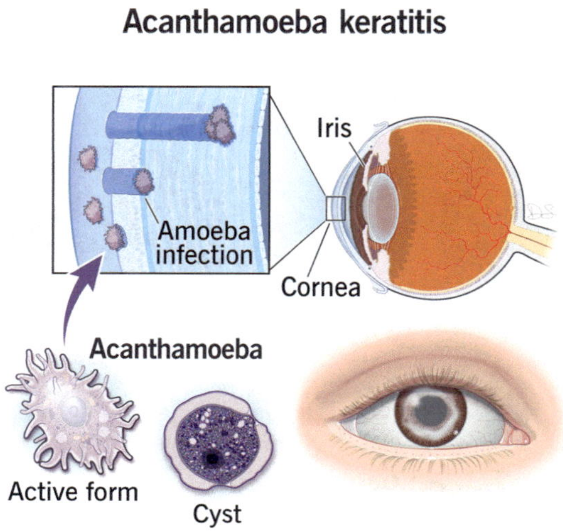

Figure 7.3. *Acanthamoeba keratitis.*

Source: https://my.clevelandclinic.org/-/scassets/images/org/health/articles/*Acanthamoeba*-keratitis.

The complexity of the parasites pathogenic mechanisms and host factors is accountable for the unpredictability of the diseases and for the inability with therapy options to overcome them, highlighting the necessity for ongoing research into effective therapeutic strategies. Understanding of the incorporation of ecological, biological, and social factors encompassed in amoebic infections is most pivotal to effective control strategies. Periodic deworming, education on infection cycles, hygiene practices, and improved access to clean water are all included in avoiding the transmission of these protozoan diseases (Unasho, 2013). Besides, the elevated incidence of *Acanthamoeba keratitis* demands special prevention programs, particularly directed at hygiene factors associated with the use of contact lenses. By the dissemination of public information regarding such infectious threats, communities will be better positioned to reduce the prevalence of amoebic infections and ultimately the broader public health consequences. Integration between research-based interventions and public participation will be essential in the battle against the disease burden associated with amoebic disease (Figure 7.3).

7.1.2. Flagellate Infections

One such well-documented example is the genus *Trypanosoma*, which comprises highly infamous pathogens for causing diseases like African trypanosomiasis, otherwise referred to as sleeping sickness, and American trypanosomiasis or Chagas disease. The complexity of these infections is further augmented by the capacity of *Trypanosoma* species to evolve and adapt in their hosts, resulting in persistent infections that can bypass the immune response. Regulatory T cells (Treg) are found to be pivotal in modulating immune responses by enabling the parasites to survive while keeping the overall homeostasis of the hosts intact, based on recent studies. These findings provide an indication of future directions in therapeutic therapy, demonstrating the fine balance between pathogen survival and host immunological integrity (Domingos et al., 2015). *Dientamoeba fragilis* is another flagellate well recognized, which contributes to our understanding of human protozoan infections by virtue of having fairly cryptic biology and questionable pathogenicity. This parasite resides within the human bowel and has been linked with gastrointestinal disturbance; however, its life cycle remains somewhat enigmatic. The advances in molecular biology during recent times have provided the avenue for newer diagnostic methods, which are important to further elucidate the role of *D. fragilis* in disease and health in humans. The pathogenicity of *D. fragilis* with controversy brings to fore the need for further studies to define its clinical significance, along with the generation of optimal treatment measures. As the scientific world continues to study this organism's intricate behaviors and modes of transmission, it offers a great opportunity to examine the host-parasite interactions dynamics in the context of flagellate infections (Barratt et al., 2016). When dealing with flagellate infections, there is also an emergent need for holistic public health strategies for prevention and control. The management of these protozoan infections not only necessitates understanding their immunological and biological aspects but also requires interventions against environmental determinants and early diagnosis. Integrated control measures, including vector control and public health education, in endemic regions of such diseases as *Leishmania*sis are required to reduce the rate of transmission. Additional research is equally necessary to determine novel therapeutic modalities in order to treat resistant populations of such parasites. The sophisticated host immune response-parasite adaptation interplay indicates the central focus of research, necessitating combined action by clinicians, public health professionals, and researchers to face the public health threat posed by flagellate infections (Domingos et al., 2015; Barratt et al., 2016) (Figure 7.4).

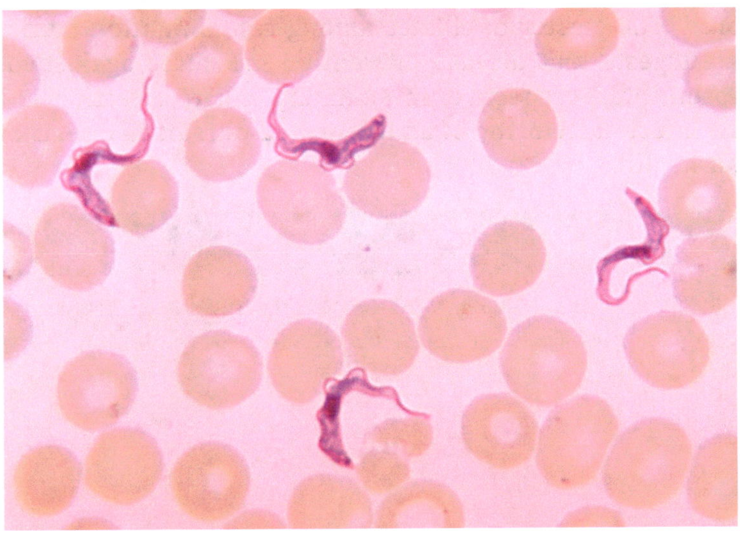

Figure 7.4. *Trypanosoma* forms in a blood smear from a patient with African trypanosomiasis.

Source: https://upload.wikimedia.org/wikipedia/commons/2/23/*Trypanosoma*_sp._PHIL_613_lores.jpg.

7.1.3. Ciliate Infections

Ciliate infections are a significant but often under-appreciated component of protozoan infections involving a broad variety of hosts, including animals, plants, and humans. Hair-like cilia-bearing ciliates are significant members of aquatic communities and possess the potential to be opportunistic pathogens. Certain free-living ciliates, for instance, have been cultured in environments where organisms are subject to microbial contamination, for instance, dishcloths used during food preparation. A recent study revealed that 47% of such cloths were ciliate-positive, indicating their intensity in ecological niches within which pathogens readily thrive. This fact underscores the efficiency of ciliate infection in being disease vectors, particularly when ingesting food or water sources infected with it, where such organisms can transmit along with more conventional bacterial pathogens, raising the chances of morbidity (Baré et al., 2014). The relationships between ciliates and other microorganisms can have intricate ecological ramifications, especially if considering the ciliates' position in the microbial food web. As predators, ciliates tend to prey on bacteria, including pathogenic ones, and thus may influence the population structure of the bacterial populations. This relationship becomes reciprocal when ciliate growth is facilitated by favorable environmental conditions, as in the case of enriched waters or polluted environments. *Pseudomonas aeruginosa* is a prime example, where pathogenic life adaptations can affect how they interact with protists, like ciliates. Research suggests environmental resilience trade-offs as a result of long-term adaptation to hosts, such that whereas ciliates have the ability to prey on pathogenic bacteria, proliferating populations under specific conditions could have unintended side effects like causing the spread of pathogens in hosts (Buckling et al., 2013). While ciliate infections are of interest to know, much remains unknown about their clinical significance and epidemiology. The study of the prevalence of ciliate infections can shed light on their nature as opportunistic pathogens, particularly where there is host immunocompromise. Ciliates , such as Colpoda, have been implicated as meaningful findings in environmental sample research, but how their occurrence forecasts the human health setting must be explored. The cluster of ciliates among contamination markers, as established in studies on dishcloths, suggests that disease prevention measures against foodborne illness take the role of such protozoa into perspective. In summary, ciliate infection is a niche discipline of study within protozoan infections worthy of an intensified pursuit to unmask their ecological roles and impacts on human health.

Test Your Knowledge

1. What are the typical diseases caused by amoebic protozoa and through what mode are they transmitted?
2. Which of the protozoan pathogens are flagellates and what infections do they typically produce?

7.2. Transmission of Protozoan Infections

Learning Outcome

1. Discuss waterborne transmission
2. Be familiar with vector-borne transmission of protozoan infections
3. Discuss direct contact transmission

Transmission of protozoan infections is by various routes, and it has significant public health impact across the world. One of the primary mechanisms is through water sources that are infested with protozoa, which multiply there and facilitate the transmission of infection in human beings. For instance, food preparation and use or ingestion of infested water may lead to gastrointestinal disease due to protozoans like *Giardia lamblia*. Moreover, climatic conditions, , such as unhygienic conditions and poor sanitation practices, increase the level of transmission. Enhancing water purification techniques and hygienic measures awareness is a major prevention strategy against such risks. Such precaution is highly necessary in developing nations where pure water lacks easy access, making individuals vulnerable to protozoan infection causing severe health problems. Another crucial mode of transmission is through vector organisms, which act as carriers for the protozoan pathogens. Mosquitoes, for instance, are the vectors of *Trypanosoma* parasites causing sleeping sickness and Chagas disease. The life cycles of such protozoa often entail complex interactions between host and vector in which the parasites have to adapt to survive under changing circumstances. All this makes control of such diseases more and more challenging while also necessitating multidisciplinary intervention to understand these interactions in a holistic sense. Interventions aimed at managing the vector population, i.e., application of insect repellent or environmental modification, can effectively manage the prevalence of these infections. Vector transmission thus remains the pillar for public health interventions targeting control of protozoan infections. Another less familiar but important mode of transmission involves contact with infected persons, which is more relevant in immunocompromised groups. *Acanthamoeba keratitis* represents a typical pathway, wherein the pathogen enters through the cornea, in most cases, in contact lens users. Poor hygiene practices, , such as improper contact lens use with contaminated water, facilitate this transmission and lead to severe ocular morbidity. The concurrent determinants of this infection are host susceptibility and environmental conditions. *Acanthamoeba* infection pathophysiology, as described in recent research, can direct prevention and care strategies essential to mitigating the accompanying risks. By creating awareness regarding proper lens care and hygiene needs, public health organizations can also assure significant reduction in the number of such infections among vulnerable populations (Khan et al., 2004; Ramesh et al., 2025).

7.2.1. Waterborne Transmission

Waterborne transmission is the most prominent mode of protozoan disease dispersal worldwide, as water is a primary vector for many pathogens. *Giardia lamblia* and *Cryptosporidium parvum* are some of the notorious protozoan parasites that cause serious gastrointestinal infections and are primarily disseminated in contaminated water supplies. The pathogens survive aquatic systems for extended durations, which aids in creating epidemics in unsanitary conditions. Moreover, climatic changes may aid in the spread of such infections, with rising temperatures and altered rainfall patterns impacting the prevalence and intensity of waterborne disease. Public health officials are better able to design strategies to counterbalance future health threats from protozoan disease, particularly in vulnerable regions without access to safe water, by understanding the ecology of waterborne transmission. Beyond point contamination of drinking water, the longevity of protozoan pathogens in the aquatic environment presents additional public health issues. The environmental persistence of the oocyst stage of protozoa, such as *Toxoplasma gondii,* allows free distribution of the parasite in surface waters and sediments. These oocysts infect not just water sources but also become part of the food chain and are incorporated in shellfish as well as other water animals that humans consume. This versatility makes full monitoring for detecting and controlling *T. gondii* and such other pathogens in their terrestrial and aquatic forms necessary. Healing the oocyst transmission channel would significantly lower the incidence of related diseases, giving added significance to intensive regulatory processes in aquaculture and agriculture for maintaining public health effectively (Bahia-Oliveira et al., 2019). With ongoing global climate change to reorder the topology of waterborne diseases, the need for ongoing surveillance and intervention is increasingly vital. It has been discovered through research that population displacement, intensified flooding, and disruption of water infrastructure facilitate the prevalence of waterborne pathogens, facilitating protozoan infection conditions (Heaviside et al., 2018).

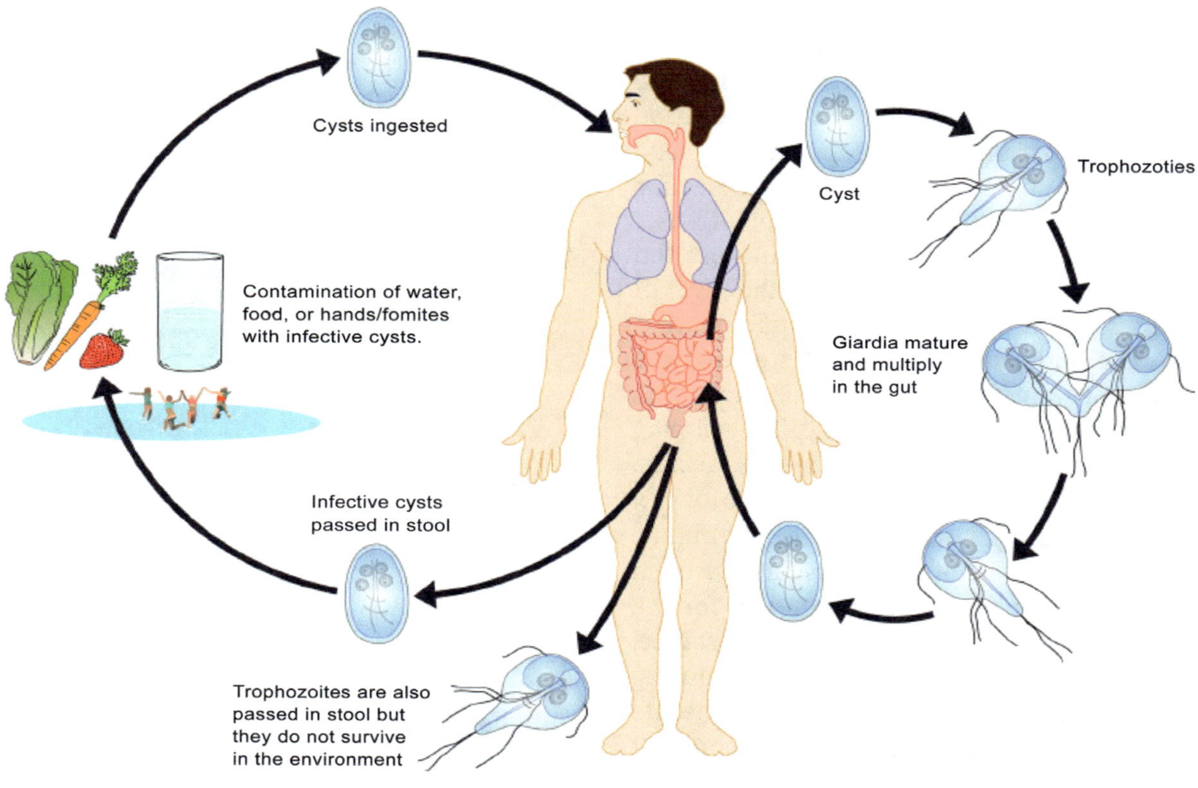

Figure 7.5. Protozoan parasites in drinking water.

Source: https://www.mdpi.com/ijerph/ijerph-15-00495/article_deploy/html/images/ijerph-15-00495-g002.png.

In most developing countries, where rapid response capacity is not present, the impact of this shift is particularly disastrous. Thus, adopting good management practices, such as better water quality surveillance and education about hygiene behaviors, is necessary. Moreover, increased cooperation between governments and health agencies can help reinforce efforts to assist at-risk groups, including ensuring the availability of clean water and reducing the negative effects of climate oscillations on waterborne transmission-related health outcomes (Figure 7.5).

7.2.2. Vector-Borne Transmission

Vector-borne transmission is of fundamental significance to the spread of protozoan disease, with certain insect species acting as vectors for the pathogens capable of disseminating serious health disorders to human populations. One such notable case of the latter is that of Chagas disease, which is disseminated by the protozoan parasite *Trypanosoma cruzi*. This disease is endemic in 21 Latin American countries and is primarily transmitted through triatomine bug feces. Triatomine bugs, also referred to as kissing bugs informally, are perfectly adapted to inhabiting human homes; hence, controlling these vectors is essential in forestalling the dissemination of the disease. Enhanced understanding of *T. cruzi,* there remain huge gaps in Chagas disease treatment and prevention, leaving millions exposed to both acute and chronic infections, and major organ systems , such as the cardiovascular and nervous systems, are especially affected (Sherman, 2019). Climate change adds yet another aspect to the vector-borne protozoan infection dynamics. Higher temperatures and shifting precipitation patterns can have major impacts on the habits and habitats of vectors, resulting in new transmission dynamics and the possibility of disease spread into previously unaffected geographical areas.

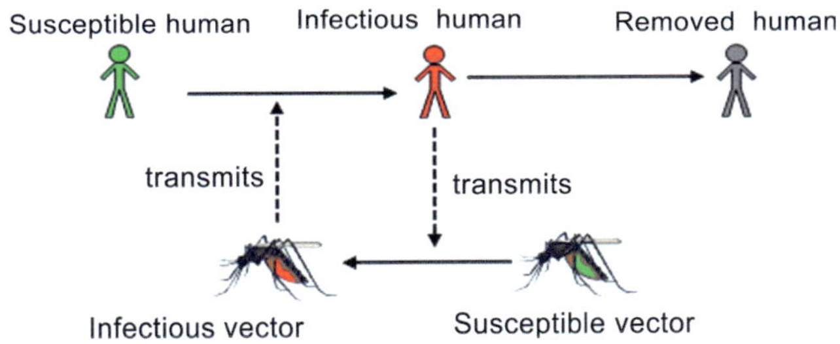

Figure 7.6. Vector-borne transmission.

Source: https://andreashandel.github.io/IDEMAbook/images/vectorborne-schematic.png.

Specifically, where there is poor infrastructure for water supply and sanitation, such regions are particularly at risk for outbreaks since they can be lacking in the resources available for proper public health intervention. The correlation between climatic change and vector distribution can exacerbate the already existing health conditions, thus complicating the epidemiological scenario. Predictive forecasts and surveillance then take center stage in this case, allowing public health planners to prepare for possible increases in vector populations as well as the related diseases , such as Chagas and others (Heaviside et al., 2018). Preventive strategies will therefore have to integrate vector control measures along with more universal public health strategies in an effort to address pressures from protozoan vector-borne disease. The implementation of effective surveillance systems can provide key information about the distribution and incidence of both vectors and their associated pathogens, thereby facilitating timely epidemiological responses to outbreaks. In addition, addressing the underlying environmental causes that enable vector multiplication—i.e., improving infrastructure, increasing sanitation, and promoting public awareness—is a buffer to transmission risk. Ensuring priority in the application of a One Health approach recognizing the interdependence of human, animal, and environmental health is essential in order to develop overarching measures for combating protozoan infection caused by vector-borne transmission. Here, international collaboration and grants are a must to ensure that the vulnerable populations are protected as well as supported (Sherman, 2019; Heaviside et al., 2018) (Figure 7.6).

7.2.3. Direct Contact Transmission

Direct contact transmission is the mechanism of protozoan infection transmission that forms the backbone of learning how they are transmitted, particularly in light of their diverse infective agent ranges. Perhaps the most common example is *Acanthamoeba*, an opportunistic pathogen responsible for causing keratitis primarily in contact lens users. The protozoan is typically spread by infected surfaces, water, or hands. Inadequate hygiene in contact lens maintenance permits the amoeba entry into the cornea from the environment, triggering an avalanche of inflammation with the potential to lead to blindness. *Acanthamoeba* pathogenicity lies in its sophistication, which accentuates the dynamics of host susceptibility, environment, and parasite virulence. Precise understanding of these factors is essential for the formulation of realistic prevention measures and treatment regimens against *Acanthamoeba keratitis*, which has gained prominence with the surge in contact lens wearers (Khan et al., 2004). *Toxoplasma gondii*, another of the primary vectors of direct contact spread of protozoal disease, is a zoonotic parasite with an intricate path of transmission. Although it is typically spread by consuming oocysts in contaminated food or water, direct contact with contaminated material—, such as soil and cat litter, is also a significant method of transmission. *T. gondii* strong oocyst form enables it to survive in different environments, infecting many intermediate hosts, , such as man. The very strong oocyst wall of the organism not only helps it survive in the environment but also gain entry into water supplies and food sources, thus making its large-scale distribution possible. The non-specificity of definitive hosts, which are primarily domesticated and wild cats, speaks volumes regarding the zoonotic nature of *T. gondii* and elevates the call for public education on direct exposure risk (Bahia-Oliveira et al., 2019). The mechanisms of transmission of protozoan infections through direct contact are of great importance to the public health initiatives aimed at declining prevalence. Public health interventions can be lowered via education for populations at risk, particularly those in agriculture or animal husbandry, to lower infection rates , such as *T. gondii*. In addition, good hygiene practice in environments , such as kitchens, gardens, and those that receive pets is the major way of preventing such infections. The incorporation of scientific understanding in outreach programs helps equip people with the ability to detect and manage risks related to direct contact transmission. With ongoing alteration of the environment and enhanced human-wildlife interface, it will be crucial to tackle these transmission routes of protozoan infections by humane public health measures and personal health practices to tackle the disease burden generated by these protozoa.

Test Your Knowledge

1. What is the contribution of waterborne transmission to the dissemination of protozoan infections?
2. Which diseases among the protozoa are transmitted by vectors, and what are the most prevalent vectors used?

7.3. Symptoms and Diagnosis

Learning Outcome

1. Describe common symptoms of protozoan infections;
2. Identify diagnostic methods used for protozoan infections;
3. Highlight difficulty in diagnosing protozoan infections.

Symptoms of protozoan infections are very varied based on the species of protozoa involved and where the infection is based in the host. *Trypanosoma cruzi*, the causative agent of Chagas disease, for instance, has an acute and a chronic phase each with distinct clinical features. The acute phase would entail mild symptoms , such as fever, weakness, and local swelling at the point of entry, while the chronic phase would lead to severe complications involving the cardiovascular system, gastrointestinal organs, and nervous system, signifying the parasite's systemic effect on the human organism (Sherman, 2019). Symptomatology knowledge plays a significant role in the initial diagnosis of such infections because it provides the first hint of likely underlying protozoan disease that would otherwise go unnoticed in endemic regions. Protozoan infection is typically hard to diagnose and will be concealed by unpredictable presentation and overlap with symptomatology for other diseases. Accurate diagnostic methods are needed for effective treatment and management of intestinal protozoa infections , such as *Giardia* intestinalis and *Entamoeba histolytica*. The standard diagnostic procedures include stool examination via direct fecal smear and concentration techniques, but they have some drawbacks with respect to sensitivity, leading to underdiagnosis (Albonico et al., 2013). The new technologies, , such as the mini-FLOTAC method, are more sensitive in detecting intestinal parasites in low-resource environments, thereby increasing levels of diagnosis and aiding in double or even triple infection detection, which might worsen the clinical prognosis. The significance of accurate symptoms and diagnosis in the treatment of protozoan infections cannot be overemphasized. Early diagnosis also significantly alters the pattern of disease and can allow for the start of a treatment that can prevent worse health outcomes associated with chronic infections. In the case of Chagas disease, for example, early detection at the acute phase allows for improved therapeutic intervention, which can potentially reduce the long-term health burden on health systems within epidemic districts (Sherman, 2019). Also, the enhancement of diagnostic techniques can facilitate epidemiological research and public health interventions for the control of protozoan disease to minimize transmission and promote improved outcomes for patients among high-risk groups. Thus, ongoing research and investment in diagnostic techniques are vital components of the mitigation of the incidence of protozoan infection worldwide.

7.3.1. Common Symptoms of Protozoan Infections

Protozoan infection involves diverse and manifold symptoms, which can significantly impact the health status of affected individuals. These infections usually manifest with gastrointestinal symptoms, such as diarrhea, abdominal pain, and nausea. For instance, infections caused by *Entamoeba histolytica*, the pathogen for amoebic dysentery, can cause blood and watery diarrhea with associated cramp and fever. Some protozoan infections can also present with systemic signs, e.g., weakness and tiredness, as the body reacts with an inflammatory response to infection. These symptoms are most often confused with other diseases, hence difficult to diagnose at an early stage and, therefore, cause delayed treatment, increasing the severity of infection. One should be aware of these symptoms both for early detection and for the use of effective therapy for the control of protozoan infections. And one further important consideration with protozoan infections is the risk of neurological presentation, particularly with such infections as *Trypanosoma brucei,* causing African sleeping sickness. Early in the disease, one may have headache, joint pains, and fever; later in the disease, though, severe neurological manifestations can develop in the form of confusion, personality alteration, or even coma.

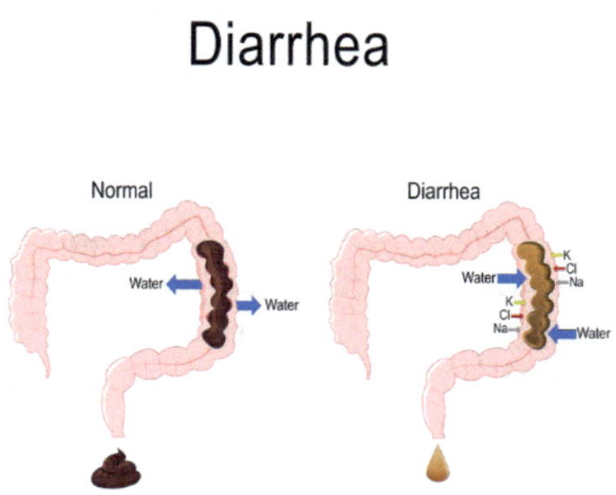

Figure 7.7. Diarrhea.

Source: https://content.health.harvard.edu/wp-content/uploads/2024/05/4c33864b-8374-4028-9351-302873e7dc40.jpg.

This evolution points to the pathological status of protozoan infections and the necessity of prompt intervention by a physician. Furthermore, parasitic infections like Toxoplasmosis, which is caused by *Toxoplasma gondii*, may lead to neurological incapacities, especially in immunocompromised individuals, where the central nervous system is also highly affected. Its control is necessary for the overall management of protozoan infections and its implications on public health. In some instances, protozoan infections can induce a spectrum of symptoms in various body systems, leading to a complex clinical syndrome. For example, in Chagas disease caused by infection with *Trypanosoma cruzi*, the symptoms range from an acute febrile illness to severe manifestations in the chronic phase affecting the cardiovascular and gastrointestinal systems. The patients may experience cardiomyopathy, arrhythmias, or gastrointestinal disorders that require intensive healthcare treatment (Sherman, 2019). Similarly, *Cytauxzoon felis*, a protozoan parasite that infects domestic cats, has symptoms ranging from fever, lethargy, to anemia, highlighting the severe health threat experienced by both animals and humans (Hickman et al., 2010). Thus, diversity in protozoan infection symptoms necessitates greater awareness and knowledge among healthcare workers for their ability to detect and treat diseases early (Figure 7.7).

7.3.2. Diagnostic Methods Used

Protozoan infections are diagnosed using a variety of methods specific to the causative agent and environmental condition. Traditional methods include the use of microscopy, whereby direct visual inspection of parasites from patient samples is enabled. For instance, the Kato-Katz method is used extensively for the identification of *Schistosoma mansoni* using stool sample analysis; the method can also analyze the intensity of infections using quantitative egg parasite quantification. The formol-ether concentration method also enhances intestinal protozoa recovery by concentrating eggs and cysts from stool samples to further boost diagnostic sensitivity. These strategies are the cornerstone in epidemic areas, where awareness of infection prevalence drives public health intervention and treatment regimens (Coulibaly et al., 2012). As these diagnostics are becoming more advanced, the need for alternatives that can differentiate more pathogens simultaneously is more pressing. Advances in diagnostic techniques in the past few years have provided higher sensitivity and more efficient approaches.

The mini-FLOTAC technique, for instance, has been recognized for its enhanced ability to detect intestinal parasitic infection, , such as protozoa. In Indian and Tanzanian research, mini-FLOTAC was found to have 90% sensitivity in detecting helminthic infection, far exceeding traditional approaches like direct fecal smear and formol-ether concentration for particular infection types (Albonico et al., 2013). This new approach allows for the examination of a number of samples within a single test and is therefore most beneficial in resource-poor settings. Further, the use of rapid diagnostic tests (RDTs) in hospital settings has minimized the detection process, such that identification of infections can be done more quickly. These improvements reflect a growing move toward employing more efficient diagnostic modalities responsive to the complexities of parasitic infections. The question of which specific diagnostic methods to apply has prevailed beyond laboratory settings, affecting public health interventions and control measures for protozoal infections. Diagnostics play an important role in adjusting treatment protocols as well as applying surveillance policies in the affected areas. For instance, the fast-screening method applied in Côte d'Ivoire enabled identifying varying levels of endemicity of *Schistosoma* spp. Across all settings, eventually informing intervention activities (Coulibaly et al., 2012). Moreover, evidence on the prevalence of co-infections, such as the evidence of dual infections within schoolchildren, points to the necessity of multivariable diagnostics. Through the application of a combination of strategies, health authorities can more accurately map the patterns of infection, measure the efficacy of treatment, and optimize the deployment of resources, thereby enhancing the overall impact of public health programs for the control of protozoan infections (Figure 7.8).

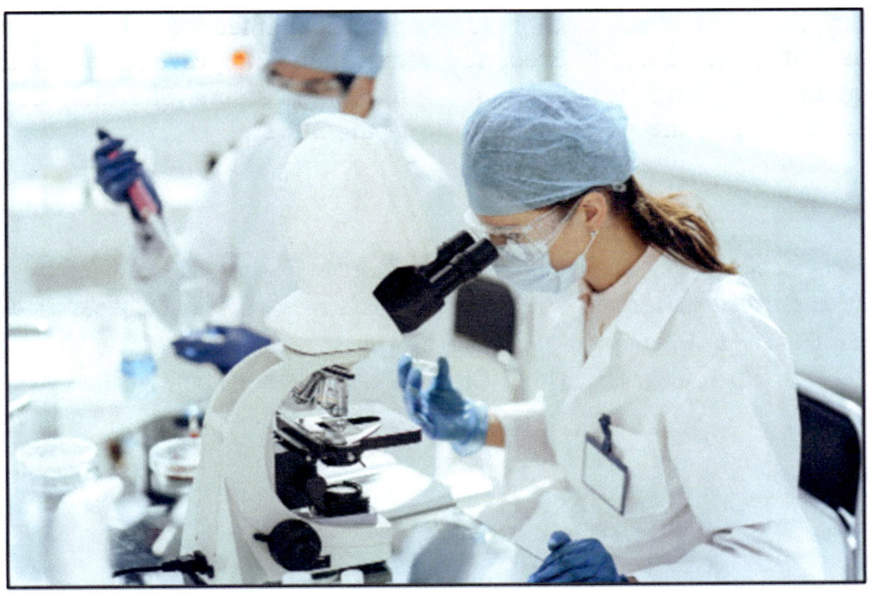

Figure 7.8. Diagnosis of protozoan infections.

Source: https://nl-lab.nl/wp-content/uploads/2023/09/stocklabfoto.png.

7.3.3. Challenges in Diagnosing Protozoan Infections

Diagnosis of protozoan infections poses significant challenges, considering the life cycles of the parasites as well as the diverse presentation of infections. For instance, the *Trypanosoma cruzi* parasite which causes Chagas disease, also has two phases of infection: acute and chronic. This uncertainty in presentation is likely to result in difficulty in the timely diagnosis, as acute presentation can be minimal or even absent, and then the chronic presentation might occur years later, causing healthcare workers to miss possible infections. Moreover, the lack of adequately sensitive and specific diagnostic tools diminishes adequate identification, as traditional methods may not always capture the nuances of infection phases, leaving millions to suffer from untreated illness (Sherman, 2019). Increased prevalence of protozoan infections across various host groups, including livestock, also complicates diagnostics. Dairy buffalo, for example, are susceptible to intestinal protozoa , such as *Giardia* and *Eimeria* that may suppress clinical signs of infection and may result in misdiagnosis or delayed treatment. Environmental problems, , such as contaminated water sources, may cause infections and make correct diagnosis outreach difficult. Present diagnostic methods also tend to overlook asymptomatic carriers; thus, the parasites are able to go undetected in populations. Hence, knowledge of the epidemiological context of infections of non-human hosts, together with novel detection mechanisms and strategies, becomes imperative to solve these diagnostic challenges (Morgoglione et al., 2021). Moreover, the emergence of drug resistance in protozoan pathogens makes the diagnosis and treatment of such infections even more challenging. Classical metaphylactic strategies have served to control infections, but their inappropriate usage has been the reason for the emergence of resistance against certain treatments as the years go by, rendering them less effective. This feature requires ongoing epidemiological surveillance and research into novel diagnostic strategies that can keep up with the evolving nature of protozoan infections. Through the utilization of cutting-edge technologies, such as molecular diagnostics and immunoassays, physicians can enhance the specificity of detection for protozoan infection, which will enhance targeted treatment and prevention in both veterinary and human medicine (Sherman, 2019; Morgoglione et al., 2021).

Test Your Knowledge

1. What are the most common symptoms for protozoan infections in humans?
2. What are the common diagnostic tests that are utilized to detect protozoan infections?

7.4. Treatment Options

Learning Outcome

1. Describe antiprotozoal drugs;
2. Discuss the importance of supportive care and management in enhancing patient outcomes;
3. Highlight the emergence of new treatments and research in the field of protozoan infections.

Treatment of protozoan infections is a multi-faceted approach that incorporates both drug therapy and public health interventions. Antimicrobial drugs, , such as antimalarials or antiparasitic medicines, remain cornerstones in the management of most protozoan infections, specifically targeting parasites like Plasmodium species and *Giardia lamblia*. For example, the use of drugs like artemisinin-based combination therapies has provided a solution to combating malaria and reducing morbidity and mortality rates associated with the disease. However, resistance development necessitates constant scrutiny and research for new drugs. Besides, preventive treatments and support interventions, , such as vaccination drives when and if available, are also needed in preventing the spread of protozoan infections. Effective treatment not only cures symptoms but also prevents transmission, hence complementing total public health intervention for the control of the infections. Environmental and sanitation improvements are also needed in reducing protozoan infection hazards, especially those transmitted through contaminated water supply. Wastewater irrigation, albeit common in the traditional systems of the majority of developing nations, remains a significant public health problem due to the potential for passing pathogens, e.g., protozoan parasites. The magnitude of consuming vegetables irrigated by untreated sewage is backed by empirical evidence linking exposure to water supplies that are contaminated with elevated disease burdens. Actions towards enhancing wastewater management and treatment, as highlighted in recent epidemiological studies, are essential in avert these risks. Through ensuring safer irrigation methods and effective wastewater treatment plants, communities are able to decrease significantly the protozoan infection load, providing the possibilities of improved food safety and public health outcomes, particularly in agricultural-dependent nations. Finally, prevention and targeted community-based health education also help avoid protozoan infection. Hygiene measures, , such as proper hand-washing, effective cooking of food, and avoidance of the use of untreated water, may be promoted by raising awareness that creates healthier practices with a high potential to lower infection rates. Special educational programs targeting individuals with increased risk of infection, particularly in areas where endemic protozoan infections are common, can empower people with preventive measures to fight transmission. In addition, combining health education with environmental policy may provide a synergistic effect through the optimization of treatment measures. By tackling both the biological and socioeconomic determinants of protozoan infections, a public health initiative arises that maximizes disease control and establishes sustainable health behavior in populations.

7.4.1. Antiprotozoal Medications

The treatment of protozoal infections relies mainly on the use of antiprotozoal drugs, which exert their action at various phases of the life cycle of the parasite to diminish their impact on the health of human beings. Some of the most important infections, , such as those caused by *Giardia* intestinalis and *Entamoeba histolytica*, are effectively cured by established drugs like metronidazole. Nevertheless, the efficacy of these classical medicines has been increasingly eroded by the possibility of drug resistance. Word has it that many protozoa species are developing mechanisms for drug resistance against antiprotozoal medication, rendering conventional treatments inefficient. This is particularly concerning in low-income countries with limited access to healthcare, thus the importance of alternative therapies that will supplement or replace conventional medicine (Ashafa et al., 2020). Expansion of our understanding of resistance patterns and exploration of new avenues of drug discovery are necessary in order to meet the growing healthcare cost burden of protozoan illness. The landscape of antiprotozoal drugs is further complexed by the heterogeneity of protozoan disease as well as the varied pharmacologic properties of the available agents. Each illness could conceivably have directed therapy to match the specific protozoan and the individual host. For example, *Leishmania*sis, caused by the *Leishmania* species, demands special antiprotozoal agents, such as amphotericin B or miltefosine. Yet even these drugs have drawbacks, including potential toxicity and parenteral administration, rendering treatment in endemic countries problematic (Jada et al., 2024). As researchers go on investigating cheaper and less toxic alternatives, research on natural products has been an exciting route. Phytoextracts of medicinal herbs may deliver bioactive substances with antiprotozoal activity useful in a comprehensive approach to the treatment of protozoan infections in populations of diverse demography. In addition, novel antiprotozoal treatments are urgently needed to counteract the drawbacks of existing treatments and to manage the resistance-arising strains. Recent studies on products based on natural sources have shown promise in combating infections , such as visceral *Leishmania*sis. A prime example is the alkaloid peganine, which has selective activity against intracellular *Leishmania donovani* stages without increased host cell toxicity. This is an illustration of utilizing bioactive products to create new therapeutic pathways, particularly where disease has been historically neglected and underfunded (Ashafa et al., 2020). The drive towards innovative drug development involves systematic optimization and testing of such compounds to increase their effectiveness and reduce side effects. As the health burden of protozoan diseases continues to weigh on the global health system, a three-pronged response of better drug forms and other therapies is needed to guarantee improved outcomes for the affected populations (Figure 7.9).

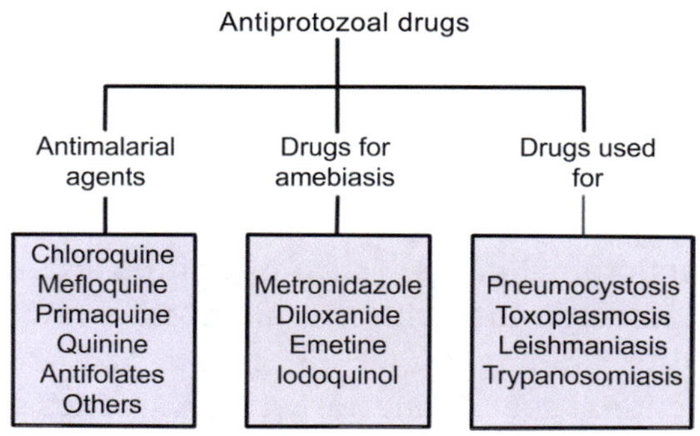

Figure 7.9. Antiprotozoal drugs.

Source: https://doctorlib.org/pharmacology/pharmacology-examination-board-review/pharmacology-examination-board-review.files/image219.jpg.

7.4.2. Supportive Care and Management

In the management of protozoan infections, supportive care and management also play significant roles in enhancing outcomes in the patients. The multifaceted nature of these infections necessitates a more holistic approach than straightforward antimicrobial therapy. Supportive care involves covering symptoms, nutrition, and psychosocial intervention, all of which factor into the quality of life of the infected persons. For instance, patients with symptomatic malaria may require not only antimalarial medication but also fluids and electrolytes to manage dehydration and re-establish metabolic equilibrium. Adapted to the broadened patient needs in this manner provides physicians with a superior method of addressing the physical and mental stress protozoal infections impose, enhancing prospects of healing and reducing complications that accompany the diseases. Besides, protozoan infections need to be managed with education and prevention as part of effective management measures. As the ongoing difficulties with sexually transmitted infections (STIs) clearly attest, behavior change and awareness programs remain the bulwark against the spread and impact of the infection. The health infrastructures worldwide must lay focus on the design of low-cost diagnostic tests and therapeutic regimens that are cost-effective and culturally tailored. For instance, when it comes to non-HIV STIs, drawing from advancements in HIV treatment and prevention also brings meaningful dividends. The use of rapid testing and point-of-care treatment is capable of controlling STIs and can be adapted to deal with protozoan infections more effectively. This proactive perspective in prevention and management underscores the vital intersection of supportive care in fostering resilient health care systems capable of beating such public health challenges (Collins et al., 2014). Ultimately, supportive care incorporation into the larger framework of protozoan infection control requires collaborative action from various stakeholders engaged, including governments, health care providers, and communities. Through joint partnerships, the stakeholders will facilitate the exchange of best practices and access to critical resources in delivering effective care. Further, having an understanding of the socio-economic and cultural barriers that patients will face will have an effect on the impact of interventions. Since it is still difficult to cure protozoan infections, dedication to training health workers and developing capacities in local health systems is required. The inclusion of behavior change interventions and ensuring prioritization of patient education are also significant aspects of this framework, capable of counterbalancing the adverse socio-economic impacts of such infections (Ramesh et al., 2025). Collective action thereby paves the way for better health outcomes in patients with protozoan infections, echoing the importance of supportive care and management in health frameworks (Figure 7.10).

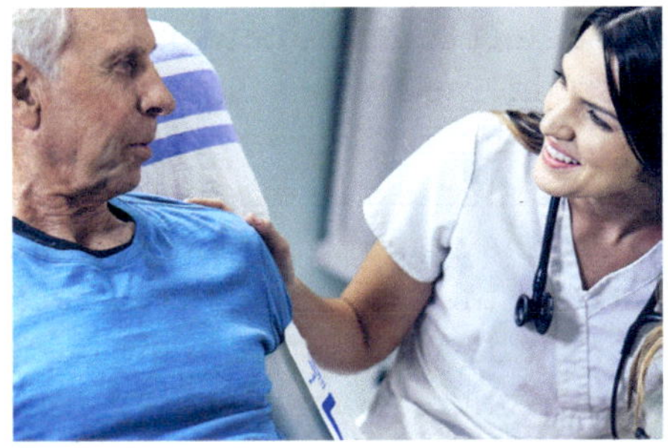

Figure 7.10. Supportive care.

Source: https://healthcare.ascension.org/-/media/healthcare/national/service-lines/hero/infectiousdisease.jpg?h=800&iar=0&w=1200&hash=7A6D937E7B38A148BE491F93FDA0DD36.

7.4.3. Emerging Treatments and Research

The advancement of novel therapies and research in protozoan infection has become increasingly important as drug resistance and lack of vaccines pose threats. New therapies aim targeted strategies which employ cutting-edge technologies to disrupt the life cycles of the protozoan pathogens. Recent work has highlighted the role of extracellular vesicles (EVs) in the host-parasite interactions and their potential as biomarkers or drugs. EVs are secreted by most cells in response to infection and stress and have the potential to carry proteins and nucleic acids with the ability to transfer information between host and parasite. This dynamic deployment of EVs can be harnessed to design diagnostic devices that improve early detection and therapeutic regimens for protozoan-induced infectious diseases and therefore revolutionize existing treatment modalities in applied translation in medical sciences (Gavinho et al., 2019). Another possible area in the research into protozoan infections is the application of systems biology for an explanation of the complexities of host-parasite relationships. Recent advances in genomic technologies, including next-generation sequencing, have presented new opportunities for understanding the biological mechanisms behind parasitic infections. They enable scientists to produce high-throughput -omics data, which can be queried to detect complex networks involved in host responses to protozoan infections. When these datasets are merged, scientists are able to identify principal pathways that may be addressed for intervention, resulting in new drug development that can circumvent existing resistance mechanisms. As the field continues to expand, increased understanding of these intricate biological processes may provide the stimulus for the creation of new antiparasitic therapeutics (Jamshidi et al., 2015). Finally, among the most notable characteristics of new treatments for protozoan infections is the discovery and development of new compounds that can penetrate drug-resistant parasite strains. Activities are increasingly focused on screening pre-existing libraries of compounds for their effectiveness against protozoan pathogens and synthesizing new molecules from natural sources. Collaborative studies, particularly international collaborative studies, are essential to provide these compounds for discovery purposes and facilitate equal access to effective medicines in endemic regions. Furthermore, the study of adjuvant therapies, which enhance the effectiveness of currently available medicines, can also enhance treatment success and reduce parasitic burden. Through concerted efforts toward understanding and improving the problems caused by protozoan infections, the potential for creating significant advances in patient treatment and public health is optimistic (Figure 7.11).

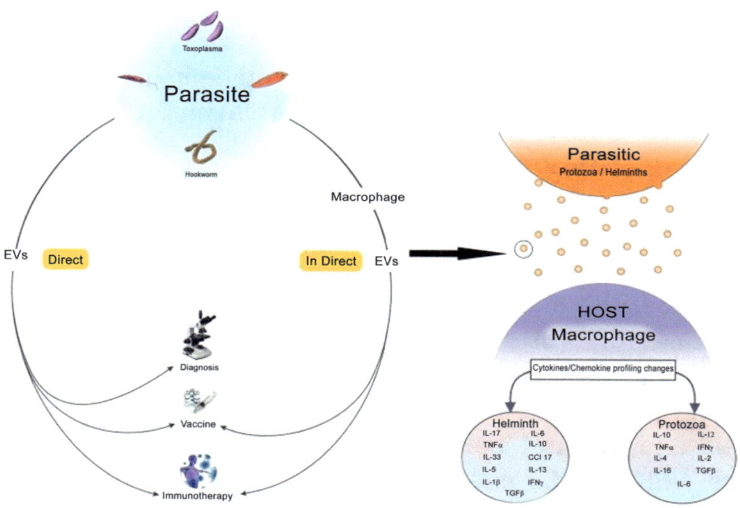

Figure 7.11. Extracellular vesicles (EVs) extracted directly from parasites or indirectly from host cells are sensed by parasites.

Source: https://www.researchgate.net/publication/340957842/figure/fig1/AS:11431281256190017@1719514471284/Extracellular-vesicles-EVs-extracted-directly-from-parasites-or-indirectly-from-host.jpg.

Test Your Knowledge

1. What are the most commonly used antiprotozoal drugs, and against what infections do they work?
2. How does supportive care complement pharmacologic therapy of protozoan infections?

7.5. Prevention Strategies

Learning Outcome

1. Identify the value of hygiene and sanitation measures in preventing protozoan infections;
2. Explain the concurrency of vaccination campaigns and protozoan infections;
3. Outline the value of public health initiatives in playing a central role in curbing the spread of protozoan infections.

Prevention of protozoan infections demands a multi-faceted approach integrating public health strategies, education, and environmental control to reduce spread. One of the most effective approaches is increasing access to clean water and sanitation facilities. When protozoan infections, , such as *Giardia* and *Entamoeba histolytica*, are prevalent, poor treatment of water tends to aggravate the problem. Educating communities on safe handling of water and fortifying hygiene measures reduces the level of infection considerably. Public health interventions must consider the environmental circumstances prevailing in the area, as exemplified by areas of high endemicity of *Schistosoma* infections, where the prevalence may vary significantly between various environments, based on sanitation conditions and water availability (Coulibaly et al., 2012). This indicates that prevention interventions tailored to local conditions are imperative to effective disease control. In addition to enhancing infrastructure, fast diagnostics become more vital for protozoan disease control and surveillance. Robust diagnostic tools enable precise identification of infection and its occurrence in a given population, rendering interventions more targeted. For instance, studies have illustrated that application of strict diagnostic procedures drastically transformed infection levels in remote schoolchildren in endemic areas (Coulibaly et al., 2012). These shifts in data bring to the fore the necessity for the integration of technological innovations in epidemiology with public health interventions to enable timely intervention. Moreover, continued surveillance by community health programs can enable the detection of outbreaks sooner and improve response programs, thereby enhancing public health resilience overall against protozoan infections. Vector control is also crucial in prevention against protozoan infections, particularly mosquito-borne and other arthropod-borne protozoan infections. Tools , such as insecticide-treated bed nets, larviciding, and environmental management to eliminate vector breeding sites are crucial. In regions , such as Lake Kainji in Nigeria, where man-induced environmental alterations have influenced the density of fish as well as their parasites, ecological processes should be comprehended for the purpose of executing effective prevention. Integrated vector management that considers ecological well-being not only reduces the transmission of disease but also promotes environmentally friendly ecosystems. Through the facilitation of interdisciplinary collaboration among ecologists, healthcare providers, and communities, prevention mechanisms can be significantly strengthened, eventually saving the public from the expense of protozoan infections and enhancing public health outcomes.

7.5.1. Hygiene and Sanitation Practices

The contribution of hygiene and sanitation practices to the control of protozoan infections cannot be overemphasized. Good hygienic habits, , such as constant hand washing with soap and handling of food in a safe condition, are the first line of defense against the transmission of many protozoan infections. Unhygienic conditions, particularly in resource-limited settings, contribute to the spread of infections , such as *Giardia* and *Entamoeba histolytica*, which thrive in dirty food and water sources. Thus, using simple sanitation measures—, such as making safe, clean drinking water available and proper sewage disposal—must be adopted.

Research emphasizes that communities with poor sanitation have high rates of protozoan infection, recalling the importance of using overall public health interventions that include hygiene as well as environmental sanitation, particularly in vulnerable groups (Coulibaly et al., 2012). The role of education and community in promoting improved hygiene practice cannot be underestimated. Large-scale education campaigns to raise awareness about the modes of transmission of protozoal infections and the importance of sanitation have proved effective in checking infection rates. Through awareness and enlightening people to proper waste disposal, boiling water, and personal hygiene practices, communities can readily lower their risk of infection. Moreover, participatory methods of engaging local populations in sanitation activities enhance ownership and responsibility, hence making hygiene practices more sustainable. Public health professionals must utilize epidemiologic tools to quantify the effectiveness of such interventions when developing guidelines and regulations aimed at enhancing levels of hygiene in different areas, especially those at risk of protozoan disease outbreaks (Blumenthal et al., 2001). Because of the difficulties in protozoan infections, adopting and keeping rigorous hygiene and sanitation practices are paramount to public health. Continuous water quality monitoring, particularly in recreational and drinking water sources, is important in identifying contamination prior to widespread health crises. Besides, it should be a priority to follow a multi-disciplinary approach encompassing the incorporation of social, environmental, and health sciences in designing interventions that will effectively fight protozoan pathogens. This not only helps with the alleviation of the disease burden but also with enhancing the quality of life in the affected population. Although protozoan infection incidence remains a significant public health concern, continued emphasis on measures of hygiene and sanitation has the potential to build on significant advances in prevention and control campaigns for diseases in the years ahead (Coulibaly et al., 2012) (Figure 7.12).

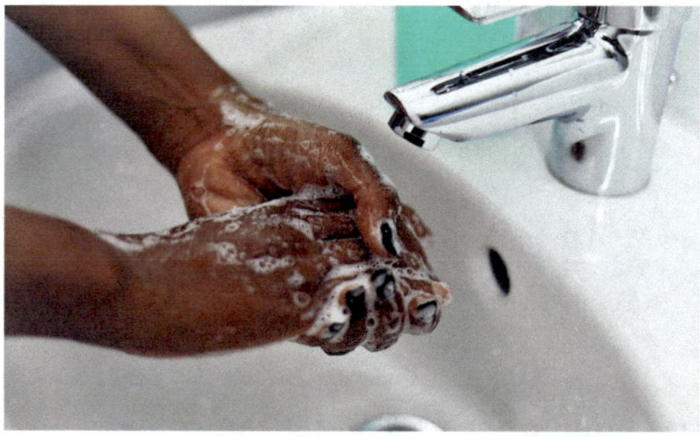

Figure 7.12. Personal hygiene.

Source: https://www.food-safety.com/ext/resources/2021/06/20/Sanitize_Img01_900.jpg?1629294586.

7.5.2. Vaccination Efforts

The intersection of vaccine development and protozoal disease is a primary area of investigation, particularly in light of the burden of diseases , such as those caused by *Trypanosoma* and *Leishmania*. These protozoa, as well as many of the neglected tropical diseases, have significant implications for health systems, especially in the developing world. Advances in genomics in the recent past have unraveled the complex biology of these pathogens, shedding light on their genetic relatedness and the diverse clinical presentations they have. Such understanding offers the opportunities for targeted vaccination strategies desperatley needed. The convergence of immunological approaches with clinical and molecular approaches is thus increasingly vital, as hinted at in recent reviews of the subject. The accelerated advances in the knowledge of these protozoal diseases provide unparalleled opportunities to transform drug, diagnostic, and vaccine development to control these diseases effectively (Stuart et al., 2008). Protozoan infection immunization programs pose unique challenges, such as the attenuated effectiveness of vaccines in chronic parasitic infection. Present evidence indicates that patients with neglected tropical diseases can deliver diminished immune responses to routine vaccinations. Studies examining the impact of chronic trematode, nematode, and protozoan infections on the immunogenicity of routine vaccinations indicate that such infections complicate routine vaccination schedules, particularly among vulnerable groups , such as pregnant women and infants. The immunomodulatory effects of parasitic infections can weaken the immune system's ability to respond effectively against vaccines and lead to suboptimal protective responses. Thus, the effectiveness of vaccination has to be augmented by a two-pronged effort that not only develops effective vaccines but also incorporates antiparasitic treatments for immunoenhancement of responses as well as public health (King et al., 2009). To provide maximal potential for vaccination programs against protozoan infections, extensive approaches must be adopted. It involves not only advancing vaccine research but also implementing effective public health practices to limit the spread of such infections. Antiparasitic medication treatment of chronic parasitic infections can enhance the effectiveness of vaccines and yield enhanced health outcomes in infected populations. Future research needs to strive to describe how various protozoan species interact with the immune system, particularly where infection loads are high. Furthermore, intervention measures must consider local epidemiological circumstances and socio-economic determinants hampering vaccination coverage. By prioritizing combined strategies encompassing both parasite control and immunization, health authorities may increase the efficacy of vaccination campaigns and ultimately reduce the incidence of protozoan infections (King et al., 2009).

7.5.3. Public Health Initiatives

Public health interventions are essential to combat the spread of protozoan infections, particularly in low-resource settings where infection poses a serious threat to health. Preventive measures like public campaigns and community health initiatives play an essential role in raising awareness among people regarding transmission modes and symptoms of protozoan infections , such as *Giardia*sis and amoebiasis. For instance, inclusion of hygiene education in school curricula can prepare children to learn healthier habits that reduce chances of infection. Moreover, such activities typically involve active participation of local communities, which is essential for their effectiveness and sustainability. By offering affordable health care and engaging residents actively, public health initiatives create a proper environment that makes individuals understand the need for preventive care, hence lowering the incidence of these infections in the long run. The difficulty in controlling protozoan infections is not merely treating them but also dealing with the socio-economic determinants of their propagation. Research indicates that lower socioeconomic status is a principal risk factor for parasitic infestation of the intestine in rural children, particularly in areas where sanitation facilities are substandard as in Mexico. The Opportunities program and the National Deworming Campaign are excellent examples of how synergistic public efforts can decrease the risks by targeting the risk groups. By initiatives focused towards enhancing mother education and availability of health care, such programs seek to address the social determinants of health causing the prevalence of protozoan infections. It is also important to evaluate such programs to determine their impact and improve on how they can be focused in reaching the most needy effectively, resulting in improved health outcomes. Finally, an integrated strategy involving treatment in addition to aggressive public health intervention can reduce the impact of protozoan disease dramatically. For example, the integration of antiretroviral therapy schemes in India is a follow-up to attempts to control intestinal parasitism through a preventive and therapeutic approach simultaneously. Such programs demonstrate the importance of a holistic public health strategy that not only cures the root immediate health concern but also encompasses broader systemic issues like education and access to clean water. Although the war against protozoan infections continues, the importance of ongoing funds, community engagement, and cross-sector collaborations cannot be overlooked. By investing in such public health initiatives, there are increased chances of achieving long-term reductions in protozoan infection rates, which ultimately lead to improved-quality living and healthier communities for the affected populace (Quihui et al., 2006) (Figure 7.13).

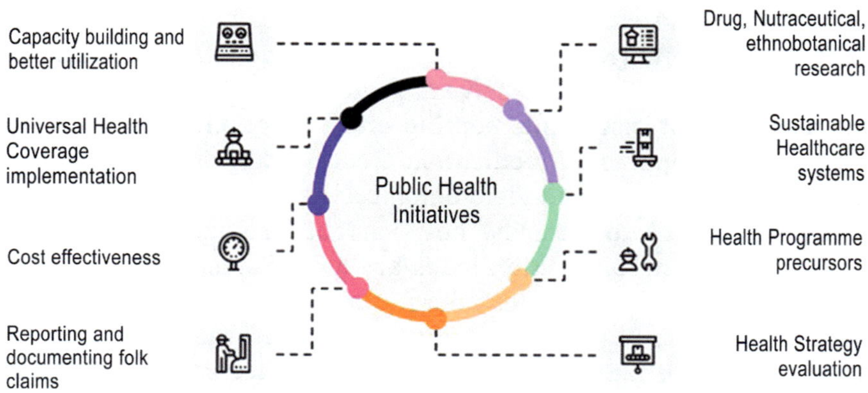

Figure 7.13. Public health initiatives.

Source: https://www.researchgate.net/profile/Karthik-K-P-3/publication/374583836/figure/fig3/AS:11431281197315779@1696963234932/Need-of-public-health-initiatives-in-Ayush.ppm.

Test Your Knowledge

1. How do hygiene and sanitation practices reduce the risk of protozoan infections?
2. What is the status of the protozoan vaccine today?

7.6. Impact on Global Health

Learning Outcome

1. Explain the burden of protozoan infections in developing countries;
2. Discuss the economic burden of protozoan infections;
3. Explain the role of public health policy in addressing protozoan infections.

The effect of protozoan infections on global health is considerable, most prominently in low- and middle-income countries where socioeconomic determinants have a significant influence on health. A. one such example is the prevalence of intestinal parasitic infection that continues to be endemic among communities located in Mexico. According to one report, over half of the rural school children have a high rate of poliparasitism and protozoan infection, reflecting the linkage of health danger with the socioeconomic condition. Specifically, maternal schooling and employment status have been associated with increasing infection rates , such as those for *Giardia duodenalis* and *Entamoeba histolytica*. The findings highlight the importance of integrating health programs into community development programs in order to address these inequalities and improve public health outcomes (Quihui et al., 2006). Public health programs should assign highest priority to education and sanitation to reduce the burden of protozoan illnesses in such a way that the future is brighter for vulnerable populations. In addition to parasitic infections, sexually transmitted diseases (STIs) are a significant global health burden whose effects are found in every layer of the population. The United Kingdom has developed heavily in terms of monitoring and managing STIs, but inequities exist across groups , such as men who have sex with men and young adults. The evolving STI epidemiology patterns throughout history demonstrate the changing nature of the public health issues and the imperative to respond flexibly. Advances in test technology, coupled with an evolving service delivery context, emphasize the requirement to deal successfully with STIs. Modern public health programming must consider the shifts in behavioral patterns and population trends in order to implement programs tailored to the specific needs of the targeted vulnerable groups, thereby promoting healthy outcomes in an equitable fashion (Field et al., 2015). Ultimately, successful decline in STIs necessitates a unified worldwide effort emphasizing education, healthcare accessibility, and participation by the community. The dynamic interplay among protozoan diseases and other issues of public health captures the holistic nature of global health outcomes. It not only involves managing the clinical aspects but also requires a proper understanding of the determinants of health. The determinants of intestinal parasitism in Mexico, such as socioeconomic status, educational level, and sanitation behavior, indicate how comprehensive approaches to public health are necessary. Similarly, the burden of STI demonstrates sexual health gaps in education and access to care which continue to disproportionately and adversely affect marginalized groups. Global health approaches, therefore, need to incorporate multi-dimensional approaches which recognize the complex interaction of the biological, social, and economic determinants of health. Since health inequalities persist, inter-disciplinary interaction and intervention are vital to tackle the worldwide burden of protozoan infections and maximize health gains for all populations (Quihui et al., 2006; Field et al., 2015).

7.6.1. Prevalence in Developing Countries

In developing countries, protozoan infection incidence is considerably high, reflecting a serious public health problem. These infections often arise due to inadequate sanitation, limited access to clean water, and low socio-economic levels. For instance, one study in Mexico conducted in rural areas discovered that intestinal parasitism significantly affects school children, as 65% of the population under study was infected with protozoa. This figure indicates the spread rate of infection, primarily in low-income areas with low education levels among mothers, who are at a higher risk of intestinal parasitism (Quihui et al., 2006). Furthermore, hygiene practices , such as open defecation aggravated the scenario, indicating massive public health interventions that include both environmental and educational factors for prevention of disease. The chronic burden of protozoan infection in Third World nations is not limited to rural areas; urban locations also have significant prevalence due to water source contamination. A study on Angke River in Jakarta mirrored the existence of *Ascaris lumbricoides* eggs and *Entamoeba histolytica* cysts, indicating severe fecal contamination of the water sources (Subahar et al., 2008). This case illustrates an expanded understanding of a problem where increased urbanization and industrialization lead to inefficient waste management and pollution. As such, communities that use contaminated water sources are highly likely to become infected with protozoan infections, compounding efforts aimed at improving public health. Preventing the spread of these diseases is highly important with clean water, which is required to address these water quality issues. Interventions in the developing world aimed at reducing the incidence of protozoan infection must be comprehensive, including health education for the community, improvement of sanitation facilities, and strict surveillance of water quality. Maternal education through public health campaigns is particularly necessary because it has been observed that educated mothers will adopt good hygiene and thereby reduce rates of infection among children (Quihui et al., 2006).

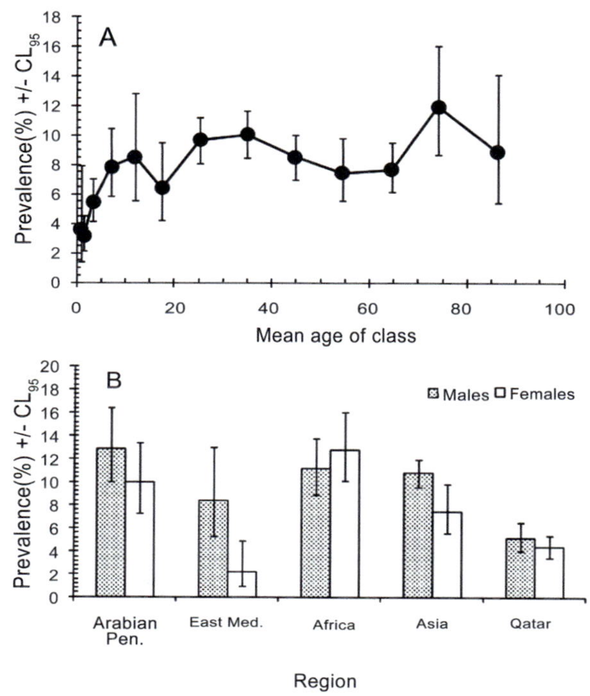

Figure 7.14. Prevalence of all protozoan infections.

Source: https://www.researchgate.net/profile/Marawan-Abu-Madi/publication/47428222/figure/fig2/AS:202530198953986@1425298370265/Prevalence-of-all-protozoan-infections-combined-For-the-goodness-of-fit-of-the-minimum.png.

Furthermore, the improvement of infrastructure for the treatment of water and the disposal of garbage can help significantly to reduce the risk of protozoan waterborne disease. Collaborative work with local governments and non-governmental organizations to facilitate health education campaigns and a suitable planning strategy to develop sustainable sanitation will be essential in reducing the prevalence of protozoan infection in these nations. Such a general strategy is essential to break the cycle of infection and facilitate improved public health benefits to developing countries (Figure 7.14).

7.6.2. Economic Burden of Protozoan Infections

The economic burden of protozoan infections in developing nations is considerable, impacting the health and productivity of infected individuals. The costs of these infections, particularly in areas with weak healthcare infrastructures, lead to high levels of healthcare spending for both governments and households. In endemic regions of protozoan infections, , such as those caused by *Giardia duodenalis* and *Entamoeba histolytica*, repeated healthcare costs for consultation and treatment cause repeated financial burdens for families. Additionally, repeated expenditure on preventive measures , such as sanitation improvement and public health awareness campaigns, becomes a financial burden on limited economic resources. As pointed out in Mexican rural communities, socio-economic status is what elevates the incidence of infections, generating increasing healthcare needs that increase the economic load on such susceptible groups. Lastly, the continuity of protozoan infections illustrates the continuity of the challenges for public health systems to overcome socioeconomic disparities. The implications of protozoan infections extend beyond immediate healthcare expense to also encompass broader economic scope, including lost productivity and reduced income. The patients with chronic infection may experience debilitating symptoms that affect work performance, thereby shortening their contribution to family earnings and overall economic production. In endemic areas, the workforce is effectively hindered because parents will be off work attending to children with diseases, thus sustaining household financial uncertainty. Furthermore, polyparasitism, or where multiple infections coexist at once, is prevalent and carries greater public health and economic stability implications. For instance, studies indicate that children living in poor households are not only more exposed to infections but that such diseases have a negative effect on their learning, perpetuating cycles of poverty and health inequalities (Coulibaly et al., 2012). To further study the economic burden of protozoan infections, one needs to consider the multifaceted interventions required to curb their impacts. Investment in public health initiatives can reverse the tide of such infections and also advance socio-economic development. Measures like increasing sanitation, enhancing access to safe drinking water, and scaling up education on hygiene are crucial to reducing infection rates. Additionally, alignment of health interventions with socio-economic development programs, such as the National Deworming Campaign for Mexico, can enhance overall impact and sustainability. Through engaging with communities and addressing the root reasons for vulnerability, it is not only possible to alleviate the immediate economic pressures but also to provide support for long-term health outcome benefits, too. Ultimately, the solving of the economic cost of protozoan infections has to be a shared endeavor that recognizes the relationship between socio-economic status and health in groups at risk (Coulibaly et al., 2012).

7.6.3. Role in Public Health Policy

Public policy has an important part to play in the fight against protozoan infections. Protozoan infections cause the greatest health burden to populations in low- and middle-income countries, and public policy can work on them very effectively with well-designed interventions. Effective interventions can be formulated to take care of the socioeconomic determinants of health that form the backbone of the transmission of these infections. Sanitation, education, and health literacy programs are required components of any proper public health strategy. In Mexico, operations of the National Deworming Campaign and initiatives like Opportunities addressing maternal care are benchmark efforts against intestinal parasitism. However, the lack of coordination among these initiatives hinders an integration strategy, thus reducing its impact in controlling protozoan infections' burden, as indicated by studies linking socio-economic determinants with children's prevalence rates within at-risk communities (Quihui et al., 2006). Secondly, public health policy must be informed by robust epidemiological data that identifies specific infection patterns in different population groups. In Cote d'Ivoire, for example, a survey of *Schistosoma* species and other protozoan infection prevalence in school settings revealed astounding diversity across school settings (Coulibaly et al., 2012). This goes to show the necessity for tailored interventions based on local endemicity and contextual transmission determinants. Policies that establish regular screening programs and enhance diagnostic facilities are paramount in the prevention and control of these infection transmissions. With each increase in empirical evidence, it can be aligned with policy-making processes to ensure optimal use and efficient targeting of resources towards high-risk groups to achieve maximum intervention strategy impact. Lastly, good public health policy should ensure multi-sectoral collaboration with government institutions, non-governmental organizations, and communities. In managing protozoan infections, it is important to stimulate an interdisciplinary front comprising healthcare, education, and sanitation sectors to tackle the underlying causes of infections holistically. Empowerment through education, accompanied by community participation in health programs, can yield remarkable health benefits, particularly among vulnerable groups. By placing first importance on public health policy based on scientific fact and on community needs, society can create sustainable solutions that not only cure current outbreaks but enhance the overall health system, which will be required to combat future public health threats from protozoan infection.

Test Your Knowledge

1. Why are protozoan infections more prevalent in developing countries compared to developed countries?
2. To what extent is the economic burden of protozoan infections on patients and the health system?

SUMMARY

Protozoan infections have significant public health, ecological, and veterinary science implications. Protozoa, often the focus of second-order consideration in infectious disease discussion, comprise a large category of agents causing serious disease in humans and animals. As recent research has shown, protozoan parasites like *Eimeria* spp. have circadian periodicities in their life cycles that make disease management difficult. It is essential to keep researching these organisms, their biology, and host interaction to come up with sufficient methods for curbing their impact. Without such information, disease control associated with protozoan infection might still remain inadequate, and the need to continue research and funding in this area, especially within conservation initiatives aimed at species like the brown kiwi, which is particularly vulnerable to such pathogens (Taylor, 2017).

In addition, the significance of protozoan infection is also forcefully highlighted through diseases like Chagas disease, caused by *Trypanosoma cruzi*. This neglected tropical disease affects millions, primarily in endemic regions of Latin America, highlighting the intersection between socio-economic factors and health. Despite advancements in understanding the pathology of the disease and improvements in diagnostic techniques, significant gaps remain in treatment accessibility and epidemiological knowledge. These deficiencies perpetuate the cycle of transmission and infection, so a holistic approach with more public health programs, education, and prevention research is the only way to help control such infections. Treating these is not just a medical imperative but also a moral one, aimed at assisting infected groups that need it desperately (Sherman, 2019). Lastly, the conclusion from the study of protozoan infections emphasizes the necessity of interdisciplinary collaboration among scientists, clinicians, and policy-makers. This collaboration is necessary for formulating multilayered, sustainable solutions to the challenges of these pathogens. The relationships among environmental determinants, host defenses, and the life cycle of protozoa must be elucidated to provide effective interventions, particularly in high-risk settings. The union of scientific research with community health programs can provide strong grounds for combating protozoan infections, not only gaining immediate health benefits but also long-term sustainability in disease management. Research in the future will have to follow these dimensions even as it lays out the socio-economic disparities that heighten the impact of protozoan infections, ultimately leading to healthier people (Taylor, 2017; Sherman, 2019).

Protozoan infections pose a public health challenge due to their complex and diverse life cycles and the mechanisms through which they interact with their hosts. Some of the most celebrated protozoan pathogens are protozoa of the genera Trypanoplasma and Plasmodium. Cyprinid fish-infected *Trypanoplasma borreli* is a classic illustration of the complex interrelationship between a protozoan and its host, triggering nitric oxide (NO) production with an immune effect. Such immune modulation, as well as having adverse effects on the host, as seen with carp that were treated with NO synthesis inhibitors having improved survival rates, *Trypanosoma carassii* adopts a different mechanism of suppression of the production of NO from infected hosts, and this indicates the diversified survival mechanisms adopted by protozoan pathogens to evade their detection by host defense. Another protozoan of public health significance is Plasmodium, which is responsible for malaria transmitted predominantly by the bite of infected mosquitoes. Plasmodium and its mosquito vector's interaction is very interesting in that speculations regarding how it originated suggest that this parasite may have evolved from non-parasitic types even algal types, so that its role in ecosystems becomes hard to describe. Plasmodium life cycle is also marked by adaptive processes that enable it to evade the immune responses of the host, a characteristic of protozoan disease pathogens. Adaptability not only enables the survival of the parasite but also complicates treatment strategies, making malaria one of the most recalcitrant diseases to be managed worldwide. It is crucial to investigate the evolutionary processes and immune evasive processes of such protozoa to make effective interventions. The protozoan infection science, therefore, entails not only identification and treatment but also the knowledge of evolutionary biology and host-pathogen interaction. The studies on the immune modulation mechanisms of protozoan parasites like *T. borreli* and *T. carassii* unveil key features of their survival strategy and impact on host health. Even though the exploration of the causes and evolutions of Plasmodium brings to the fore the evolutionary forces that govern disease prevalence,. Knowledge learned from these studies can inform public health interventions and improve treatment approaches, so the function of interdisciplinary research in responding to protozoan infections becomes more critical. As the infectious disease ecology of the globe continues to evolve, discoveries derived from these take-home points are as crucial as ever to construct effective and inclusive health responses.

KEY TERMS FROM THIS CHAPTER

- Alkaloid peganine
- Antiprotozoal agents
- Ciliate infections
- Cryptic biology
- Epidemiological surveillance
- Flagellate infections
- Health programs
- Human medicine
- Intensive healthcare treatment
- Preventive measures
- Amoebic infections
- Chagas disease
- Colitis
- Environmental resilience
- Extracellular vesicles
- Genomic technologies
- Health sciences
- Immunological integrity
- Microfluidic real-time PCR technology
- Protozoan illness

CRITICAL THINKING QUESTIONS

1. **Which of the following is NOT a type of protozoan infection?**
   a. Malaria
   b. *Giardia*sis
   c. Amoebiasis
   d. Tuberculosis
2. **Through what mechanism are most intestinal protozoan infections, like *Giardia*sis, generally transmitted?**
   a. Airborne droplets
   b. Contaminated food or water
   c. Direct blood contact
   d. Insect bites
3. **Which of the following symptoms is generally associated with malaria, a protozoan infection?**
   a. Rash on the skin
   b. Chills and high fever
   c. Sputum with cough
   d. Pain in joints
4. **What is the proper way of preventing tropical protozoan infection?**
   a. Wearing thick clothes
   b. Not taking dairy foods
   c. Using insecticide-treated bed nets
   d. Daily consumption of antibiotics
5. **What is the most common symptom of *Entamoeba histolytica* infection?**
   a. Rash
   b. Diarrhea with blood and mucus
   c. Dry cough
   d. Night sweats

Short Answer Questions

1. What are the primary groups of protozoan infections that infect humans?
2. How are protozoan infections most typically spread from host to host?
3. What are the common symptoms of protozoan infections like malaria, amoebiasis, and *Giardia*sis?
4. What are the treatment options for common protozoan infections, and how effective are these?

5. How do individuals and communities prevent protozoan infections, particularly in high-risk areas?
6. What is the role of vectors , such as mosquitoes and dirty water in causing protozoan diseases?
7. How do protozoan infections contribute to disease burden globally, particularly in developing countries?
8. What are some diagnostic and control challenges of protozoan infections internationally?

Answer to Critical Thinking Questions

1. (d); 2. (b); 3. (b); 4. (c); 5. (b)

REFERENCES

1. Stuart, K., Brun, R., Croft, S., Fairlamb, A., Gürtler, R. E., McKerrow, J., Reed, S., & Tarleton, R. (2008). Kinetoplastids: related protozoan pathogens, different diseases. *The Journal of clinical investigation*, *118*(4), 1301–1310. https://doi.org/10.1172/JCI33945(accessed on 13th June 2025).
2. Albina, E., Aprelon, R., Delannoy, S., Devillers, E., et al. (2020). *Upscaling the Surveillance of Tick-Borne Pathogens in the French Caribbean Islands*. https://core.ac.uk/download/288641885.pdf (accessed on 13th June 2025).
3. Albonico, M., Barda, B. D., Clementi, M., Cringoli, G., et al. (2013). *Mini-FLOTAC, an Innovative Direct Diagnostic Technique for Intestinal Parasitic Infections: Experience from the Field*. https://core.ac.uk/download/pdf/20046407.pdf (accessed on 13th June 2025).
4. Ashafa, A. O., & Ojuromi, O. T. (2020). *An Overview of Some Medicinal Plants and Isolated Active Compounds with Potential Antiprotozoal Activity*. https://core.ac.uk/download/478320863.pdf (accessed on 13th June 2025).
5. Bahia-Oliveira, L., de Wit, L. A., Dixon, B., Dumètre, A., et al. (2019). *Environmental Transmission Of Toxoplasma Gondii: Oocysts in Water, Soil and Food*. https://core.ac.uk/download/286729987.pdf (accessed on 13th June 2025).
6. Bahri, A., Drechsel, P., Raschid-Sally, L., Redwood, M., et al. (2025). *Wastewater Irrigation and Health: Assessing and Mitigating Risk in Low-Income Countries*. https://core.ac.uk/download/pdf/6405282.pdf (accessed on 13th June 2025).
7. Baré, J., Chavatte, N., Houf, K., Lambrecht, E., et al. (2014). *Co-Occurrence of Free-Living Protozoa and Foodborne Pathogens on Dishcloths: Implications for Food Safety*. https://core.ac.uk/download/55886934.pdf (accessed on 13th June 2025).
8. Barratt, J., Chan, D., Ellis, J. T., Stark, D., et al. (2016). *Dientamoeba fragilis, the Neglected Trichomonad of The Human Bowel*. https://opus.lib.uts.edu.au/bitstream/10453/87542/1/Clin.%20Microbiol.%20Rev.-2016-Stark-553-80%20%282%29.pdf (accessed on 13th June 2025).
9. Bhat, R., Maheshwari, S. K., & Saha, S. (2025). *Treating HIV/AIDS Patients in India with Antiretroviral Therapy: A Management Challenge*. https://core.ac.uk/download/pdf/6443480.pdf (accessed on 13th June 2025).
10. Blumenthal, U., Esrey, S. A., Fleisher, J. M., Peasey, A., et al. (2001). *Epidemiology: A Tool for The Assessment of Risk*. https://core.ac.uk/download/13110839.pdf (accessed on 13th June 2025).
11. Buckling, A., Buckling, A., Casadevall, A., Folkesson, A., Jousset, A., Kunert, A., Zaborin, A., et al. (2013). *Pseudomonas aeruginosa Adaptation to Lungs of Cystic Fibrosis Patients Leads to Lowered Resistance to Phage and Protist Enemies*. https://core.ac.uk/download/19503793.pdf (accessed on 13th June 2025).
12. Quihui, L., Valencia, M. E., Crompton, D. W., Phillips, S., Hagan, P., Morales, G., & Díaz-Camacho, S. P. (2006). Role of the employment status and education of mothers in the prevalence of intestinal parasitic infections in Mexican rural schoolchildren. *BMC public health*, *6*, 225. https://doi.org/10.1186/1471-2458-6-225(accessed on 13th June 2025).

13. Caramia, G., Coman, M. M., Silvi, S., Verdenelli, M. C., et al. (2015). *Treatment of Acute Diarrhea: Past and Now*. https://core.ac.uk/download/pdf/54655355.pdf (accessed on 13th June 2025).
14. Collins, L., Ortayli, N., Ringheim, K., Sladden, T., et al. (2014). *Sexually Transmitted Infections: Progress and Challenges Since the 1994 International Conference on Population and Development (ICPD)*. https://core.ac.uk/download/pdf/82755161.pdf (accessed on 13th June 2025).
15. Domingos, A., Domingues, N., Ferrolho, J., Santos-Gomes, G., et al. (2015). *An Overview*. https://core.ac.uk/download/187231188.pdf (accessed on 13th June 2025).
16. Field, N. M., & Hughes, G. (2015). *The Epidemiology of Sexually Transmitted Infections in The United Kingdom: Impact of Behavior, Services and Interventions*. https://core.ac.uk/download/29410608.pdf (accessed on 13th June 2025).
17. Gavinho, B., Combes, V., Dlugonska, H., Hart, E., Evans-Osses, I., Rossi, I. V., Inal, J., et al. (2019). *A New Landscape of Host–Protozoa Interactions Involving the Extracellular Vesicles World*. https://core.ac.uk/download/287580982.pdf (accessed on 13th June 2025).
18. Gillen, Alan L. and Sherwin, Frank, "The Genesis of Malaria: The Origin of Mosquitoes and Their Protistan Cargo, Plasmodium falciparum" (2013). *Faculty Publications and Presentations*. 136. https://digitalcommons.liberty.edu/bio_chem_fac_pubs/136(accessed on 13th June 2025).
19. Groeneveld, A., van Muiswinkel, W. B., Saeij, J. P. J., et al. (2002). *Immune Modulation by Fish Kinetoplast Parasites: A Role for Nitric Oxide*. https://core.ac.uk/download/pdf/29297473.pdf (accessed on 13th June 2025).
20. Heaviside, C., Lake, I., & Nichols, G. (2018). *Climate Change and Water-Related Infectious Diseases*. https://core.ac.uk/download/322490318.pdf (accessed on 13th June 2025).
21. Hickman, E., Kreider, D., Powell, J., Reynolds, K., et al. (2010). *Studies into Cytozoon and Helminth Infections of Bobcats (Lynx rufus) of Northwest Arkansas*. https://core.ac.uk/download/148340648.pdf (accessed on 13th June 2025).
22. Jada, S. (2024). *Scaffold Hopping for The Lead Optimization of The Orally Active Antileishmanial Pyrrole-Quinazoline Alkaloid Natural Product Pegamine*. https://core.ac.uk/download/603978348.pdf (accessed on 13th June 2025).
23. Jamshidi, N., Lewis, N. E., Swann, J., Winzeler, E. A., et al. (2015). *Systems Analysis of Host-Parasite Interactions*. https://core.ac.uk/download/323077861.pdf (accessed on 13th June 2025).
24. Khan, N. A. (2004). *The Pathogenesis of Acanthamoeba Infections: Current Status and Future Implications*. https://core.ac.uk/download/7518.pdf (accessed on 13th June 2025).
25. King, C. H., King, C. L., King, M. J., LaBeaud, A. D., et al. (2009). *Do Antenatal Parasite Infections Devalue Childhood Vaccination?* https://core.ac.uk/download/pdf/8287064.pdf (accessed on 13th June 2025).
26. Lee, J. S., & van der Putten, W. (2011). *Soil Borne Human Diseases*. https://core.ac.uk/download/38621779.pdf (accessed on 13th June 2025).
27. Morgoglione, M. E. (2021). *Ozonated Water for Parasitic Control in Buffalo Farms (OZO-PAR)*. https://core.ac.uk/download/574199266.pdf (accessed on 13th June 2025).
28. Obiekezie, A., Okaeme, A. N., & Olufemi, B. E. (2001). *Parasites and Non-Fish Predators of Tilapia with Particular Reference to The Sustainable Management of Fisheries of Lake Kainji Nigeria*. https://core.ac.uk/download/11019315.pdf (accessed on 13th June 2025).

29. Sherman, Emily, "Review of Chagas Disease and Treatment Obstacles to Eradication" (2019). *Senior Honors Theses*. 890. https://digitalcommons.liberty.edu/honors/890(accessed on 13th June 2025).

30. Coulibaly, J. T., Fürst, T., Silué, K. D., Knopp, S., Hauri, D., Ouattara, M., Utzinger, J., & N'Goran, E. K. (2012). Intestinal parasitic infections in schoolchildren in different settings of Côte d'Ivoire: effect of diagnostic approach and implications for control. *Parasites & vectors, 5*, 135. https://doi.org/10.1186/1756-3305-5-135 (accessed on 13th June 2025).

31. Subahar, R. (Rizal), & Sutanto, L. (Lisawati). (2008). *Ascaris Lumbricoides Eggs and Human-Intestinal Protozoan Cysts Found in River Water of Angke River, Jakarta*. https://media.neliti.com/media/publications/148041-EN-ascaris-lumbricoides-eggs-and-human-inte.pdf (accessed on 13th June 2025).

32. Taylor, H. S. (2017). *The Eimeria Species Affecting Brown Kiwi: Host-Parasite Interactions and Conservation Implications: A Thesis Presented in Partial Fulfilment of The Requirements for The Degree of Master of Science in Conservation Biology at Massey University, Manawatu, New Zealand*. https://core.ac.uk/download/186668377.pdf (accessed on 13th June 2025).

33. Unasho, A. (2013). *An Investigation of Intestinal Parasitic Infections Among the Asymptomatic Children in Southern Ethiopia*. https://core.ac.uk/download/544387414.pdf (accessed on 13th June 2025).

HELMINTHIC INFECTIONS

8

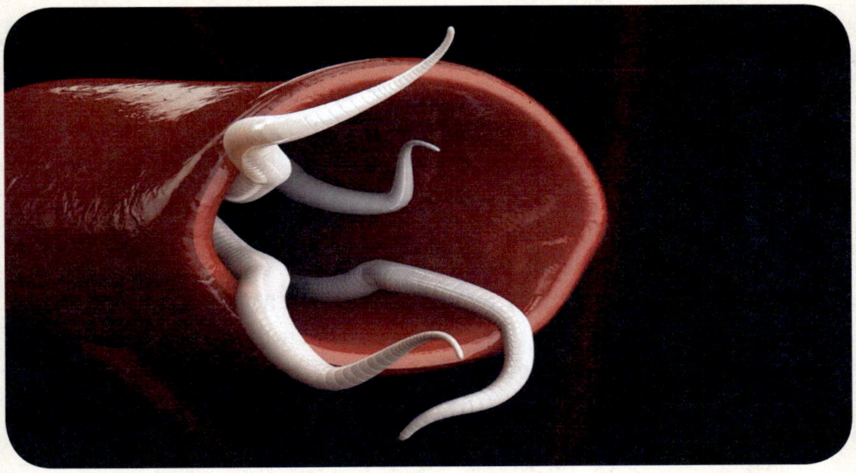

LEARNING OBJECTIVES

After studying this chapter, you will be able to:

1. Explain the types of helminths;
2. Explain about transmission and life cycle of helminthic infections;
3. Explain the symptoms of helminthic infections;
4. Identify effective treatment methods of helminthic infections;
5. Handle prevention and control of helminthic infections;
6. Discuss the global impact of helminthic infections.

Introduction

Helminthic infections, particularly intestinal helminths, are public health issues of great concern, more so in developing nations. These parasitic infections are most commonly linked with poor environmental sanitation and low socio-economic conditions, that create a good environment for their transmission. The prevalence rates are proven as high among the most affected, particularly school children, who are likely to be most affected on account of poor exposure to health education and inadequate hygiene practices. For instance, the infection rate among rural Indian school children was found to be 17.8% and untrimmed nails and not washing hands properly were the high-risk factors for the infection (Boratne et al., 2008). The research indicates the critical need for intervention programs in raising hygiene levels and providing health education to decrease helminthic infection burdens in rural populations. In regions where the dominant form of infection is helminthic, the public health consequences are widespread. Extensive levels of infection not only result in short-term illnesses , such as malnutrition, anemia, and impaired cognitive ability in infected children, but also in cumulative socio-economic disadvantage. For example, a prevalence of 13.8% of intestinal helminths was documented among school children from a survey in Ethiopia, illustrating the need for ongoing health information communication and periodic treatment to combat these infections (Mitiku et al., 2015). If not controlled, these infections turn into poverty and health inequality. Therefore, good strategies involving both medical treatment and participatory learning are the solutions to putting an end to this malignant cycle and enhancing overall well-being of the people. Hygiene education coupled with medical intervention seems to be a vital strategy towards combating helminthic infections. Participatory strategies that involve the people and emphasize personal hygiene can significantly reduce the incidence of these infections among vulnerable people. The aforementioned study in India showed the effectiveness of child-to-child hygiene education in enhancing better practices, and this resulted in enhanced nail cleanliness and hand washing among school-going children (Boratne et al., 2008). Hence, incorporating these educational measures along with frequent preventive treatment is of utmost significance to sustain health gains. This two-pronged approach can effectively lower infection rates, improve the health status of children, and eventually lead to socio-economic growth in communities afflicted by helminthic infection.

Definition of Helminthic Infections

Helminthic infections are illnesses brought about by parasitic worms, which are further classified primarily into three classes: nematodes (roundworms), cestodes (tapeworms), and trematodes (flukes). Such pathogens have complicated life cycles involving two or more hosts and environmental forms, making them superior in transmission between environments. Helminthes like *Ascaris lumbricoides*, *Schistosoma* spp., and *Taenia solium* produce significant morbidity among the infected populations. Infection is typically acquired through ingestion of faecally contaminated food and water, through the skin, or via a vector , such as an insect. Identification of the diverse methodologies employed by these parasites to colonize hosts is crucial in the effective prevention of public health problems and the delivery of preventative interventions for these infections, especially in regions where socioeconomic factors result in increased prevalence. The global burden of helminthic disease is most forcefully felt in the developing world, where compromised health care and sanitation infrastructure further enable transmission. For instance, such infections are prominently visible among children, who are more susceptible because of poor hygiene and nutritional inadequacies. In line with public health research, most such infections occur among children aged below five years and school-going children, showing the role of targeted interventions (Amanda et al., 2023). Effective control of helminthic disease can be dependent on community education and hygiene promotion, as well as the application of prophylactic drugs. In designing targeted strategies effective in reducing the risk of transmission and health benefits maximization for vulnerable populations, understanding the specific populations identified as affected by helminths becomes important. Recent epidemiological research has also enlightened the complex relationship of helminthic infections with various diseases, particularly with regard to allergic disease. Although in the past they have been thought of as harmful, recent work shows that helminths play a multifaceted role in modulating immune responses. As an example, some research has reported a possible protective function of helminth infection with regard to the development of allergic conditions, although evidence remains contradictory and under investigation (Arrais et al., 2020). Such dual comprehension of helminths as pathogen and as potential immune modulators underscores the necessity for a full understanding of their environmental and biological impacts. While the investigators go on to investigate this intricate relationship, it is important that they grapple with its implications for public health interventions and control strategies for helminthic infections keeping in mind their overall contribution to human health (Figure 8.1).

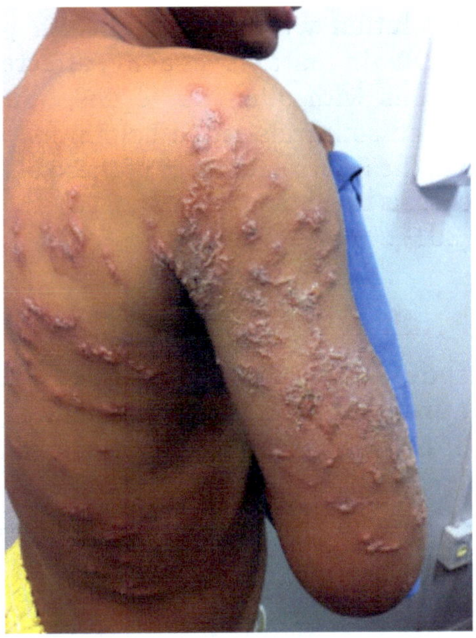

Figure 8.1. Helminthic infection.

Source: https://ars.els-cdn.com/content/image/1-s2.0-S0190962214023159-gr3.jpg.

Importance of Studying Helminthic Infections

It is important to investigate helminthic infections in public health and disease control, particularly in low- and middle-income countries where the parasites are endemic. Helminth research can shed light on the complex interaction between disease prevalence, environment, and human behavior. These diseases impact not just the health status of individuals but also result in serious socio-economic consequences. Helminthic illnesses in regions with poor sanitation and limited healthcare access can limit productivity and schooling, and create a cycle of poverty. By looking at the distribution and prevalence of helminthic infections, researchers can design specific interventions and policies that improve health benefits as well as minimize the disease burden on the health system. Studying helminthic infections also yields information on the immune system and its evolutionary dynamics. Certain helminths were discovered to be therapeutically valuable in altering immune responses and promoting health. For instance, hookworms, which have long been thought of as virulent parasites, are today being researched as potential treatments for diseases like autoimmune disorders and allergies. This change in thinking about how helminths affect human health can be applied to new forms of treatment that take advantage of the body-protective properties of such organisms. Comprehension of the intricate relationship between humans and helminths can open up new avenues for therapeutic development, advocating the core role of these infections as a public health problem as well as in evolutionary medicine (Strosberg, 2014). Research on helminthic infections also helps in evaluating the effectiveness of public health interventions, i.e., mass drug administration (MDA) programs. Such programs tend to reduce the prevalence of soil-transmitted helminthiasis and related diseases, particularly in co-endemic regions. A recently published study conducted in India in Alappuzha compared pre- and post-MDA incidence of soil-transmitted helminthiasis against lymphatic filariasis and offered useful information regarding the impact of such intervention (Bhagat et al., 2018). Identification of the success or failure of such initiatives enables health authorities to modify strategies based on this information, resulting in effective control. By continuously monitoring helminthic infections, scientists and public health organizations can ensure interventions are modified as conditions change and therefore result in better health in vulnerable populations.

8.1. Types of Helminths

Learning Outcome

1. Define nematodes (roundworms);
2. Describe cestodes (tapeworms);
3. Define trematodes (flukes).

Helminths are parasitic worms that come in a wide variety and are, for the most part, divided into three major types of helminths: nematodes, cestodes, and trematodes. Nematodes, also called roundworms, have cylindrical bodies that taper at one end, differentiating them from other helminth types. Nematodes harbor some of the significant human pathogens, , such as *Ascaris lumbricoides* and hookworms. Ascaris, in particular, can increase to an enormous size and cause severe intestinal complications, while hookworms are notable for causing anemia due to resulting blood loss. The prevalence of these infections is especially vexing in regions with poorer sanitation facilities and weaker healthcare access, which continue to fuel a disease-poverty cycle. Cestodes or flatworms have ribbon-shaped and segmented bodies. Tapeworms, belonging to this category, stay primarily in the intestines of their host and can absorb nutrients directly through their skin, making them highly effective parasites. Such infections are mostly observed in humans due to the consumption of uncooked or infested meat. Some of these species like *Taenia saginata* and *Taenia solium* carry the risk of causing serious health issues like malnutrition and intestinal blockage. Also, infection has more general health implications, particularly in developing countries where access to adequate nutritional resources is already compromised. Trematodes, commonly referred to as flukes, constitute another large group of helminths that have complex life cycles, typically with intermediate hosts, e.g., snails. *Schistosoma* species, the etiologic agents of schistosomiasis, are significant causes in the tropics and subtropics. These infections are caused when free-swimming larval cercariae invade human skin in infested water. Chronicity of trematode infections typically leads to longstanding health impairment, including liver damage, and increased susceptibility to other infections. The virulence of such helminthic infection is a testament to the urgency of their resolution within public health policy, particularly in nations heavily affected by co-infections with other pathogens, , such as malaria and soil-transmitted helminths, which speaks to the interrelatedness of these diseases as discussed by Futagbi et al. (2016) and Mak et al. (2017.

8.1.1. Nematodes (Roundworms)

Nematodes, commonly referred to as roundworms, form a significant helminth group that poses health risks in various populations of people, particularly in developing countries. Nematodes are multicellular parasites inhabiting various ecosystems and can infest the human body via contaminated water, soil, or food. Unhygienic and unsanitary living conditions are usually found to be directly related to the development of nematode infestations, thereby indicating the role of socio-economic determinants. In particular, the circumstances on which they are passed on—, such as overcrowding, lack of waste disposal, and lack of access to clean drinking water, unequally affect vulnerable populations, like children and pregnant women. It would be useful to learn the life cycle and modes of transmission of nematodes so as to devise effective public health interventions to address these parasitic diseases, especially in regions where such situations are prevalent. The impact of nematode infection on health is severe, especially in maternal and child health. The facts are that geohelminthiasis, which is brought about predominantly by nematodes, may lead to a decrease in cell-mediated immunity among pregnant women. Their susceptibility to the occurrence of severe complications , such as maternal anemia, preterm delivery, and even stillbirth is enhanced because of the compromised immune system, reflecting on the severity of health outcomes of these infections (Lal et al., 2019). Besides, the presence of nematodes has the potential to adversely affect the growth of children's cognitive skills, aggravating their education and well-being. Since nematode infections have the potential to delay physical and mental development, there is a need to address these health issues through the application of specific interventions for the purpose of improving sanitation conditions and access to health care. Based on the enormous health burden presented by nematodes, intense prevention and control measures are urgently required. Proper steps consist of education regarding personal hygiene, environmental sanitary conditions, and preventive community health programs to reduce the prevalence of such infections (Futagbi et al., 2016). The role of public health policies in facilitating access to antihelminthic medications cannot be downplayed either; regular screening and treatment can mitigate the severity of infections in vulnerable populations. By increasing awareness and understanding of the socio-economic drivers of nematode transmission, the stakeholders will be in a position to use integrated and sustainable control measures to combat helminthic infection. Lastly, solving these issues will not only improve the health outcome of individuals but also the quality of life of those communities infested with nematodes and other helminths (Figure 8.2).

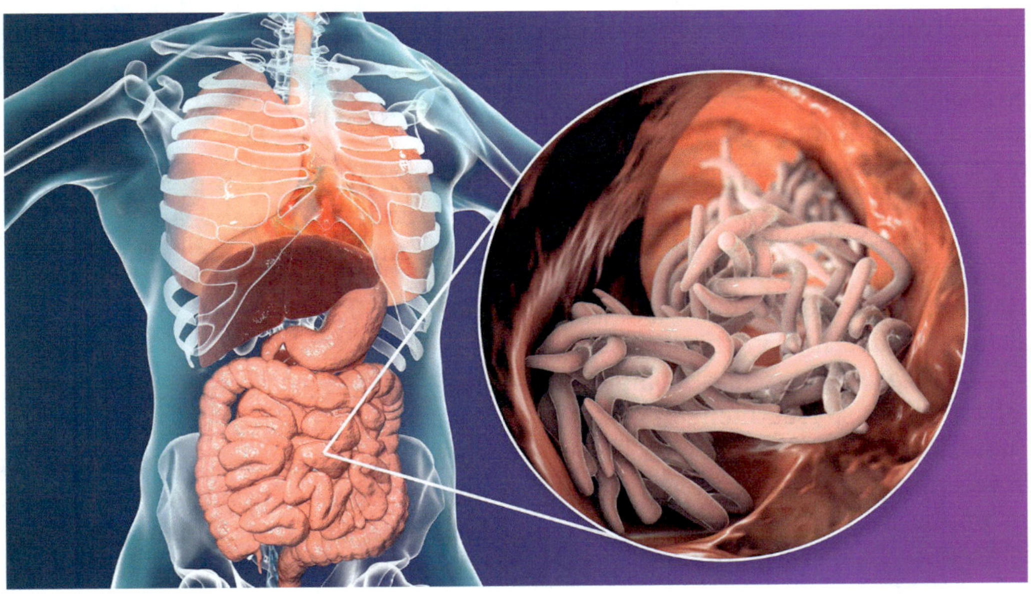

Figure 8.2. Round-worms in human intestine.

Source: https://cdn.hswstatic.com/gif/shutterstock-1837076626.jpg.

8.1.2. Cestodes (Tapeworms)

Cestodes, or tapeworms, represent a varied group of helminthic parasites that share a flat, elongated, and segmented body. Cestodes infect the intestines of many vertebrate hosts, including humans, and result in a wide range of health issues. The life cycle of the cestodes typically involves many hosts, where eggs or proglottids are expelled via feces and subsequently ingested by intermediate hosts , such as livestock or rodents. After they become adults in the definitive hosts' intestines, the larvae develop tapeworms that can lead to malabsorption of nutrients and cause diseases like abdominal pain and diarrhea. This complex life cycle suggests the importance of understanding environmental and social determinants that create conditions for tapeworm transmission, as discussed in many studies that document their prevalence among populations. The prevalence of tapeworm infections differs significantly with geography and host species. For instance, a cross-sectional survey of small ruminants in Ghana identified that 94.4% of goats were infested with tapeworms, which illustrates the high prevalence of these parasites among livestock herds (Futagbi et al., 2016). These findings demonstrate the risk to human consumers who may consume undercooked or infected meat. Apart from livestock, stray animals—, such as dogs and cats, are significant in cestode infection epidemiology. Another research in Iraq also highlighted that stray cats are highly infected, particularly with Dipylidium caninum, with zoonotic significance to humans (Aqeele et al., 2024). Detection of these infection patterns is essential for effective intervention in public health and knowledge of potential transmission pathways of tapeworms. Treatment of cestode infections must be pursued on various fronts, including in veterinary medicine practice, human health, and public health education. Effective deworming practice in animals, proper pet care, and proper food handling are the most important factors required to help reduce the incidence of tapeworm infection. Publicity efforts can also educate the population regarding symptoms and signs of helminthic infection and alert them to seek medical treatment when necessary. As zoonotic potential is ever-present, constant monitoring of parasitic infestation in domestic and wild animals is critical. The enforcement of such measures not only does much to control the frequency of cestodes but also supports broader insight into helminthic infection within a public health context. With the collaboration of veterinarians, epidemiologists, and public health officials, initiatives towards the prevention of the impact of such parasites on the health of animals and humans can be taken (Figure 8.3).

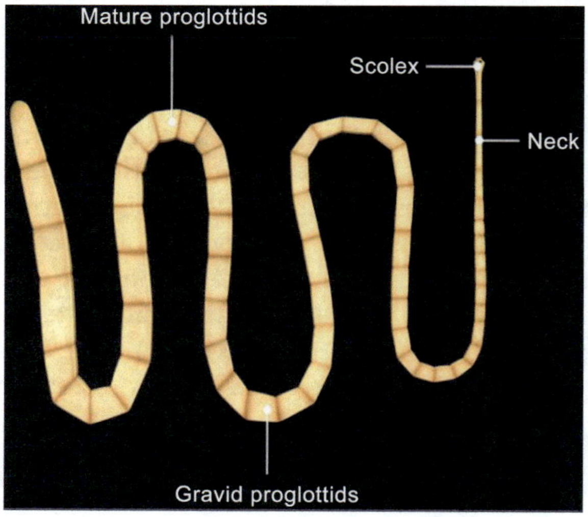

Figure 8.3. Tapeworm.

Source: https://cdn-prod.medicalnewstoday.com/content/images/articles/170/170461/the-taenia-solium-tapeworm.jpg.

8.1.3. Trematodes (Flukes)

Trematodes or flukes are a suborder of parasitic flatworms that form the class Trematoda. These pathogens are characterized by their leaf-shaped morphology, soft-tissue consistency, and complex life cycles with one or more intermediate hosts, often mollusks and fish. Characterization of their epidemiology has led to the discovery of approximately 18,000 species, of which only a few are recognized as significant human pathogens. Significantly, these infections are more widespread in low-resource settings where environmental and socioeconomic conditions facilitate transmission. The high incidence of infections by trematodes points to the high need for public health interventions due to their association with significant morbidity and long-term conditions, including liver and gastrointestinal disease. Furthermore, other liver fluke species have been identified as being biological carcinogens, highlighting the level of awareness and effective prevention and control measures (Harrington et al., 2017). The transmission dynamics of trematode infections are greatly influenced by human behavior, including agricultural practices and feeding habits. Areas with irrigation facilities have the possibility of creating very conducive environments for intermediate hosts, which facilitate the transmission of these pathogens. Additionally, dietary habits , such as the consumption of raw or uncooked fish have been shown to enhance infection risk from trematode species like *Clonorchis sinensis* and *Opisthorchis viverrini*. The global helminthic infection situation is also compounded by the movement of people from endemic to non-endemic regions, where exposure to reintroduction of such parasites to new regions is enabled. There is evidence that an understanding of the complex interplay among human activities, environmental features, and trematode life cycles is required to manage the infection burden, particularly in poor-resource settings (Teimoori et al., 2019). Diagnosis and treatment of trematode infections have become quite sophisticated with advances in molecular tools and epidemiological studies. Traditional tests may be the detection of adult flukes in host material or eggs in fecal material, but the sensitivity of the traditional methods is usually not adequate for low-burden infections. Recent studies through polymerase chain reaction (PCR) and sequencing of specific genetic markers have revolutionized the field of diagnostics, enabling more precise detection of known and unknown trematode species. For instance, molecular analysis of jackals infected with trematodes revealed high molecular similarities to *Haplorchis taichui*, suggesting cross-species transmission and also denoting complex ecological relationships (Teimoori et al., 2019). These developments not only help achieve better diagnostic precision but also emphasize the importance of continuous monitoring in an attempt to effectively control helminthic infections and decrease their impact on public health (Figure 8.4).

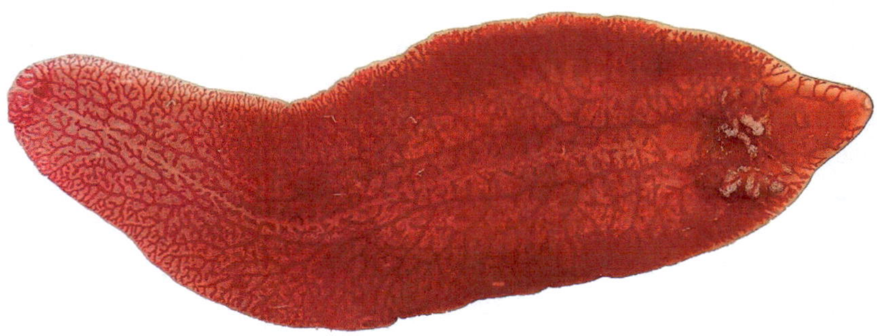

Figure 8.4. Liver fluke.

Source: https://cdn-prod.medicalnewstoday.com/content/images/articles/319/319479/liver-fluke-br-image-credit-veronidae-2013-br.jpg.

Test Your Knowledge

1. What are the main characteristics and examples of nematodes (roundworms) that infect humans?
2. In what respects do cestodes (tapeworms) differ in structure and life cycle from nematodes and trematodes?

8.2. Transmission and Life Cycle

Learning Outcome

1. Understand modes of transmission of helminthic infections;
2. Outline the life cycle stages of helminths;
3. Outline environmental factors affecting the transmission dynamics of helminthic infections.

Transmission and life cycle, particularly that of soil-transmitted helminths (STHs), are important in understanding why they are so common and the associated health consequences. The life cycle of STHs like *Ascaris lumbricoides*, hookworms, and *Trichuris trichiura* typically consists of both human and environmental components. Consumption of eggs through contaminated food or soil initiates the life cycle for Ascaris, whereby the larvae are released and migrate through the body of the host to develop in the intestines. The hookworm larvae, however, penetrate the skin, enter the bloodstream, and reach the lungs, where they migrate to the gastrointestinal tract. This complex human-environment interaction reinforces the importance of sanitation and hygiene in controlling transmission rates. Interruption of these life cycles can be achieved through preventive interventions, like the building up of public health infrastructure, leading to a reduction in infection rates eventually. The life cycle stages of the helminths also demonstrate their survival and reproduction adaptation mechanisms. Within the host, the parasites can survive for years, taking the host's nutrients while evading the immune system. For *Ascaris lumbricoides*, the adult worms can produce a thousand eggs a day, which ensures their dissemination within endemic communities. Above all else, the geographical extent of such infections is marred by problems since conditions for transmission , such as poor sanitation and poor access to healthcare, are prevalent in the majority of developing nations. Besides, environmental determinants , such as soil and humidity affect the survival of helminth eggs in the environment outside a host. As the literature observes, increased investments in research are needed to advance understanding of these dynamics and develop effective interventions for controlling transmission and its health impact (Lamberton & Jourdan, 2015). Effective control initiatives rely on a clear understanding of transmission dynamics alongside life cycle complexities. While preventive therapy has been established to reduce the morbidity of helminthic infection, equal access among vulnerable groups remains a challenge (Jourdan et al., 2018). Furthermore, the efficacy of mass deworming campaigns raises doubts, questioning whether they can eliminate disabling clinical manifestations of helminthiasis without improving environmental and socio-economic status at the same time. In addressing these problems, diagnostic aids and public health interventions come first. The development of sensitive testing techniques for helminth infection detection and promoting hygiene awareness can influence helminth transmission levels and the life cycle of the parasite considerably, resulting in better world health.

8.2.1. Modes of Transmission

Modes of transmission for helminthic infections are varied and play a significant role in public health. One of the principal routes is ingestion of contaminated food and water, particularly in conditions of poor sanitation standards. For instance, populations with less access to clean drinking water are more at risk for helminthiases , such as *Ascaris lumbricoides* and *Trichuris trichiura*. Poor habits of personal hygiene, especially among food handlers, augment the risks since contaminated food is used as a vehicle for transmission. Research identifies food handlers as central to intestinal parasite transmission with an estimated 6.6% of such employees being helminth carriers, as indicated by surveys of pathogen prevalence. Therefore, there is a need to appreciate and intervene in these modes of transmission in order to succeed. Direct handling of soil or surfaces contaminated with filth is another primary mode of helminthic infection, a route of transmission generally referred to as soil-transmitted helminths. This mode is particularly prevalent in the tropical and subtropical regions where the conditions for helminth egg or larva survival and infectivity are favorable. Farm workers who play on contaminated soil or who engage in farming without proper protective gear are more likely to be infected. Environmental contamination may occur through fecal contamination in unsanitary settings, leading to increased transmission of helminths , such as hookworms and whipworms. Moreover, studies have found that seasonal variations in the environment, e.g., increased rainfall, influence helminth infection prevalence through increased contamination of water and soil sources (Brown et al., 2008).

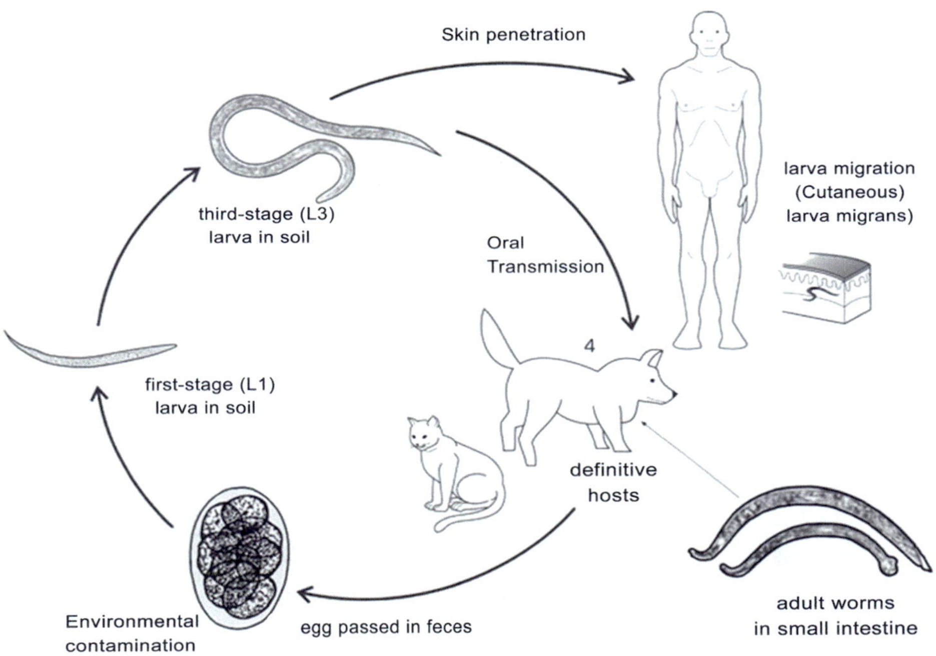

Figure 8.5. Transmission of helminthic infections in humans.

Source: Alvares V, Rubinsky-Elefant G, Urbano M. Soil-Transmitted Helminthic Zoonoses in Humans and Associated Risk Factors [Internet]. Soil Contamination. InTech; 2011. Available from: http://dx.doi.org/10.5772/23376

Therefore, effective public health measures must aim at augmented sanitation and hygiene measures to prevent this transmission route. Vector transmission of helminthic infections, even though less common, is yet another important mode, particularly for certain species that require an intermediate vector or host to complete their lifecycle. Certain helminths like schistosomes are reliant upon freshwater snails to complete their lifecycle and can be transmitted to man in contact with infested water bodies. The prevalence of such infections can be particularly prevalent among groups engaged in activities , such as fishing or bathing in water known to be infected. On the other hand, travelers and migrants may present different risks of exposure from those of indigenous communities, a reality demonstrated on a study where the lower incidence of helminthic infections observed in travelers coming back from their trips, compared with immigrants and refugees who tend to get exposed to such infections in endemic areas (Brown et al., 2008). Intervention against these specific vectors of transmission requires tailored education and preventive actions, especially among risk communities (Figure 8.5).

8.2.2. Life Cycle Stages of Helminths

Life cycle stages of the helminths are significant to understand for a clear insight into their transmission and their role in human health. They are sophisticated animals with a complicated life cycle involving different developmental phases that can include intermediate and definitive hosts. First, environmental factors beyond the parasites are involved in the transmission since most helminth eggs or larvae are passed into the feces of infected hosts.

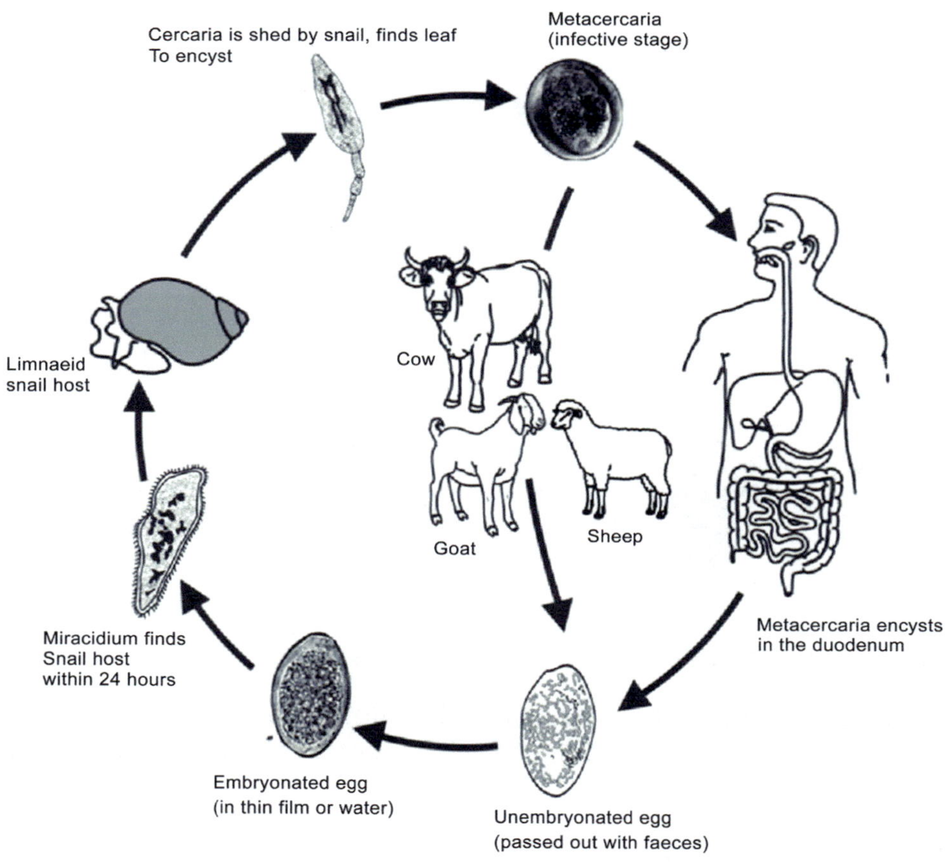

Figure 8.6. Life cycle of liver flukes.

Source: https://www.researchgate.net/profile/Omotosho-Lawal/publication/343718557/figure/fig1/AS:933791040274435@1599644541583/Life-cycle-of-liver-flukes.png.

These life stages can survive in water or in the soil before being ingested by the next host. Soil-transmitted helminths like *Ascaris lumbricoides*, for example, require specific atmospheric conditions to survive and finish their life cycle, which indicates the intricate interactions between these parasites and their environments. An appreciation of these life cycles underpins their prevalence and longevity and ultimately public health interventions to limit helminthic infection. Once ingested, the larvae of helminths continue to mature in the host organism, evolving through various growth stages and stages of maturity. This stage often involves travel through the body systems of the host, whereby parasites adapt to their respective niches. For example, while *Ascaris larvae* migrate initially through the lungs, adult worms develop in the intestines, where they are quite sensitive to host immune responses. These adaptations of types, from evading detection by the immune system to compatibility with host responses, are largely responsible for the long-term survival of helminths (Ambrosio et al., 2018). In addition, the excretory-secretory products discharged by these parasites throughout their life cycle stages have the potential to affect the host's immune system and induce a Th2-dominant response that tends to promote the host's survival with the helminths.

The transmission dynamics vary among different species of helminths. For instance, soil-transmitted helminths primarily transmit via contaminated soil and food, and the infections are high where there is poor sanitation (Lamberton & Jourdan, 2015). Others, however, , such as those that transmit via secondary hosts, have more complex interactions that can involve various transmission vectors. By delineating the various stages of life cycles, researchers can employ particular control techniques, i.e., drug therapy and reinforced sanitation regulations, that are aimed at transmission rates. In total, detailed knowledge of such life cycle phases not only enhances our helminth biology but also plays an important role in devising good public health strategies for combating helminthic infections (Figure 8.6).

8.2.3. Environmental Factors Affecting Transmission

The epidemiology of transmission of helminthic infections is inextricably linked with a variety of environmental determinants that affect the prevalence and distribution of the parasites. Climatic characteristics matter as temperature and humidity control the life cycle of the helminths and their intermediate hosts. For instance, the survival of soil-transmitted helminths (STH) is strongly promoted by hot and damp conditions, typically found in tropical and sub-tropical regions. These environmental conditions can lead to increased infection rates among vulnerable populations , such as children residing in rural areas where they are exposed to faecally contaminated water sources and soil. Thus, it is crucial to have an understanding of the special environmental conditions that promote helminth transmission to come up with apt intervention measures that could mitigate their contribution to public health and economic growth (Ajjampur et al., 2014). Socio-economic determinants are intertwined with environmental factors, adding to the epidemiological scenario of helminthic infections. Lower socio-economic status (SES) populations are observed to have higher rates of infection in most regions due to poor sanitation and hygiene. For example, high co-infections among the population in coastal Kenya rural communities have been reported to be driven by shared risk factors, including household crowding and inadequate access to clean water (Ajjampur et al., 2014). Unfavorable environmental degradation, including deforestation and wrong disposal of waste, increases the risks that make transmission of parasites easier. Therefore, in view of the socio-economic determinants of health as well as environmental factors, becoming essential while formulating inclusive public health interventions against helminthic infections. Spatial analysis has also been identified as a powerful tool in the research on environmental determinants of transmission of helminths. Spatial aggregation of infection has been found to be prevalent in some villages and hence localized interventions with the specific environmental characteristics in view become a necessity. For instance, a study in coastal Kenya categorized specific single and co-infection clusters due to socio-demographic and environmental risk factors with a heterogeneous prevalence pattern in different landscapes (Bisanzio et al., 2014). Using a local level of analysis, it can inform health policy makers where to deploy the resources and how to best prioritize intervention efforts. Thus, the incorporation of spatially informed approaches ensures a particular response to the complexity of helminthic infections, thereby enhancing the efficacy of public health interventions for the control of these endemic diseases (Figure 8.7).

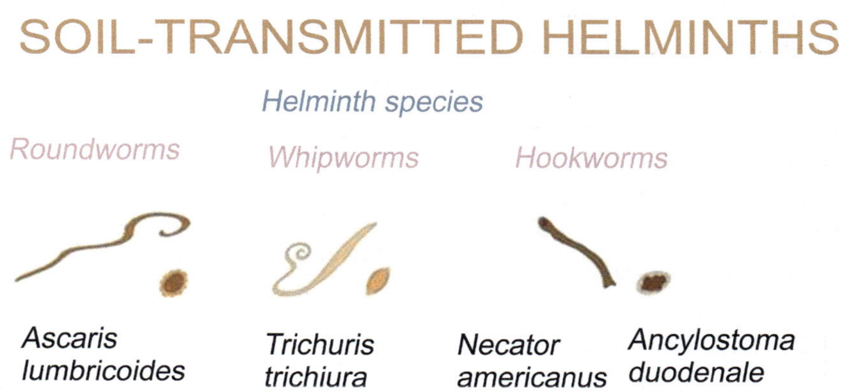

Figure 8.7. Soil-transmitted helminths (STH).

Source: https://www.who.int/images/default-source/departments/ntd-library/soil-transmitted-helminthiases/soil-transmitted-helminths-deadly-worms.tmb-549v.jpg?Culture=en&sfvrsn=f06cc6e0_2.

Test Your Knowledge

1. What are the main modes of helminth infection transmission in humans?
2. How does the life cycle of helminths enable them to remain in the environment?

8.3. Symptoms and Diagnosis

Learning Outcome

1. Explain the common symptoms of helminthic infections;
2. Explain diagnostic methods involved in infection identification;
3. Highlight challenges in the diagnosis of helminthic infections.

Symptoms of helminthic infections may be extremely nonspecific, with variation tending to depend on the specific helminth involved and the host's response. Common presenting complaints in infected persons include gastrointestinal disturbances, i.e., abdominal pain, diarrhea, and nausea, and these will have a similar presentation to other intestinal pathologies. In particular, *Ascaris lumbricoides* infections have the potential to result in serious complications, including intestinal obstruction that occurs when there is a heavy burden of worms, resulting in an intussusception. The obstruction is extremely painful and requires surgical intervention, which indicates the necessity for early diagnosis and treatment of these infections, especially where helminth burdens are high (Ciardi et al., 2016). Therefore, the separation of everyday gastrointestinal issues from those caused by helminthic infections is crucial to ensure timely intervention and prevention of serious consequences. Helminthic infection diagnosis is primarily laboratory testing of stool, whereby ova, larvae, or adult worms may be identified. This method is considered to be the gold standard in the diagnosis of most intestinal helminths, including hookworms, tapeworms, and pinworms. However, not all helminthic infections yield eggs in stool examination in the acute phases, and in some parasites, a few of them have diagnostic markers, and therefore, for them, serological tests have to be utilized. For example, the diagnosis of schistosomiasis can be made through the detection of particular antibodies in the blood, thus allowing more extensive utilization of diagnostic techniques best tailored to the suspected causative helminth. DDS. With the diverse presentation of such infections, the clinicians need a high degree of suspicion as well as a good knowledge of the symptomatology of different helminths (Brown et al., 2008). With travel all over the world, the diagnostic picture of helminthic infections makes clinical assessment more complicated. Travelers from endemic regions can have symptoms that are easily attributable to other causes, for example, travelers' diarrhea or respiratory illness. Of particular interest is the fact that studies have established that travelers are less likely to be diagnosed with helminthic infections compared to immigrants and refugees, who are more likely to have a greater burden because they spend more time exposed to infected environments (Brown et al., 2008). This difference highlights the importance of considering travel history in diagnosis and also pretravel medical consultation to prevent risks by preventive measures, including vaccination and prophylactic medications. In general, a general awareness of symptoms, diagnostic techniques, and exposure history enhances helminthic infection management, leading to improved patient outcomes.

8.3.1. Common Symptoms of Helminthic Infections

Helminthic infection, which is caused by parasitic worms, will often present with a wide range of signs and symptoms based on the helminth species and the patient's immunity. The most frequently encountered symptoms are abdominal pain, gastrointestinal distress, and significant weight loss. The patient may have an interplay of diarrhea and constipation, typically secondary to intestinal obstruction due to the mass effect of the worms. Specifically, *Ascaris lumbricoides* has been linked with severe infections that include complications , such as intestinal intussusception, showing the potentially severe consequences of helminthic infestation on gastrointestinal well-being. Also, the resulting nutritional deficiencies from helminthic parasitosis can exacerbate symptoms and lead to more generalized health complications, particularly in populations with limited access to healthcare and sanitation. With the higher worm burden, the onset of symptoms also becomes more severe, further emphasizing the importance of good prevention and treatment regimens (Ciardi et al., 2016).

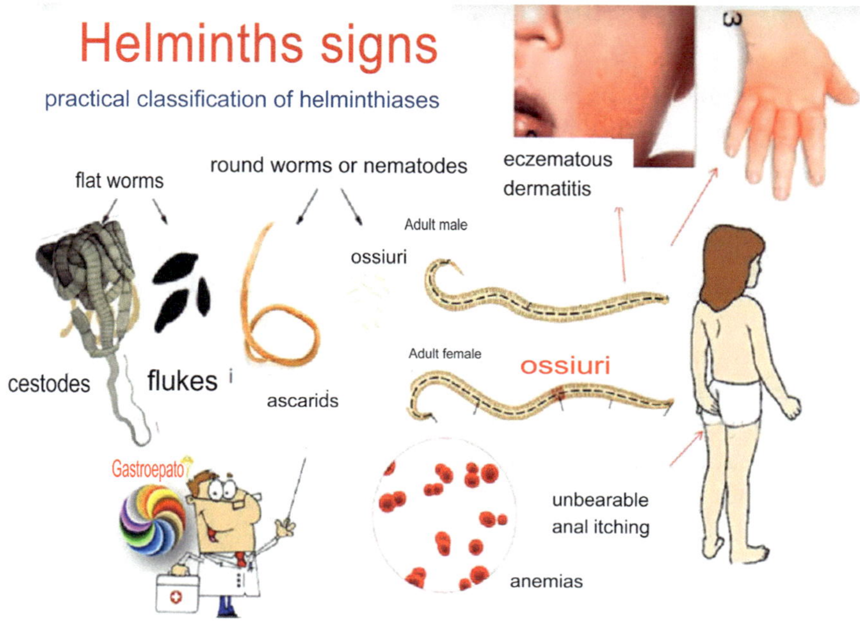

Figure 8.8. Helminth signs.

Source: https://www.gastroepato.it/en_helminths-signs.webp.

Besides the gastrointestinal signs, helminthic infections may also elicit systemic responses that worsen a person's general health status. These are fever, weakness, and malaise, which are indicative of the body's immune reaction to the parasites. Some of the helminthic infections, especially those involving *Schistosoma* species, might also result in more severe symptoms , such as hepatosplenomegaly and anemia. Systemic effects of these infections may be seen through secondary complications , such as eosinophilia, where an increase in the levels of eosinophils can reflect an inflammatory response to the presence of the helminth within the body. Infection with helminths can also cause overlapping symptoms with other diseases, which makes their diagnosis even more challenging. Hence, knowledge of the different symptoms of such infections is essential for healthcare workers so that they can deliver treatment at the right time and effectively (Brown et al., 2008). The relevance of such symptoms goes beyond the health of an individual and affects public health outcomes and health systems, especially in high-helminth prevalence regions. The chronicity of helminthic infections has a tendency to result in long-term health issues, disrupting children's development and mental functions, and inducing school and workplace absenteeism. The resultant socioeconomic effects are likely to perpetuate and generate poverty and destabilize community development. Therefore, health interventions in the form of enhanced sanitation, education, and access to health care are critical not only for decreasing the burden of helminthic infections but also for improving the overall health of communities. The treatment of these infections involves a multi-faceted approach, integrating medication, health education, and public health infrastructure strengthening to alleviate the symptoms and related long-term complications of helminthic infections (Ciardi et al., 2016) (Figure 8.8).

8.3.2. Diagnostic Methods Used in Identifying Infections

Diagnosis of helminthic infections calls for the application of a number of diagnostic methods capable of detecting these parasites accurately. The Kato-Katz thick smear is one traditional method employed in the diagnosis of infections like ascariasis. Although the method is being employed as a comparison detection tool, it lacks high sensitivity. Increased stool sampling can enhance this sensitivity, yet still below that of other microscopy techniques, , such as FLOTAC, with improved diagnostic capability. The ongoing application of Kato-Katz is still prevalent for mapping and monitoring national control programs, pointing to the strategy's utility despite its flaws. Thus, research investment in more efficient diagnostic tests is critical because current methods must improve to be able to meet the challenges posed by helminthic infections (Lamberton & Jourdan, 2015). In addition to conventional microscopy methods, antibody detection serological tests have been useful for diagnosis. The tests offer the advantage of having higher sensitivity, particularly in assessing transmission dynamics in regions to be targeted for elimination. Their utility is often constrained by the inability to deliver a clear diagnosis, therefore limiting their use in clinical practice. Molecular diagnostics represent a step beyond this, ushering in a new era of specificity and sensitivity to the diagnosis of helminthic infection. Even though the application of molecular methods is still limited due to expense, they provide unparalleled possibilities for individual diagnosis, drug effectiveness, and the correct determination of individual helminth species like *Ascaris suum*. All of these diagnostic improvements are key to helminth control and in eliminating human suffering associated with parasitic diseases (Lamberton & Jourdan, 2015). The existence of zoonotic helminths, , such as *Baylisascaris procyonis,* poses another challenge for the diagnostics community. With raccoons increasingly invading the city, the potential for human infection via environmental exposure to their eggs increases, and this is a priority public health issue. *B. procyonis* eggs can remain viable in the environment for extended periods of time, posing a genuine threat to unsuspecting individuals, especially young children who may unknowingly ingest them. Rapid and accurate diagnosis of this infection is critical, as it could lead to severe complications in the form of neurological damage. Advanced diagnostic tests to detect *B. procyonis* infections are hence required to inform public health guidelines and mitigate the risk of this emerging zoonosis. As helminthic infections and our understanding of them evolve, so do the diagnostic tests that help combat them effectively.

8.3.3. Challenges in Diagnosing Helminthic Infections

Diagnosis of helminthic infections presents serious challenges because of a blend of conditions that affect the precision and accessibility of diagnostic tests. Conventional diagnostic methods, e.g., the Kato-Katz method, are still common but have low sensitivity for diagnosing infections with aetiology produced by soil-transmitted helminths like *Ascaris lumbricoides*. Even though it is usually used for public health investigations, its drawbacks require greater sampling and inspection approaches to enhance detection rates. Additionally, the crossing of symptoms with other conditions of the gastrointestinal tract makes clinical diagnoses more challenging, and therefore, once more demands the search for more precise diagnostic methods. Consequently, the urgent necessity of investment and research in more sensitive diagnostics has become increasingly apparent, particularly in regions that are greatly impacted by helminthic infections (Lamberton & Jourdan, 2015). Molecular diagnostics are a turning point in the fight against helminthic infection, with technology offering greater sensitivity and specificity than conventional practice. For example, polymerase chain reaction (PCR) assays have been highly promising but are costly and useful mainly in research settings rather than routine clinical practice. In addition, diagnostic tests based on antibodies, while probably sensitive enough to pick up infections, are cumbersome in practical application, especially for the assessment of transmission dynamics in areas that aim for the elimination of the infections. The trade-off between cost-effectiveness and diagnostic performance is a point of contention, which poses challenges to combat such infections at the global scale (Lamberton & Jourdan, 2015). In order to identify the economic forces at play, it is important to create sustainable diagnostic solutions that are directed towards the development of public health. Additionally, epidemiological studies on helminthic infections are necessary to address inconsistencies in prevalence data, as discussed in studies with special populations. For example, a cross-sectional study revealed low intestinal helminth prevalence among children experiencing diarrhea and emphasized the need for having strict data collection procedures. Environmental determinants , such as sanitation and hygiene practices, also play a very important role in infection rates, whose diagnosis accuracy and control measures are challenging. It is challenging to determine risk populations and implement successful control measures due to interactions among these determinants. Thus, overcoming the diagnostic challenges will need a multi-faceted approach, including technology and extensive field research with a focus on prioritizing environmental circumstances and individual health patterns.

Test Your Knowledge

1. Enumerate the common symptoms of helminthic infections in human beings.
2. Enumerate the main issues faced in accurately diagnosing helminthic infections.

8.4. Treatment Options

Learning Outcome

1. Recognize the role of anthelmintic drugs in the treatment of helminthic infections;
2. Enumerate other treatment practices;
3. Explain the importance of appropriate treatment compliance.

The management of helminthic infections, to a large degree, depends on effective treatment, which plays a central role in the disease burden control of such parasitic infections. Anthelmintic agents , such as albendazole and mebendazole have been found to be first-line drugs for soil-transmitted helminthiasis and are found to possess substantial efficacy in worm burden reduction and the alleviation of clinical manifestations. But despite these effective and safe drugs being available, disparities in access to treatment remain present, particularly where endemicity is most prevalent. Statistical data indicates that only up to half of children in high-risk groups were treated in 2016, indicating a broad gap in public health measures aimed at treating these infections among vulnerable populations (Jourdan et al., 2018). Thus, enhancement of access to anthelminthic therapy along with increased knowledge of treatment necessity is important for morbidity reduction and ultimately better quality of life in those affected. In addition to routine pharmacological regimens, other treatment modalities have been studied and present a new frontier in the treatment of helminthic infections. The evolving landscape of molecular medicine represents new approaches, including the identification of druggable targets through next-generation omics and bioinformatics technologies. Such approaches are likely to lead towards personalized medicine, which has the prospect of optimizing therapy specific to individual patients. With improved understanding of the genomics and pathophysiological mechanisms underlying helminthic infections, the medical community is now able to utilize more refined and effective treatment modalities that are superior to the standard practices that are suboptimally effective in each patient (Singh et al., 2020). With these ongoing research pursuits, they will work to supplement existing treatment regimens, leading ultimately to better overall treatment of helminthic disease. Public health interventions must also counterbalance medical interventions by emphasizing prevention and control in addition to treatment. Mass deworming has been able to reduce helminthic infections in most endemic regions, but programs must have a larger scope that includes better diagnostics and education at the community level. There is a need for healthcare professionals to not just administer treatment but to also get involved in educating patients and populations on hygiene, diet, and environmental control in order to prevent reinfection. Furthermore, maximization of diagnostic tools will be critical in exactly identifying those who will gain from treatment and bolstering the effectiveness of public health interventions in reducing helminthic infections (Jourdan et al., 2018). By adopting a multi-faceted approach through the treatment and prevention of helminthic infections, the medical community can actually attempt to safeguard the populations at risk as well as the impact of helminthic infections on public health.

8.4.1. Anthelmintic Medications

The role of anthelmintic drugs is central in managing helminthic infections caused by various parasitic worms. These infections, being significant public health concerns, significantly weigh down on the vulnerable groups, particularly in developing nations where the socio-economic status is poor. Anthelmintic medications constitute a major front line of defense against such helminths as flukes, tapeworms, and nematodes, which thrive well within human hosts. Therapies like albendazole and mebendazole are widely used because of their effectiveness against soil-transmitted helminths, showing the significant impact that these drugs have on reducing morbidity from infection with such parasites. The treatment of helminthiasis not only promotes health but also economic development through increased productivity and standards of living of infected people, as these infections have been linked in the past to stunted growth, anemia, and low cognitive function in children, as reported in Lamberton & Jourdan (2015) . The reliance, however, on a limited portfolio of anthelmintic drugs is a serious concern, particularly the development of drug resistance. Repeating administration of such drugs as albendazole and mebendazole is the cause behind this phenomenon, and it has been observed largely in veterinary medicine, with growing concerns about similar trends in human health. The World Health Organization emphasizes combating neglected tropical diseases but acknowledges that the threat of resistance prevents them from carrying out control and eradication programs for helminthic infections. Thus, it is important to investigate new drug strategies and design new compounds that have pan-helmintic efficacy against various helminth strains. Repurposing drugs research and identification of new pharmacological agents from natural sources are of extreme importance in finding alternatives, as highlighted in Tewelde & Tadesse (2022). Vaccine development for helminthic infection is also a long-term possibility. The new concept of a pan-anthelmintic vaccine is centered on providing broad protection against different helminth species and thus reducing dependency on drugs as well as resistance risks. Despite the daunting vaccine development challenges, including the complexity of helminth biology as well as immune evasion mechanisms, available work portends promising potential. Integration of methods like employing high-tech immunological tools and recombinant technologies can enhance vaccine performance. There should be collective efforts from researchers, health practitioners, and global health institutions in a bid to make these goals a reality and, finally, improve global health outcomes for helminthic infections as argued in the ongoing debates regarding the need for new anthelmintic measures in Tewelde & Tadesse (2022) (Figure 8.9).

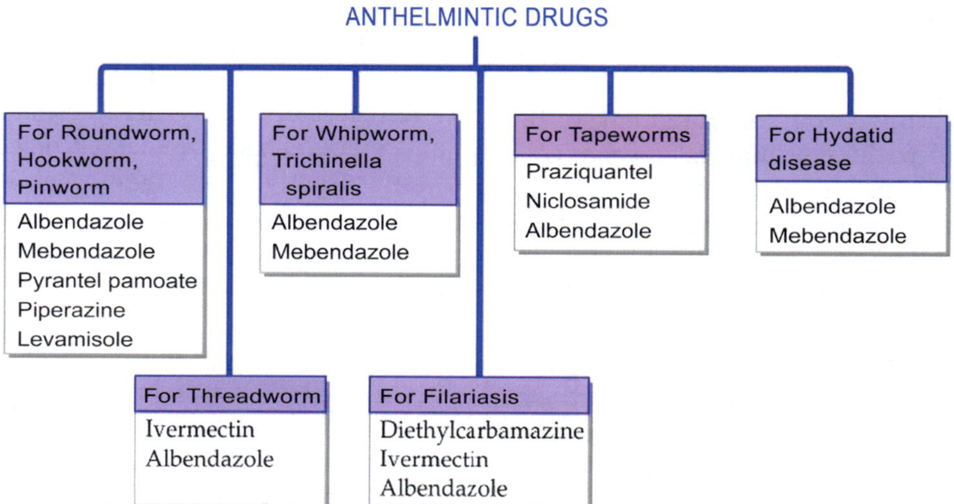

Figure 8.9. Anthelmintic drugs.

Source: https://pharmacyfreak.com/wp-content/uploads/2025/05/CLASSIFICATION-OF-ANTHELEMETIC-DRUGS.jpg.

8.4.2. Alternative Treatment Approaches

Investigations into novel treatment modalities of helminthic infections have gained appreciable momentum, especially against the background of the limitations of conventional pharmacologic therapies. Conventional anthelmintics, while effective, are often plagued with problems, such as poor coverage in the endemic areas, prohibitively high costs, and vulnerability to resistance. In response, researchers have looked for substitute methods , such as food therapies, probiotics, and immunomodulatory therapies that leverage the host's immunity instead of relying purely on chemical agents. These alternatives are promising not only in filling current treatment gaps in accessibility but also in reducing side effects associated with chemical drugs. Investigating these options is crucial in populations at risk of infection, particularly children residing in endemic regions where helminthic infections are most prevalent and often remain untreated due to logistical challenges in providing healthcare (Jourdan et al., 2018). Immunotherapy, using the body's own immune response processes, is a notably attractive strategy for the treatment of helminthic infections. The highly polarized immune responses induced by helminthic infections, like increased IgE production, could provide hints at potential therapeutic directions. For instance, specific immunotherapies aimed against the Th2 immune response, typically upregulated in infected patients with co-infections like malaria and helminthiasis, are under investigation. Recent studies indicate that helminth co-infections are capable of increasing total serum IgE levels significantly, and in so doing, suggest a mechanistic link between helminth infections and immune modulation within the context of co-infectious environments (Belyhun et al., 2014). On the basis of this evidence, it can hopefully be possible to formulate targeted interventions that will possess the ability to limit the effects of both malaria and helminthic infection, doubled through enhanced immune response modulation. Another potential alternative treatment is employing classical and indigenous medicining practices that have been employed for centuries throughout various cultures. Herbal remedies and plant remedies have been utilized in most societies to cure helminthic infections, most of which have been handed down through generations. Modern ethnopharmacological research has only just begun to look into how effective such classical medicines would be when coupled with formal medicine. These integrative approaches, besides offering effective treatment, can actually increase patient compliance and acceptability. As public health policy continues to search for cost-effective, socially acceptable alternatives in helminthic infections, proper studies on these alternative modalities become essential to determine their efficacy and safety, culminating ultimately in a more integrative approach in the control of helminthic infections in endemic populations (Jourdan et al., 2018).

8.4.3. Importance of Proper Treatment Adherence

The importance of proper adherence to treatment in the management of helminthic infections cannot be overstated, particularly if one considers the burden of these infections to vulnerable groups , such as children. Proper treatment is not merely crucial to alleviate symptoms but also to prevent long-term health consequences that follow from untreated infections. Where the prevalence of helminthic infection is high, particularly in children under five years of age, strict adherence to drug treatment is necessary. The mother study in Kuwaluhan Village recognizes the correlation between knowledge and levels of drug treatment adherence to the use of helminthic drugs. The findings were consistent in that most mothers manifested medium levels of adherence despite having adequate knowledge in terms of treatment, and the need for specific education in order to enhance adherence. This inconsistency implies that even with sufficient information, both healthcare access and socioeconomic status can hinder uniform treatment patterns, which can exacerbate the public health impact of helminthic infections (Amanda et al., 2023). Compliance with appropriate treatment is further underscored by the deleterious effects of untreated helminthic infections, which can cause severe health issues , such as anemia and stunted growth. The link between helminths and anemia in postpartum women unveils the symbiotic relationship between parasitic illness and general health. Research in Mbarara Regional Referral Hospital indicates that failure to adhere to hematinic drug is largely responsible for the incidence of postpartum anemia, with other factors including conditions like helminthic infestations (Anwar et al., 2016). The significance of this data extends to the health of children, too; straightforward helminthic infection can lead to cognitive impairment and malnutrition, thus perpetuating disease and poverty cycles. Ensuring appropriate adherence, then, not only cures immediate short-term health consequences of helminthic infection but also serves as a critical approach to improving long-term health benefits and breaking the cycle of disease transmission in infected groups. Public health interventions to combat helminthic infections must put a strong emphasis on treatment compliance as an integral component of their efforts. It needs a co-related approach that includes education, availability of drugs, and outreach in the community for creating required health attitudes. Stakeholders must get together to undertake comprehensive programs working on the determinants of treatment compliance which are socioeconomic and cultural. Long-term follow-up and support interventions can also facilitate adherence by reminding individuals that continued treatment regimens are necessary. Through the formation of an adherence culture, communities can effectively combat the prevalence and intensity of helminthic infections, leading to the overall improvement in the quality of life of infected persons. Dedication of the health care providers, governments, and families will be essential towards ensuring treatment guidelines are adhered to on a consistent basis, leading the way towards healthier futures and reducing helminthic disease burden (Amanda et al., 2023).

Test Your Knowledge

1. Which are the most commonly used anthelmintic drugs for the treatment of helminthic infections?
2. What complementary or alternative treatment modalities can be used for the management of helminthic infections?

8.5. Prevention and Control

Learning Outcome

1. Be familiar with the public health prevention of helminthic infection;
2. Explain sanitation and hygiene as a role;
3. Make education and awareness campaigns the top priority in combating helminthic infections.

Prevention and control of helminthic infections are essential not only for public health but also for socioeconomic development in infected areas. Effective measures largely rely on community participation and education, taking into account hygiene and sanitation measures. Among the primary measures is the promotion of hand washing with soap, which has been demonstrated to have a substantial impact in reducing rates of transmission of gastrointestinal pathogens, , such as helminths. An intervention in low- and middle-income countries indicates the favorable impact of hand washing, such that chronic compliance and behavior change interventions can lead to better health outcomes for populations infected by these pathogens. Handling hygiene-related practices, therefore, forms a fundamental component in the overall helminthic infection control management (THE STATE OF HANDWASHING IN 2016, 2017). Vacination is also a critical component in the preventive measure against helminthic infection, supporting that integrated healthcare practices are required. For instance, handling cervical cancer risks due to human papillomavirus (HPV), research shows that vaccination coverage among adolescent girls is overcome by various factors, including access barriers. Low-resource settings are often beset with obstacles, , such as transportation to health centers, that can significantly reduce completion rates of vaccinations (Mabeya et al., 2018). It is thus essential to utilize innovative delivery models and education for children and parents in order to address barriers to vaccination. With improved availability and delivery of vaccinations with complete education on their importance, the likelihood of protection for younger populations against preventable diseases significantly increases. Moreover, mass deworming programs also represent another significant strategy in helminthic infection control and prevention.

The programs are most effective among schoolchildren, who are the most exposed to the parasites. Regular deworming combined with health education can lead to improved physical well-being, enhanced mental development, and educational attainment. The World Health Organization has also recommended systematic deworming programs in the endemic regions, given its effectiveness in reducing the infection levels as well as the associated morbidities. Constant monitoring and evaluation of the programs are critical to the scalability and sustainability, which can ultimately contribute to the significant reduction of helminth burdens among the population (Mabeya et al., 2018). A multi-modal approach that unites hand washing, vaccination, and deworming interventions can greatly enhance prevention and control of helminthic infections globally.

8.5.1. Public Health Strategies for Prevention

Prevention public health measures for helminthic infections must be multi-dimensional, including vaccination, education, and increased access to healthcare services. Preventive immunization, particularly in those settings where the prevalence of helminthic disease as well as other diseases is present, can have such priceless public health impacts. As an illustration, the inclusion of the HPV vaccine within general health programs can serve as a case study that can demonstrate success and issues. In sub-Saharan Africa, where the proportion of cervical cancer cases attributable to HPV is very high, geographical access and ignorance are big barriers to uptake of vaccination. This is clearly demonstrated in a study where only 39.1% of schoolgirls completed the three doses recommended due to logistical factors as well as lack of appropriate health education, as identified in the study findings (Mabeya et al., 2018). Conquering such setbacks through novel delivery mechanisms is crucial for enhancing public health results overall. Aside from vaccination, promotion of behavior change through effective health education efforts is a key feature of averting helminthic infection. Hand washing with soap has been repeatedly shown to be effective in curbing the transmission of parasitic infection, including helminths. Public health practitioners must therefore place first priority on activities ensuring hygiene awareness and compliance, especially in settings of low resources. From studies in this area, the success of handwashing interventions relies on understanding determinants of behavior and social culture about cleanliness (THE STATE OF HANDWASHING IN 2016, 2017). This discovery necessitates placing health messages within local contexts and situating interventions within the specific needs of populations. Incorporating knowledge of local customs and traditions into education campaigns can help public health efforts more effectively reach people and foster lasting behavior change to reduce helminthic transmission. Lastly, strengthening healthcare systems to deliver equal access to treatment and prevention interventions is the backbone of any successful public health initiative against helminthic disease. This involves not just expanding physical infrastructure but expanding healthcare worker training and resource allocation to rural areas where helminthic infection is prevalent. Strategic partnerships between governments and non-governmental organizations can assist in dispersing necessary medication and conducting routine deworming programs in schools.

In these interventions, public health agencies are able to target risk groups where the burden of the helminthic disease is most severe. Besides, continuous research and surveillance activities are necessary in evaluating the effectiveness of such public health interventions and introducing corrective modifications depending on new data. A strong focus on enhancing healthcare access and quality is thus part of an overall prevention strategy against helminthic infection (Figure 8.10).

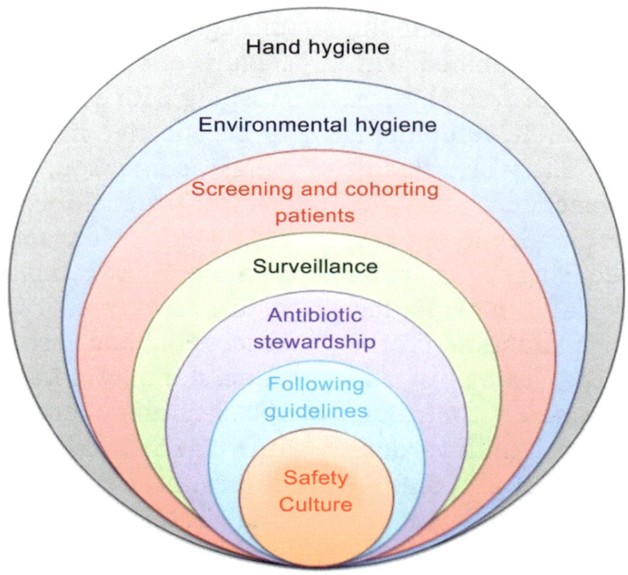

Figure 8.10. Strategies to prevent healthcare-associated infections.

Source: https://infectionsinsurgery.org/wp-content/uploads/2019/02/prevention-1.jpg?w=863.

8.5.2. Role of Sanitation and Hygiene

The interaction of sanitation and hygiene with endemicity of helminthic infections is important in the understanding of public health policy more broadly. Poor sanitation and unhygienic conditions are significant facilitators of intestinal parasites spreading, which target sensitive groups, for example, children in developing nations. As highlighted in a recent publication of hand hygiene literature, effective hand washing with soap has been shown to reduce the occurrence of infection caused by pathogens, like helminths, by disrupting the transmission chain (THE STATE OF HANDWASHING IN 2016, 2017). Moreover, communities that spend money on improved sanitation facilities normally observe a decline in parasitic illnesses, and that's why sanitation programs should be part of overall health plans. Results of studies conducted in rural India also provide more insight into the role of hygiene education in combating helminthic infections.

The research revealed a significant prevalence of intestinal parasite infection among children who had poor hygiene practices in which they failed to wash their hands and left their nails uncut (Boratne et al., 2008). The use of targeted hygiene education was effective in changing behavior patterns, with a significant rise in the prevalence of correct handwashing after defecation and good nail care. This two-fold approach of drug treatment alongside participatory hygiene education proved to be vital in reducing parasite loads in infected groups, and education could be an effective tool to combat helminthic diseases. Overall, establishing a culture of sanitation and hygiene is essential to disease prevention and public health. Integrating holistic hygiene practices into daily life can really minimize the disease burden of helminth infection and other infectious diseases. Activity to improve infrastructure, , such as provision of clean water and adequate sanitation facilities, must also go on in tandem with campaign activities. By making these interventions a top priority, communities can construct a healthier environment that is supportive of the well-being of their population, and put an end to the cycle of infection, paving the way for continued improvement in health on the long term.

8.5.3. Education and Awareness Programs

Education and awareness programs are of special significance in the fight against helminthic infections, particularly where such parasitic diseases are endemic. Infections of this nature thrive in low-resource settings where socio-economic factors limit access to healthcare and sanitation. Properly educating the population on sanitary practices , such as regular washing using soap, is effective in preventing the transmission of helminths and other disease-producing agents. Evidence indicates that informed practice change is inversely related to disease prevalence reduction; for instance, an in-depth review of hand hygiene practices documented consistent gains in preventing infection among low- and middle-income countries and placed educational outreach as a major strategy first (THE STATE OF HANDWASHING IN 2016, 2017). Through community outreach and targeted programming, one can encourage a culture of health awareness with a priority on hygiene as a main force towards preventing helminthic infections. In addition to promoting elementary hygiene behaviors, educational programs must also address the specific health risks helminthic infections present, particularly to the vulnerable child population. Infection can undermine physical and cognitive development, and if continued, contribute to malnutrition, thus greatly affecting educational outcomes. Awareness programs, particularly in the Sub-Saharan region, have established the need for access to preventive care interventions, , such as sanitation and health care services, which are pivotal in helminthic disease burden control. Understanding these relationships can equip the community with the ability to advocate for better public health policies and resource allocation. A Kenyan research identified some major challenges to HPV immunization among girls, directly related to access to health care, therefore highlighting the interdependence of health education and other public health objectives (Mabeya et al., 2018). Furthermore, integration of educational courses into immunization campaigns can also further enhance health benefits for at-risk groups of helminthic infections. Collaboration among public health officials and communities in the sharing of information on vaccination as well as hygiene can be an integrated approach to disease prevention. Effective strategies include workshops, school health education, and local leadership coalitions to foster community acceptance. These programs can lead to better turnout for vaccination campaigns, raising coverage rates and overall public health. As shown in cervical cancer and HPV immunization awareness campaigns, informed communities will tend to minimize stigmatization of health interventions and maximize practice adherence. In line with this, sustainable health education and awareness programs are essential in reducing the impacts of helminthic infections and developing resilient, health-conscious communities.

Test Your Knowledge

1. What are the most useful public health practices for preventing and controlling helminthic infections in the community?
2. How do sanitation and hygiene habits reduce the spread of helminthic infections?

8.6. Global Impact

Learning Outcome

1. Recognize the burden of helminthic infections throughout the world;
2. Educate about the socioeconomic consequences of helminthic infections on affected populations;
3. Explain the impact on public health systems.

The global impact of helminthic infections extends far beyond individual health, influencing economic and social conditions in infected areas. The disease burden of these infections, particularly in low- and middle-income countries, results in an extreme loss of productivity because they often result in chronic illness and diminished capacity to work. The connection between socio-economic status and helminthic infections is extremely important; residents of poor neighborhoods tend to suffer from polyparasitism, which deteriorates their health status and hinders economic growth. In order to mitigate such effects, integrated strategies incorporating education and healthcare accessibility must be applied as they can improve not only the health status but also economic resilience among these groups (THE STATE OF HANDWASHING IN 2016, 2017). In the majority of coastal regions, as well as in Kenya, the prevalence of helminthic infection is highly spatially heterogeneous, and environmental and socio-demographic conditions interact to produce heightened exposure. Research has indicated that in some Kenyan villages, over 50% of screen-tested individuals have one or more parasites infecting them, with co-infection reaching levels of nearly 20% (Bisanzio et al., 2014). These findings underscore the need for context-sensitive intervention approaches that incorporate local patterns of infection and risk factors at the population level. Helminth infection management not only benefits public health but also contributes to economic opportunities by allowing communities to utilize their resources more efficiently and reduce the costs to the health system. The global reaction to helminthic infections must also respond to global health policies as well as disease prevention and control efforts. Education and collaboration across national boundaries are needed in the battle against the spread of these diseases. Activities , such as improved sanitation, hygiene, health education, and establishment of additional health care centers can all help curb the infection rates. In addition, global health programs to educate communities about the importance of preventive interventions, including hand washing and waste disposal, have the potential to reap long-term benefits. By encouraging sustainable behaviors and the implementation of multi-component intervention strategies, helminthic infection burdens can be significantly reduced in the long term, ultimately contributing to global health, economic prosperity, and quality-of-life improvements (THE STATE OF HANDWASHING IN 2016, 2017).

8.6.1. Prevalence of Helminthic Infections Worldwide

Helminthic infections are one of the most significant public health concerns globally, particularly in low- and middle-income countries where socio-economic determinants account for a significant proportion of disease burdens. Soil-transmitted helminths (STHs) infect over one billion people worldwide. *Ascaris lumbricoides*, the causative organism of ascariasis, is one of the most common STHs infesting human populations. Diagnostic work on helminthic infections is typically reliant on methods , such as the Kato-Katz technique, although this is low in sensitivity, but remains the gold standard for mapping and control program monitoring. The shortcomings of low diagnostic abilities continually lead to underreporting of the infection rates, highlighting a pressing demand for better detection tools and increased research expenditures to accurately portray the occurrence of such infections, thereby driving effective intervention strategies (Lamberton & Jourdan, 2015). Geographically, helminthic infections largely thrive in tropical climatic areas, where environmental factors enhance the survival and dissemination of parasitic eggs. Poor sanitation zones, lack of clean potable water, and inadequate access to healthcare are most at risk. Sub-Saharan Africa, endemic for diseases like schistosomiasis and lymphatic filariasis, illustrates the intersection of poverty and helminthic disease. This group is further complicated by co-infection with diseases like malaria that may impact vaccination efficacy, , such as the HPV vaccine. The worldwide prevalence of cervical cancer, in these settings compounded, is a reflection of the need for synergistic solutions that can concurrently address multiple threats to health and tackle the underlying social determinants of health that drive such infections (Mabeya et al., 2018). Furthermore, the impact of helminthic infections does not just impact individual health but also economic and societal costs. High morbidity levels from these infections can lead to decreased productivity, affecting educational outcomes and workforce participation within infected populations. Children tend to be the most affected and may experience stunted development and mental disability, which can have a lasting impression on their development and subsequent prospects. Further, the cost of treating helminthic infections burdens healthcare facilities, particularly in impoverished environments. Therefore, reducing the incidence of helminth infections becomes important not only for increasing public health outcomes but also in generating economic growth and stability in developing nations. Granting adequate funding and political will to control measures is important in reducing the impact of such infections on global health (Lamberton & Jourdan, 2015; Mabeya et al., 2018) (Figure 8.11).

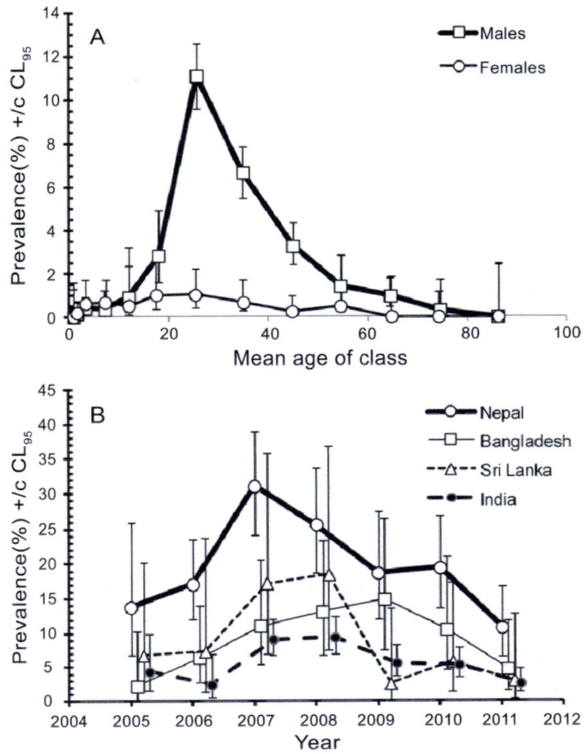

Figure 8.11. Prevalence of helminth infections. (A) Age-prevalence profiles of helminth infections in male and female subjects (all regions, years, and age classes combined); and (B) Changes in prevalence of helminth infections over the period of 7 years in male subjects (all age classes) from the four countries showing overall the highest prevalence rates in the study population.

Source: https://www.researchgate.net/profile/Marawan-Abu-Madi/publication/235905528/figure/fig2/AS:393848917381154@1470912307501/Prevalence-of-helminth-infections-A-Age-prevalence-profiles-of-helminth-infections-in.png.

8.6.2. Socioeconomic Effects on Affected Populations

Socioeconomic consequences of helminthic infections in infected populations are huge, having a tendency to reinforce present vulnerabilities in poor communities. In the majority of developing countries, the infections are rampant in regions ravaged with inadequate sanitation, inadequate health care, and poor access to clean water. The conjoined barrier of poverty and parasitic disease gives rise to a cycle of descent in which the infected are at a higher probability of having difficulty gaining employment and are often unable to function within family and societal structures. Furthermore, the economic burden of curative treatment for chronic infection has the potential to induce household economic instability, diverting resources from essential requirements , such as education and nutrition. Helminthic infection is particularly dangerous in the case of children, whose intellectual and educational progress is adversely impacted, establishing a poverty cycle and inhibiting later opportunities for development and prosperity, as indicated by the geohelminthiasis and socioeconomic research (Lal et al., 2019). In addition to personal misery, helminthic infections also have social and population-level implications for public health and solidarity. The simultaneous presence of parasites like *Schistosoma haematobium* and hookworm is likely to lead to co-infections, which create the condition in which not only are health problems rampant but also interconnected (Bisanzio et al., 2014). This complexity demands understanding of converging risk factors like economic underdevelopment and overpopulation that characterize the majority of affected countries. The resulting health disparities undermine community efforts to improve overall wellness because higher levels of disease reduce productivity among employees and strain local health services. Communities can therefore suffer from lower economic growth alongside increased difficulty in addressing other significant social issues. Efforts to address helminthic infections will therefore need to address not just medical measures, but also economic and social development initiatives to break the cycle (Bisanzio et al., 2014). The psychosocial impact of helminth infections on infected communities should not be downplayed since it further worsens the socioeconomic condition. Individuals suffering from chronic infections may become helpless, stigmatized, and socially ostracized, diminishing their general well-being. Where health awareness and literacy are low, the disease stigma leads to discrimination and exclusion, undermining social solidarity. Furthermore, the weight of chronic illness on mental health can also result in increased levels of depression and anxiety, further weakening the ability to engage in positive social and economic activities. This health-mental well-being interface highlights the requirement for overall socioeconomic interventions that not only address helminthic infections but also provide mental health care, education, and empowerment at the community level, which are key to reversing the adverse effects of such infections on such populations (Lal et al., 2019).

8.6.3. Impact on Public Health Systems

The impact of helminthic infections on public health systems is pronounced and multifaceted, with direct implications for disease burden and healthcare resources. Helminths have been proven to cause high morbidity, particularly in low- and middle-income countries where public health infrastructure may be underdeveloped. Intestinal parasitic infection often leads to debilitating chronic health impairments , such as stunted growth in children and anemia, with the potential to have lasting impacts on a person's development and productivity. The exacerbation of health inequalities associated with helminthic infestations is a challenge to public health systems, and hence, advanced management and prevention approaches are required. Effective intersectoral coordination between various fields of intervention, including agriculture, sanitation, and education, is essential to minimize the risk determinants for transmission and to enhance overall health status among populations at risk of these infections. Environmental persistence and transmission dynamics of certain helminths are a sign of the challenges that public health systems are likely to encounter in order to cure these infections. For instance, the re-emergence of the zoonotic helminth *Baylisascaris procyonis* is a sign of the risk imposed by wildlife habitat encroachment. Raccoons, now rampant in urban settings, leave eggs that are environmentally persistent for weeks or months, and thus exposure and infection become highly probable among humans. As has been observed, the infective dose of *B. procyonis* is rather low, thus public knowledge and prevention become critical in curtailing its spread. This puts into question public health intervention, as publics need to be educated on the dangers of helminthic infections, particularly where human and animal populations closely interact with each other, thus potentially overwhelming already strained public health systems with additional complications. Furthermore, the relationship between helminthic infection and hygiene practice cannot be ignored when creating public health policy and intervention strategies. In accordance with a 2016 study, the practice of handwashing with soap has been proven to limit the transmission of various infectious diseases brought about by helminths. Behavior change focus is essential in developing long-term public health interventions that encourage compliance with hygiene behaviors. Targeting hand washing determinants, , such as availability of water and soap, is an important step toward establishing the setting for health-promoting conduct. Linking sanitation education and prevention interventions with disease prevention activities, public health systems can potentially decrease incidence of helminthic infections and enhance health outcomes. The combined strategy here emphasizes the interrelatedness of behavior, environmental determinants, and health system capacity to tackle the burden of helminthic diseases among vulnerable populations.

Test Your Knowledge

1. What is the world burden of significant helminthic infections today, and where do they occur most frequently?
2. In what ways do helminthic infections affect the socioeconomic status of the population and communities?
3. How have global health programs and policies addressed the global burden of helminthic infections?

SUMMARY

Helminthic infection studies have interesting results concerning their burden and impact on health, particularly in resource-poor settings. In addition to malnutrition and anemia, helminthic infections complicate treatment for other diseases, , such as HIV/AIDS. Co-infections with malaria parasites have added to the risk of exacerbating the health problem for vulnerable populations, as shown in various research reports, which need to be addressed with comprehensive health measures to control various infections simultaneously. The issue of high prevalence of helminthic infection among the Sub-Saharan African population emphasizes the necessity of health-focused public health interventions with a focus on education, treatment access, and prevention. Lacking suitable schemes incorporating all these aspects, the disease burden cycle will persist, impeding further progress toward enhanced health in affected regions. In addition, the coincidence of helminthic infection and vaccine uptake, particularly in the case of HPV, also indicates health system and environmental determinants of health outcomes. Scientific evidence indicates that endemicity for infections , such as malaria and helminths is likely to have an effect on vaccine immune response, potentially requiring vaccination protocols to be adjusted in such populations. Results of Kenyan research demonstrate that supply-side challenges like access distance to the point of vaccination greatly affect completion of vaccine doses. Innovative methods to enhance access and health education about HPV and screening for cervical cancer are critical to empower the community to overcome these obstacles and to promote better public health. Interventions that tackle both infectious diseases and vaccination strategies are required in order to reduce overall disease burden. Overall, intervention against helminthic infection is of crucial importance in global public health, namely the management of co-morbidities and increasing health outcomes among infected populations. Focused deworming treatment and immune function implications will be an area of concern for future research, with data from studies indicating enhanced CD4 counts and hemoglobin levels in HIV-positive patients after albendazole treatment. With a multi-faceted approach involving prevention, treatment, and education, stakeholders can create robust health systems that can combat the dual threats of helminths and other infectious diseases. As a whole, progress toward eliminating infection by helminths will not only enhance individual outcomes but will also facilitate more general public health efforts to promote healthier communities and diminish the socioeconomic impact associated with infection.

The relationship with other conditions , such as malaria and HIV infection, is significant in understanding the broader epidemiological context. Co-infections, for instance, have been shown to exacerbate health complications , such as anemia among susceptible groups , such as pregnant women. For instance, a study conducted in Rwanda proved that a significant number of HIV-positive pregnant women were co-infected with malaria and helminths, and the importance of these dual infections was realized in a resource-poor setting. Data , such as these strengthen the need to understand the interplay of such infections as a method of obtaining better public health programs tailored specifically to the setting. Through targeted interventions, e.g., deworming and enhanced education programs, the health status of these vulnerable groups would be significantly improved, illustrating the significant interdependence of alleviating multiple infectious disease burdens concurrently (Emil et al., 2017).

In addition, the research on helminthic infections reveals that certain parasite strains of parasites , such as hookworms, have particular associations with malaria, and this impacts the intensity and prevalence of anemia. Research shows that pregnant women infected with hookworm are far more likely to develop malaria than those who are not infected with hookworm (Kilian et al., 2017). Such evidence suggests the ability of helminths to weaken individuals' immune systems, making them susceptible to other infections , such as malaria (Mak et al., 2017). The character of these interactions necessitates comprehensive studies that not only treat solitary infections but also the prevalence in combination and the resultant health effects. Such an approach can be fruitful in providing insights that make an additional contribution to a fuller understanding of how helminthic infections operate in the context of greater infectious disease paradigms. Lastly, the contribution of deworming interventions is particularly notable in the case of controlling helminthic infections among HIV-positive individuals. The research has shown that albendazole treatment significantly affects immune markers, which in turn leads to increased CD4 counts and viral load decrease among the infected subjects. This implication shows the beneficial effect of intervention against helminthic infections, particularly among subjects who are already subtracting from their health status, for instance, those on antiretroviral therapy. In addition, the deworming strategy, whether targeted or untargeted, has proved to be equally effective in reducing helminth prevalence and improving overall better health outcomes. The complementarity between helminth treatment and other comorbid diseases , such as HIV and malaria, indicates the necessity of integrative health practices with consideration of the multi-dimensional nature of infectious diseases (Emil et al., 2017).

KEY TERMS FROM THIS CHAPTER

- Allergic disease
- CD4 counts
- Co-infection clusters
- Conventional diagnostic methods
- Geohelminthiasis
- Helminthic infections
- Immune function implications
- Inadequate sanitation
- Intestinal blockage
- Molecular analysis
- Antihelminthic medications
- Cestode infections
- Constant monitoring
- Gastrointestinal disease
- Health awareness
- Holistic hygiene practices
- Immune modulators
- Infectious disease paradigms
- Intestinal helminths
- Molecular diagnostics

Critical Thinking Questions

1. **What is a common mode of transmission for helminthic infection?**
   a. Inhalation of spores
   b. Contact with infected water through the skin
   c. Ingestion of contaminated food or water
   d. Direct blood transfusion
2. **Which of the following parasites is known to cause anemia due to blood loss?**
   a. *Necator americanus*
   b. *Ascaris lumbricoides*
   c. *Enterobius vermicularis*
   d. *Taenia saginata*
3. **The "scotch tape test" is used to diagnose infection by:**
   a. *Trichuris trichiura*
   b. *Enterobius vermicularis*
   c. *Strongyloides stercoralis*
   d. *Schistosoma mansoni*
4. **Which of the following helminths is transmitted by freshwater snails and causes schistosomiasis?**
   a. *Schistosoma haematobium*
   b. *Taenia solium*
   c. *Ancylostoma duodenale*
   d. *Echinococcus granulosus*
5. **A distinguishing feature of *Taenia solium* infection, as opposed to *Taenia saginata*, is:**
   a. Larger proglottids
   b. Lack of intermediate host
   c. Transmission via uncooked beef
   d. Risk of cysticercosis

Short Answer Questions

1. What are helminthic infections and which organisms cause them?
2. How are helminthic infections typically transmitted to human beings?
3. What are the common symptoms of intestinal helminthic infections?
4. How is a diagnosis of helminthic infection typically made?
5. What role does eosinophilia play in helminthic infections?
6. What drugs are used to treat common helminthic infections?
7. What public health practices prevent helminthic infections?
8. What are the complications that follow chronic helminthic infections?

Answer to Critical Thinking Questions

1. (c); 2. (a); 3. (b); 4. (a); 5. (d)

REFERENCES

1. Futagbi, G., Abankwa, J. K., Agbale, P. S., & Aboagye, I. F. (2015). Assessment of helminth infections in goats slaughtered in an abattoir in a suburb of accra, Ghana. *West African Journal of Applied Ecology*, *23*(2), 35-42. (accessed on 13th June 2025).

2. Jourdan, P. M., Lamberton, P. H. L., Fenwick, A., & Addiss, D. G. (2018). Soil-transmitted helminth infections. *Lancet (London, England)*, *391*(10117), 252–265. https://doi.org/10.1016/S0140-6736(17)31930-X(accessed on 13th June 2025).

3. Ajjampur, S. S. R., Kang, G., Kattula, D., Levecke, B., et al. (2014). *Prevalence & Risk Factors for Soil Transmitted Helminth Infection Among School Children in south India*. https://core.ac.uk/download/55800525.pdf (accessed on 13th June 2025).

4. Amanda, S. R., Hadi, I., Haresmita, P. P., Wardani, N. A., et al. (2023). *Description of Mother's Knowledge and Adherence to Use of Helminthic Drugs in Kuwaluhan Village, Magelang Regency, Central Java*. https://core.ac.uk/download/654628895.pdf (accessed on 13th June 2025).

5. Ambrosio, L. F., Celias, D. P., Cervi, L. A., Chiapello, I., et al. (2018). *Helminth Infections: Recognition and Modulation of The Immune Response by Innate Immune Cells*. https://core.ac.uk/download/286535343.pdf (accessed on 13th June 2025).

6. Anwar, Z., Bulus, L., Ndenge, C., Andrew, J., et al. (2016). *Incidence and Factors Associated with Postpartum Anemia at Mbarara Regional Referral Hospital*. https://core.ac.uk/download/234691696.pdf (accessed on 13th June 2025).

7. Aqeele, G. (2024). *Traditional Detection of Intestinal Helminths in Stray Cats in Wasit Province, Iraq*. https://core.ac.uk/download/618209136.pdf (accessed on 13th June 2025).

8. Arrais, M., Brito, M., Cooper, P., Gama, A. C., et al. (2020). *Helminth Infections, Atopy, Asthma and Allergic Diseases: Protocol for A Systematic Review of Observational Studies Worldwide*. https://core.ac.uk/download/323385702.pdf (accessed on 13th June 2025).

9. Ash, L. R., Berlin, O. G. W., Morse, S. A., Sorvillo, F. J., et al. (2002). *Baylisascaris procyonis: An Emerging Helminthic Zoonosis*. https://core.ac.uk/download/323062358.pdf (accessed on 13th June 2025).

10. Belyhun, Y., Elias, D., Erko, B., Kassu, A., et al. (2014). *Helminths and Malaria Co-Infections Are Associated with Elevated Serum IgE*. https://core.ac.uk/download/pdf/50697116.pdf (accessed on 13th June 2025).

11. Bhagat, H., Dwivedi, A., Garg, A., Garg, R., et al. (2018). *Effect of Multiple Rounds of Mass Drug Administration Under Lymphatic Filariasis Elimination Program on Prevalence of Soil-Transmitted Helminthiasis in One of The Co-Endemic Districts of India*. https://core.ac.uk/download/354381796.pdf (accessed on 13th June 2025).

12. Bisanzio, D., Bustinduy, A. L., King, C. H., Kitron, U., et al. (2014). *Cross-Sectional Study of The Burden of Vector-Borne and Soil-Transmitted Polyparasitism in Rural Communities of Coast Province, Kenya*. https://core.ac.uk/download/29469451.pdf (accessed on 13th June 2025).

13. Biwott, G. K., Ngeiywa, M. M., & Wanjala, P. M. (2014). *Prevalence of Gastrointestinal Parasitic Infections Among Food Handlers in Eldoret Municipality, Kenya*. https://core.ac.uk/download/234660479.pdf (accessed on 13th June 2025).

14. Boratne, A. V., Deshmukh, P. R., Dongre, A. R., Garg, B. S., et al. (2008). *An Approach to*

Hygiene Education Among Rural Indian School-Going Children. https://core.ac.uk/download/pdf/86989.pdf (accessed on 13th June 2025).

15. Brown, G. V., Leder, K., Matchett, E., O'Brien, D. P., et al. (2008). *Illness in Returned Travelers and Immigrants/Refugees: The 6-Year Experience of Two Australian Infectious Diseases Units*. https://core.ac.uk/download/pdf/9416725.pdf (accessed on 13th June 2025).
16. Ciardi, G., Ogwang, D. M., Okello, T. R., Opira, C., et al. (2016). *Intestinal Intussusception in An Adult Caused by Helminthic Parasitosis*. https://core.ac.uk/download/188828822.pdf (accessed on 13th June 2025).
17. Ekanem, E. E., Eyong, K., Ikobah, J. M., Uhegbu, M., et al. (2021). *Helminthic Infestation in Children Aged 6 To 59 Months with Diarrhea in Calabar*. https://core.ac.uk/download/478392701.pdf (accessed on 13th June 2025).
18. Emil, I. (2017). *The Prevalence of Helminth and Malaria Infections and The Effects of De-Worming on Disease Progression Markers in HIV-1 Infected Pregnant Women on Antiretroviral Therapy in Rwanda*. https://core.ac.uk/download/188775605.pdf (accessed on 13th June 2025).
19. Harrington, D., Lamberton, P. H. L., & McGregor, A. (2017). *Human Liver Flukes*. https://core.ac.uk/download/96882191.pdf (accessed on 13th June 2025).
20. Lamberton, P. H., & Jourdan, P. M. (2015). Human Ascariasis: Diagnostics Update. *Current tropical medicine reports*, *2*(4), 189–200. https://doi.org/10.1007/s40475-015-0064-9 (accessed on 13th June 2025).
21. Mabeya, H., Menon, S., Weyers, S., Naanyu, V., Mwaliko, E., Kirop, E., Orango, O., Vermandere, H., & Vanden Broeck, D. (2018). Uptake of three doses of HPV vaccine by primary school girls in Eldoret, Kenya; a prospective cohort study in a malaria endemic setting. *BMC cancer*, *18*(1), 557. https://doi.org/10.1186/s12885-018-4382-x(accessed on 13th June 2025).
22. Lal, S. S., Mohan, A. J., & Upmanyu, N. (2019). *Pregnancy, Children and Inter-Relating Factors Affected by Geohelminthiasis*. https://core.ac.uk/download/322445222.pdf (accessed on 13th June 2025).
23. Mak, J. W., Naing, C., Nyunt-Wai, V., Reid, A., et al. (2017). *Malaria and Soil-Transmitted Intestinal Helminth Co-Infection and Its Effect on Anemia: A Meta-Analysis*. https://core.ac.uk/download/85215062.pdf (accessed on 13th June 2025).
24. Mitiku, H., Mohammed, J., & Tefera, E. (2015). *Intestinal Helminthic Infections Among Elementary Students of Babie Town, Eastern Ethiopia*. https://core.ac.uk/download/478429091.pdf (accessed on 13th June 2025).
25. The State of Handwashing in 2016: Annual Review What we learned about handwashing in 2016; https://globalhandwashing.org/wp-content/uploads/2017/03/The-State-of-Handwashing-in-2016.pdf. (accessed on 13th June 2025).
26. NSingh, B. (2020). *Molecular Medicines for Parasitic Diseases*. https://core.ac.uk/download/322580845.pdf (accessed on 13th June 2025).
27. Teimoori, S., Mowlavi, G., Arimatsu, Y., Sripa, B., Mobedi, I., Sharifdini, M., Massoud, J., & Naddaf, S. R. (2019). Infection of the Jackal (*Canis aureus*) by *Haplorchis taichui* (Trematoda: Heterophyidae) in Southwestern Iran: A Clue for Potential Human Infection. *Iranian journal of parasitology*, *14*(1), 120–126.(accessed on 13th June 2025).

28. Strosberg, S. A. (2014). *The Human–Hookworm Assemblage: Contingency and The Practice of Helminthic Therapy*. https://core.ac.uk/download/232563064.pdf (accessed on 13th June 2025).

29. Tewelde E, Tadesse S. Drug Discovery and Development for Soil-Transmitted Helminthiasis: Current Anthelmentics and Compounds in the Pipeline [Internet]. Roundworms - A Survey From Past to Present. IntechOpen; 2023. Available from: http://dx.doi.org/10.5772/intechopen.106830 (accessed on 13th June 2025).

HOSPITAL-ACQUIRED INFECTIONS (HAIS) AND INFECTION CONTROL

9

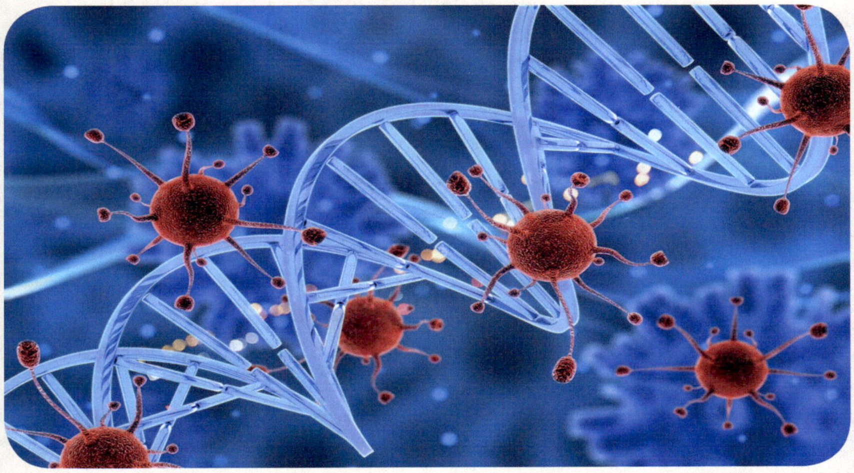

LEARNING OBJECTIVES

After studying this chapter, you will be able to:

1. Define the types of hospital-acquired infection;
2. Describe the causative pathogens and risk factors for hospital-acquired infections;
3. Understand the impact of HAIs on patient outcomes;
4. Highlight implementation of effective infection control measures for control of hospital-acquired infections (HAIs);
5. Describe the role of healthcare workers in the control of hospital-acquired infections (HAIs);
6. Manage challenges in infection control.

Introduction

The question of hospital-acquired infections (HAIs) has also become a central concern in the healthcare sector, with public health officials, practitioners, and researchers all redirecting their focus to the issue. The infections the patient attains by being treated for another purpose pose direct challenges to conducting safe patient care in many types of medical settings. Millions of HAIs infect patients worldwide every year, and they cause extra morbidity, mortality, and financial cost to the health systems. The difficulty of controlling these infections is further amplified by the growing issue of antimicrobial resistance, and prevention and control measures are now more crucial than ever. Understanding the spread of HAIs is the foundation on which successful interventions are designed, as well as the high patient safety standards. Owing to the prevalent problems of HAIs, a comprehensive description of causes, effects, and control is justified. Moreover, the role of environmental factors in enhancing the rate of HAIs cannot be overlooked. Hospital environments act as reservoirs for infectious pathogens due to a number of reasons, including the presence of susceptible patient populations along with inadequate infection control practices. Strict adherence to proper cleaning and disinfection procedures is essential in the quest to prevent the hazards of contaminated surfaces and equipment. According to published literature, correct hand hygiene practice and disinfection regimen have been established to be required in the transmission of HAIs in health care facilities. Some of the suggested recommendations are the routine use of soap and water for handwashing, coupled with the application of alcohol-based disinfectants, with emphasis on compliance with set guidelines.

Thus, it is necessary to study the various strategies adopted in infection control to develop strategies overall against HAIs and ensure patient safety. The dynamicity of HAIs also demands continuous research and innovation in infection control. Recent advancements, as mentioned by the Technology Strategy Board (TSB) and Department of Health (DH), also suggest the use of sophisticated diagnostic tests in the detection. Priority areas , such as Methicillin-resistant *Staphylococcus aureus* (MRSA) and *Clostridium difficile* are mentioned in the study, emphasizing the economic advantage of point-of-care testing to be used for the early diagnosis and treatment. Such developments not only expand existing knowledge but also bring about the identification of loopholes in existing procedures and economic effects of new technologies. Despite the efforts of the medical centers to reduce the incidence of HAIs, the adoption of multi-dimensional practice as stringent research, advanced diagnosis processes, and strict infection control practices becomes inevitable in upholding patient health as well as enhancing healthcare outcomes.

Definition of Hospital-Acquired Infections (HAIs)

Hospital-acquired infections (HAIs) are a source of considerable worry in hospitals, namely, infections that patients have contracted while in the hospital or residing in a health care facility and were neither present nor incubating on admission. This would be applicable to most types of infections, including urinary tract infection, surgical site infection, and bloodstream infection. The presence of HAIs emphasizes the scope of effective infection control measures. For instance, a Scottish national point prevalence survey reported that HAIs were found in 9.5% of acute hospital patients, and the most common presentations of HAIs included surgical site infection and urinary tract infection (Allardice et al., 2008). The outcomes reveal not only the incidence of such infections but also all the different facets of their impact on the health of patients, and hence necessitate an integrated approach towards prevention and control. The effects of HAIs are not only the direct impact on the health of patients. They immensely escalate the rates of morbidity and mortality, and they place a heavy economic burden on the healthcare systems. HAIs result in a considerable cost of treatment in the form of increased length of hospital stay, additional diagnostic tests, and increased antibiotic use, all adding to the rising healthcare expenditure. In addition, HAIs are one of the top causative agents of antimicrobial resistance, which complicates treatment and hinders public health initiatives (Cammalleri et al., 2019). The complexity of HAIs and their relevance to healthcare economics demands strict infection control in hospitals. Infection control strict policies are central in ensuring not only the health of the patients but also the sustainability of healthcare resources. Proper infection control is central to proper HAIs management. Severe disinfection and cleaning measures, supplemented by aggressive hand hygiene practices, form one of the main pillars of infection control. Proof does exist to show that an intervention bundle, all of which are practiced simultaneously, is capable of reducing HAI occurrence by more than half (Cammalleri et al., 2019). Classification of medical devices based on the risk of infection transmission also serves to inform adequate sterilization protocols, thereby increasing standards of safety. The application of these controls within the contexts of hospitals is critical because hospital contexts have the potential to serve as reservoirs for pathogen agents responsible for HAIs. It is consequently an increased demand centered on prevention and sensitization of health workers that is necessary in the mitigation of hospital-acquired infections, which ultimately translates into improved patient outcomes and maintenance of public health standards (Figure 9.1).

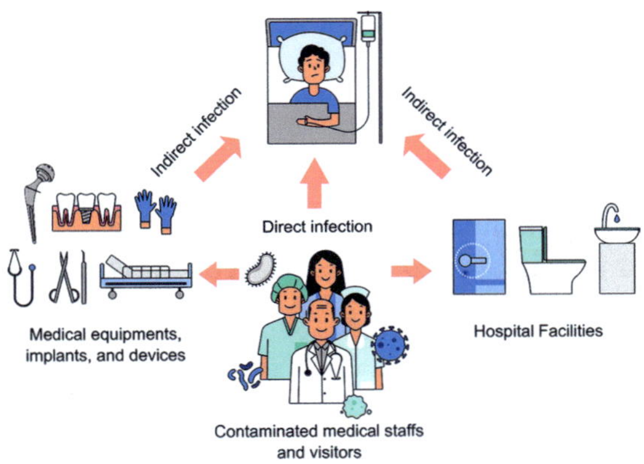

Figure 9.1. Schematic illustration of transmission routes of hospital-acquired infections (HAI) or nosocomial infection.

Source: https://www.researchgate.net/publication/360825411/figure/fig1/AS:11431281360750071@1744104123867/Schematic-illustration-of-transmission-routes-of-hospital-acquired-infections-HAI-or.png.

Importance of Addressing HAIs in Healthcare Settings

Hospital-acquired infections (HAIs) are a very important healthcare system threat and so the demand for an effective communication and reporting mechanism is required. Incorporation of safety culture in healthcare institutions, emphasized by the European Federation of Nurses Associations, is highly important in the fight against HAIs. This culture includes early reporting of blunders, best practice sharing, and bi-directional sharing of research evidence. Through facilitating openness among health workers, organizations can identify trends and mitigate risks from HAIs. Additionally, heightened awareness through training and education enforces such a culture so that all members of staff feel responsible for preventing infection. These steps not only guarantee patient safety but also lower healthcare costs associated with prolonged hospitalization and mismanagement of HAIs, thus maximizing general community benefits (Burke et al., 2008). The resolution of the HAI problem is not only paramount to patient safety but also has crucial implications for HCWs' safety themselves. There is evidence that HCWs stand a high risk of infection via occupational pathways, particularly with blood and other body fluid exposure. There is evidence in Tanzania that HIV is spread via needle stick injuries, thus making prevention intervention within health facilities a priority (Kilale et al., 2013). Without the right guidelines and adequate health and safety guidelines, the risks to HCWs are further exacerbated. For this to be verified, the health facilities ought to provide the necessary training in infection control protocols, as well as the provision of personal protective equipment (PPE). Procuring appropriate materials for HCWs not only protects them but also makes the environment safer for patients, thereby resulting in the alleviation of HAIs. With the exceedingly complicated problems of HAIs, having standard infection control protocols in place is crucial. Widespread practice, ranging from diligent hand hygiene policy to accurate sterilization policy, is demanded in any healthcare facility. Adhering to best practice learned from successful European interventions tells volumes about the worth of evidence-based intervention to prevent HAIs.

Moreover, systematic reporting and examination of infection data enable targeted intervention and continuous improvement of infection control policies. Yet, effectiveness in these measures is contingent upon a commitment from healthcare leaders to ensure adequate resources for training and monitoring compliance. By strongly emphasizing war against HAIs through infection control practice that is well-coordinated and well-educated, healthcare facilities can contribute significantly to patient safety, reduce healthcare-related expenses, and create a culture of health and safety among both patients and providers (Burke et al., 2008) (Figure 9.2).

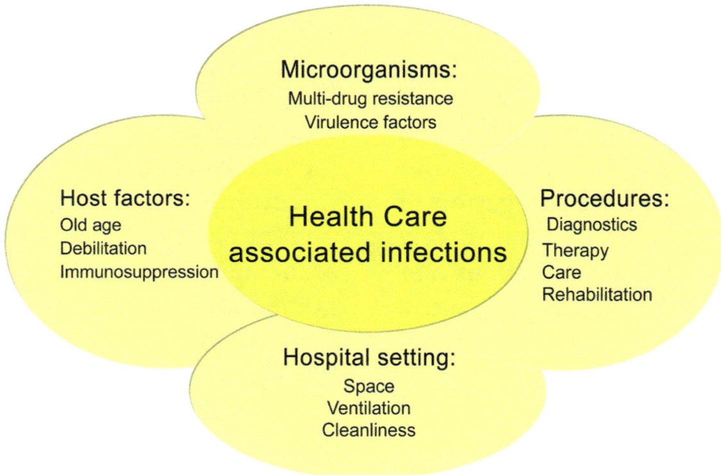

Figure 9.2. Factors determining health care associated infections.

Source: https://www.researchgate.net/profile/Hans-Kolmos/publication/221925213/figure/fig4/AS:668677443690514@1536436534912/Factors-determining-health-care-associated-infections.png.

Overview of Infection Control Measures

Infection control measures play a critical role in an effort to curb the prevalence of hospital-acquired infections (HAIs) that are very deleterious to patient safety and healthcare systems. At the forefront of infection control measures is the practice of enforcing strict hand hygiene measures. Hand hygiene comprises a variety of rituals, including soap and water bathing and alcohol-based disinfection, each of which is specifically tailored to specific clinical environments. Evidence highlights the proportion with which adherence to these protocols is matched with decreasing infection rates, lowering the risk of HAIs, particularly in intensive care units where HAIs are more common. Evidence-based practice of hand hygiene not only protects patients, but also health care providers and creates a safer health care environment. Therefore, revitalizing hand hygiene training and compliance is the answer to today's battle against HAIs, the backbone of effective infection control initiatives and ultimately better health facility patient outcomes. Another aspect of infection control, with much planning surrounding environmental disinfection and cleaning, is the second. Hospital environments are typically reservoirs of microbes, and thus, stringently applied cleaning practices are necessary to prevent cross-transmission. The application of polyphenolic and chlorine disinfectants against environmental surfaces and close adherence to cleaning routines are critical in prevention against HAIs. Inclusion of these practices with hand hygiene provides an overall infection prevention program from the available literature. The development of bundles, or concurrent practices embraced together, has also increased as a cost-saving infection control intervention. For instance, a package can encompass not only disinfection of surfaces but appropriate sterilization of equipment and instruments—a combination that optimizes patient safety and reduces potential rates of infection. Last but not least, antimicrobial stewardship practice cannot be sidestepped in the guise of infection control interventions. With growing concern over antimicrobial resistance (AMR), the rational use of antibiotics is most crucial. Antimicrobial prescribing pattern monitoring allows for the detection of inappropriate use that culminates in the emergence of resistant forms of microbes. Interventions that raise awareness among healthcare providers about prudent prescribing patterns can greatly enhance the utility of available antimicrobial agents. In addition, policy implementation through hand hygiene, environmental cleaning, and antimicrobial stewardship to specific sites offers a multifactorial treatment to control HAIs. Encouraging such a culture prioritizing such interdependent control measures, the health institutions are then able to greatly reduce the occurrence of HAIs, thereby enhancing patient care on an individual level as well as public health outcomes in general (Cairns et al., 2018; Cammalleri et al., 2019).

9.1. Types of Hospital-Acquired Infections

Learning Outcome

1. Discuss surgical site infection (SSI);
2. Identify catheter-associated urinary tract infections (CAUTIs);
3. Discuss ventilator-associated pneumonia (VAP).

Of all of the various classes of hospital-acquired infection (HAI), urinary tract infection (UTI) is the most prevalent. UTIs normally develop due to catheter use, and device placement in the urinary tract offers an entry point for pathogens. As quoted, UTIs contribute to 17.9% of the total HAIs in acutely hospitalized patients, a figure that reflects the significance of monitoring as compared to the use of catheters and personal cleanliness to prevent such occurrences. Having even the most minimalistic of prevention procedures in place, , such as the guarantee of aseptic practice, does go a long way in keeping the occurrence of UTIs at bay. In addition, improved training and sensitization of healthcare providers are necessary since improper catheter management can lead to increased infections, besides increasing patient distress and healthcare costs. Certain HAIs, , such as UTIs, are hence pivotal to examine in developing effective infection prevention interventions in the health sector (Bocicor et al., 2016). Surgical site infections (SSIs) are yet another form of serious HAIs with negative patient outcomes. These infections can be post-operative, commonly secondary to intra-operative contamination, and account for approximately 15.9% of HAIs in the hospital. Conditions that predispose to SSIs include intrinsic patient conditions, type of surgical technique employed, and asepsic practices compliance. The effect of SSIs on hospital management is enormous because they not only increase mortality but also lead to increased hospitalization and runaway healthcare expenses. For instance, adherence to surgical sterilization and prophylaxis antibiotics before, during, and after surgery can be integrated into clinical practice to lower the prevalence of SSIs. Elimination of these factors enhances patient safety and lowers the wide-reaching consequence of HAIs in hospitals (Bocicor et al., 2016). Gastrointestinal infections are a type of HAIs resulting from other environmental and procedural sources that aggravate patients' condition in hospitals. They are responsible for 15.4% of all nosocomial infections. Pathophysiology of these infections is broadly associated with transmission through contaminated water, food supply, or poor hygiene among healthcare providers. Hospitals can minimize the occurrence of gastrointestinal infections with strict infection prevention measures, including high levels of hand cleanliness, proper disinfection of medical equipment, and food safety surveillance in hospital dining halls. As shown through a national survey, these infections have disproportionately affected vulnerable patient groups, , such as elderly or immunocompromised patients. This raises the importance of patient-specific infection control strategies to meet the specific needs of different patient groups without endangering safety culture in healthcare organizations (Allardice et al., 2008).

9.1.1. Surgical Site Infections (SSIs)

SSIs rank among the greatest priorities in the grand plan of hospital-acquired infections (HAIs). SSIs not only prolong hospital stays but also increase morbidity and mortality in surgical patients. Pathogenesis of SSIs is often a multifactorial association between patient, environment, and surgical technique.

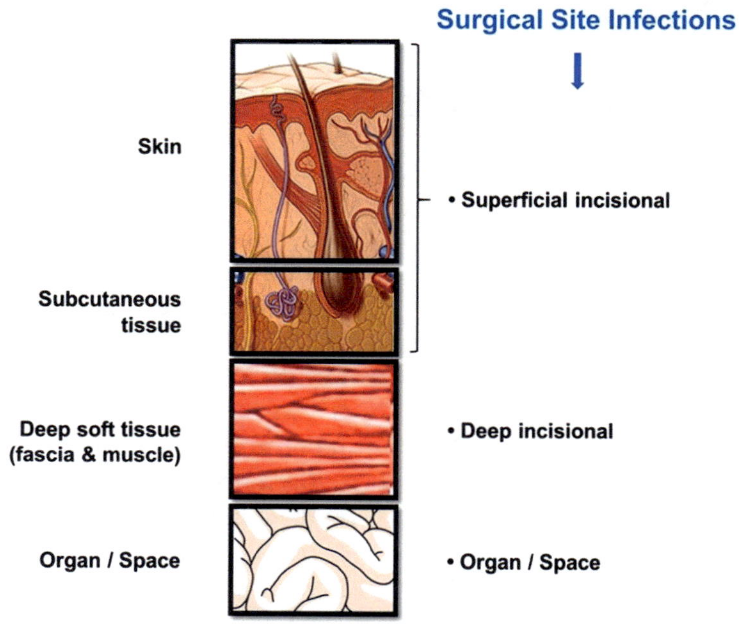

Figure 9.3. Anatomy of surgical site infections and their classification.

Source: https://www.researchgate.net/publication/339826667/figure/fig1/AS:873756780138498@1585331258606/Anatomy-of-surgical-site-infections-and-their-classification-adapted-from-CDC-1.jpg.

For instance, comorbidities of patients, nutritional status, and use of foreign objects like sutures and implants are major causative factors for SSIs. Sterilization of the operative site as well as the timing of surgery are equally vital in preventing SSIs. Effective infection control practices need to counteract these variables in an organized manner to avert the threat of SSIs in the hospital setting, improving patient outcomes and reducing healthcare costs. Thorough Infection Control Risk Assessments (ICRAs) are one of the key control measures of SSI. According to the literature, the most critical risk assessment of HAIs is surgical site infection, and it is given a top priority for infection control practices in healthcare facilities (Listiowati et al., 2019). The integrated strategy is intended for detection and risk analysis with different types of surgery. Disruption of the transmission cycle of pathogenic microorganisms is a major contributor to the decline in SSI incidence. With evidence-based antibiotic regimens, for example, the rate of bacterial infection among postoperative patients has been demonstrated to decrease. Lastly, regular review and continued surveillance of infection control policies may help enhance the effectiveness of the preventive measures and, in turn, create a culture of safety within operating theaters. Besides the use of preventive measures against SSIs, evidence-based practice and trained teams play an important role in infection control. Having specialized staff perform surgery may aid in the maintenance of infection control measures, as has been reported by effective programs in reducing central line-associated bloodstream infections (Silow-Carroll & Edwards, 2011). These staff can deliver facilitating infection rates to be tracked, best practices to be shared, and feedback for continuing improvement to be recorded. Moreover, engaging surgical staff in team-based approaches fosters an active infection control culture. Routine training, communication, and adherence to protocol-based practices can guarantee optimal patient care and further minimize the risks of surgical procedures. Last but not least, the management of SSIs in HAIs and infection control ensures a safer health environment, improved patient safety, and therapeutic outcomes (Figure 9.3).

9.1.2. Catheter-Associated Urinary Tract Infections (CAUTIs)

CAUTIs are a high-risk issue in the hospital-acquired infection (HAI) category. The Centers for Disease Control and Prevention (CDC) estimates that CAUTIs are causative of approximately 40% of all HAIs in the US, and it is therefore an indicator of the necessity of proper infection control. Indwelling catheters, utilized for several clinical indications, can become a vehicle for disease-producing pathogens by virtue of inappropriate placement or handling. Since CAUTIs have the greatest probability of resulting in extended hospital stays and negative patient outcomes, health care centers are interested in providing education and compliance with protocols to avoid attendant risk. It is grounded on determinants of CAUTI development that call for a pluralistic approach involving clinician education, patient education, and strict infection control policies to facilitate effective management within health care centers (Ali et al., 2018). Apparently, to effectively reduce the occurrence of CAUTIs, evidence-based practices , such as prevention and response should be implemented. This undertaking has part of its contribution in the Post Foley Removal Guideline (PFRG), developed with the aim of reducing unnecessary catheter reinsertion with high infection risk. Literature reveals that the majority of the CAUTIs are preventable, and catheter insertion time and catheter usage duration are risk factors. Thus, the creation of organizational forms that help to diffuse the obstacles to the implementation of EBPs into all the medical facilities can enhance the quality of care significantly. Measures to promote adherence to the guidelines, along with rigorous nurses' training in catheter care, have been found effective in preventing the incidence of CAUTI. With the implementation of such measures as a priority item, hospitals can ensure utmost patient safety and overall success in healthcare (Gabbard, 2016). Comparing the impact of organized interventions on CAUTI incidence illustrates the efficacy of infection prevention measures. A practice study project to reduce the incidence of CAUTI proved that intervention with targeted education sessions to nursing staff resulted in dramatic reductions in infection rate. By utilizing a CAUTI maintenance tool and staff training that ensued, CAUTI reporting dramatically dropped, illustrating how education impacts clinical practice. These findings also mean that there is a need to empower nursing staff to understand the nuances of indwelling catheter utilization and complications. This is not only one method of building safety culture in healthcare organizations but ultimately results in the enhancement of patient care quality, avoidance of hospitalization rates, and quality of life for patients. Therefore, improving the knowledge base among healthcare professionals is an essential component of preventing CAUTIs and improving infection control practices (Ali et al., 2018) (Figure 9.4).

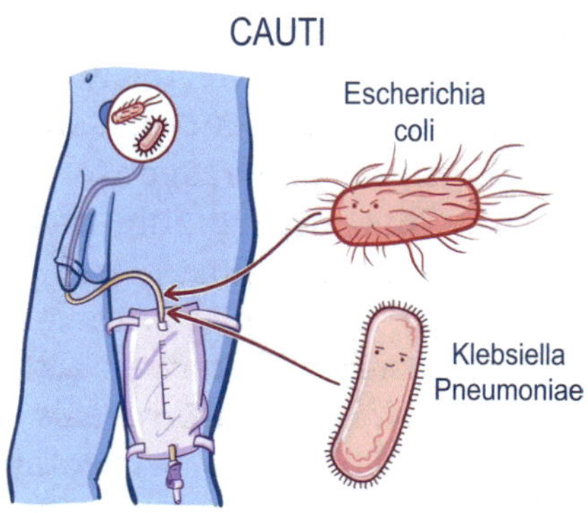

Figure 9.4. Catheter-associated urinary tract infections (CAUTIs).

Source: https://www.osmosis.org/_next/image?url=https%3A%2F%2Fd16qt3wv6xm098.cloudfront.net%2FyEaRWOZiRtudrdVBOW9jevhiSQKLgu2j%2F_.jpg&w=3840&q=75.

9.1.3. Ventilator-Associated Pneumonia (VAP)

VAP is a severe complication among mechanically ventilated patients, particularly in hospital-acquired infections (HAIs). Even though more than 48 hours of mechanical ventilation, VAP is most commonly caused by aspiration of oropharyngeal or gastric pathogens. There are numerous risk factors, not only prolonged ventilation, endotracheal tube use, and patient immobilization, but also the immunocompromised nature of the vast majority of patients requiring ventilation and thus susceptible to bacterial colonization and infection. VAP prevention is crucial not just to optimize patient outcomes but also to minimize the cumulative burden of HAIs in healthcare settings, highlighting the importance of strict infection prevention measures specifically for this vulnerable patient group. VAP can only be prevented through evidence-based interventions focused on airway hygiene and avoidance of exposure to pathogens. Evidence-based standardized guidelines—derived from interprofessional research—have been demonstrated to prevent this infection. For instance, semi-recumbent position with mechanical ventilation effectively decreases aspiration likelihood, whereas stringent oral care is required to prevent bacterial colonization. Also, pathophysiologic insights govern the use of standard suctioning strategies and selective application of antibiotics for the maintenance of respiratory tract health. The addition of specific teams to oversee compliance with the protocol reveals the possibility of major decreases in the occurrence of VAP when medical professionals are accountable for infection precautions (Silow-Carroll & Edwards, 2011). Additionally, continuous education of the medical and nursing staff in VAP prevention is required in order to have infection precautions enforced. As with most healthcare systems, the increasing number of patient safety interventions highlights and reinforces the necessity of hands-on training methods more likely to limit procedural errors with VAP development. Simulation training has proven to enhance the effectiveness of the healthcare workforce, thus lowering VAP rates. Evidence-based goal-setting strategies that offer concrete goals and take into account compliance with best practices have the potential to empower settings with a patient safety orientation. Through collaborative efforts and lifelong learning, healthcare organizations can alter their practices, which in turn reduces

VAP rates and enhances patient morbidity and mortality (McCarthy et al., 2011). This concentrated dedication to infection prevention serves to benefit not only the patient individually but also to establish a system-wide reduction in hospital-acquired infection (Figure 9.5).

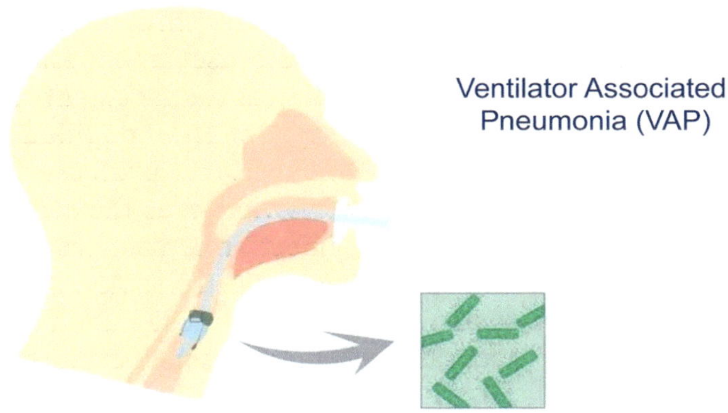

Figure 9.5. Ventilator-associated pneumonia (VAP).

Source: https://stgaccinwbsdevlrs01.blob.core.windows.net/newcorporatewbsite/blogs/June2024/2dQb3MjKXmtujgKSkoY5.webp.

Test Your Knowledge

1. What are surgical site infections (SSIs), and how do the most common risk factors lead to their development?
2. What is the pathogenesis of catheter-associated urinary tract infections (CAUTIs) and how can prevention reduce their incidence?

9.2. Causes and Risk Factors

Learning Outcome

1. Describe patient-related factors;
2. Describe healthcare-related factors;
3. Recognize the relationship between environmental factors related to hospital-acquired infections (HAIs).

Hospital-acquired infections (HAIs) are the most important complication in healthcare institutions, primarily due to their multifactorial causes and risk factors. A very important cause of HAIs is colonization of patients with pathogenic microorganisms at the time of hospital admission. Already being infected or having colonization of soft tissues at admission leads to patients being susceptible to the carriage of infection agents. Furthermore, the invasive procedures that are given to patients, , such as catheterizations or surgeries, compromise their body because it allows pathogens a direct route to sterile fields. Thus, understanding these pathways supports the fundamental need for rigorous infection control measures in hospital settings to the point that health workers come at rigorous sterilization and hygiene protocols as a patient safety bulwark in accordance with the position of the European Federation of Nurses Associations on establishing a culture of safety to minimize medication mistakes and HAIs (Burke et al., 2008). Additionally, risk factors of HAIs extend beyond patient individual factors to environmental and procedural hospital factors. The presence of multi-drug resistant organisms, oftentimes aggravated by improper use of antibiotics and poor sterilization, poses a challenging environment to control infection. Patients with compromised immune systems, either due to underlying disease or longer-than-anticipated hospital stay, are most vulnerable to HAIs. The increasing cost of healthcare for HAIs, highlighted in a number of studies, emphasizes the significance of a framework for infection prevention. Methodologies used to estimate excess LOS attributable to HAIs also indicate the additional burden on healthcare systems, demonstrating the importance of accurate calculations for informing resource distribution and maximizing patient outcomes (Giraldi et al., 2019). Lastly, employee alertness and adherence to infection prevention protocols are still the key in lowering HAIs. Training initiatives that aim to support a culture of vigilance among health care workers actually has an effect on infection rates. Institutional support for continuous learning and the creation of bundles of best practices can enhance the capacity of health care workers to recognize and respond to potential infection risks. Furthermore, encouraging a culture of openness will allow healthcare professionals to report near misses or errors without fear of reprisals to facilitate the improvement of patient safety. Such an approach is aligned with the EFN guidelines for creating highly reliable organizations with care provision safety as their number one priority (Burke et al., 2008). By addressing individual and system risk factors, hospitals can make concerted efforts to largely eradicate HAIs and make the environment healthier for every patient.

9.2.1. Patient-Related Factors (e.g., Age, Comorbidities)

The influence of patient-specific factors, particularly age and comorbidities, is a leading actor in the causation of hospital-acquired infection (HAI). The older patients become, the more their immune systems weaken, reducing their ability to resist infections and leaving them susceptible to numerous pathogens. Older patients tend to present with multiple comorbidities, , such as diabetes, chronic respiratory conditions, and cardiovascular illnesses, that complicate their clinical management and the risk of HAIs is higher. This population trend necessitates healthcare professionals to acquire good knowledge, as the elderly may require tailored infection control programs to reduce risks with prolonged hospital stay and the compromised state of these patients to infection. Hence, the combination of comorbidities and age can serve as a potent combination for the complications of HAIs, thereby adding to patient morbidity and healthcare costs as a whole. Moreover, the rate of comorbidity among inpatients can also contribute significantly toward increased HAI risk. Multiple-patient histories are more prone to prolonged hospitalization due to treatment-related complications of their underlying conditions. The existence of over a single comorbid condition has the tendency to be associated with a higher rate of invasive procedures , such as catheterizations and surgery, serving as avenues for opportunistic infections. As highlighted in the literature, patient complexity and length of stay are central to comprehending the dynamics of HAIs within hospital settings (Hauck et al., 2025). These adverse interactions between hospital environment and patient condition of health point to the value of infection control policy that specifically responds to the comorbid vulnerabilities. Apart from age and comorbidities, recent studies have established how previous use of antimicrobials adds to the complexity of HAIs. The antibiotic use, while significant in the case of treating established infection, has the unwanted consequence of encouraging resistance among bacterial populations, particularly among complicated-infection patients. Research has indicated that previously used antimicrobials significantly influence subsequent-isolate rates of susceptibility and thus compromise the effectiveness of empirical treatment regimens (Epstein et al., 2015). This relentless cycle of infection and resistance calls for higher surveillance among healthcare professionals regarding proper medication handling, especially in vulnerable categories of patients. Therefore, understanding these patient-related factors is crucial to formulating efficient infection control practices in reducing the incidence of HAIs and thereby improving patient outcomes along with saving healthcare resources (Figure 9.6).

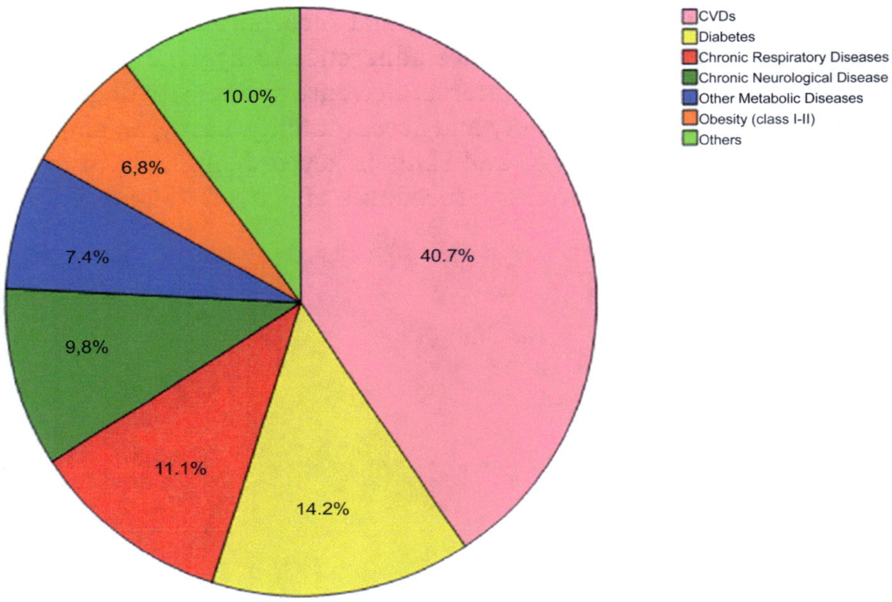

Figure 9.6. Proportions of comorbidities of patients. The pie chart shows the proportion of each comorbidity among the total of 2295 comorbidities recorded in the study population.

Source: https://www.researchgate.net/publication/372196752/figure/fig3/AS:11431281176627579@1690215230784/Proportions-of-comorbidities-of-patients-included-in-the-study-The-pie-chart-shows-the.png.

9.2.2. Healthcare-Related Factors (e.g., Invasive Procedures)

The healthcare environment encompasses various invasive procedures that have a key role in hospital-acquired infections (HAIs). Surgical interventions, catheter insertion, and intravenous line placement, while at times requisite to treat a patient, represent an immediate conduit for microorganisms into the body. When entering the sterile environments, such microorganisms can multiply and lead to surgical site infection complications or sepsis. The studies have indicated that the infectious diseases resulting from such invasive treatments are typically due to multi-resistant bacteria among patients accustomed to healthcare settings. It accentuates the need to monitor infection rates continuously and implement strict infection controls directed at specific interventions to reduce HAIs' risks (Ceccarelli et al., 2015). Excessive and improper use of antibiotics, particularly among patients with invasive devices, within the hospital setting, creates a cycle of resistant infections. Multi-drug-resistant organisms pose a dangerous threat because empirical antibiotic coverage may fail, leading to treatment failures, longer stays in the hospital, and death. For example, one study highlighted that empirical therapy was largely inappropriate in hospital-acquired infections, indicating the urgency of enhanced diagnostic processes that enable quick detection of the pathogen and its resistance pattern. This highlights the necessity for the inclusion of antibiotic stewardship programs that educate healthcare providers on the correct and responsible use of antibiotics, particularly for the treatment of infections resulting from invasive interventions (Ceccarelli et al., 2015). Moreover, education and training of healthcare workers play a vital role in avoiding HAIs that are invasive. The implementation of intense educational interventions can reinforce adherence to infection control practices in a big way to minimize the incidence of HAIs. For instance, specially developed training programs that incorporate motivational strategies with application methods have been found to enhance adherence to hygiene practices and preventive measures among health care workers. These interventions are in line with ongoing hospital demand for infection prevention and a culture of safety and accountability. Lastly, an empowered healthcare workforce that has the relevant knowledge and skills is key to being able to manage HAIs' risks, particularly those related to invasive medical procedures effectively (Figure 9.7).

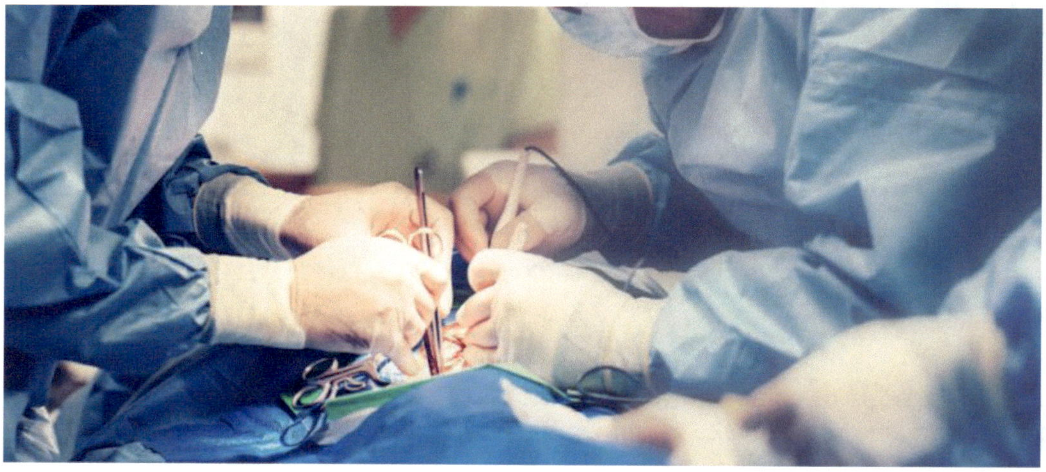

Figure 9.7. Invasive procedure.

Source: https://yashojyotfetalmedicine.com/wp-content/uploads/2020/10/AdgDr8BJ2L-768x342.jpg.

9.2.3. Environmental Factors (e.g., Hospital Cleanliness)

The interaction between environmental conditions, in this case, hospital cleanliness, and the occurrence of hospital-acquired infection (HAI) is a cause for concern in infection control. The evidence suggests that there must be high cleanliness levels in healthcare facilities to minimize the risk of HAI. Hospitals adopting rigorous cleaning protocols exhibit lower infection rates, which have been further supported by an increasing body of research highlighting the importance of cleaning the environment. A key area missing is proper assessment of cleanliness through current performance measures, where visual checks prove inadequate. Depending on such subjective results fails to provide a balanced picture of hospital environments. Therefore, healthcare facilities should adopt more objective techniques of cleaning verification so that infection control can be demonstrated to be effective, as highlighted in the review by May et al. (2012). Moreover, the effect of public perception of cleanliness in healthcare facilities cannot be overlooked. Generally, the public associate cleanliness with safety, and it is an important consideration in their confidence in healthcare facilities. Such frequent concerns regarding hygienic environments may discourage patients from acquiring the required medical care, and thus their health status may deteriorate. Interestingly, while public areas—, such as public transport, are usually regarded as not being hygienic, studies suggest that the risk of infection through pathogens in those spaces may be overestimated, as noted by Bernard et al., (2014). Such disparity between reality as perceived and reality as it is highlights the need for healthcare facilities not only to carry out cleanliness standards but also to be capable of communicating these efforts to the general public. Educating both the patients and employees regarding the tight cleaning protocols and their impact on infection control can enhance the overall perception of hospital safety. Finally, hospital cleanliness is not solely an institutional policy issue but also requires coordination of efforts from a range of stakeholders, including facility management and members of the clinical team. Literature exists that indicates that facilities underestimate the complex, multi-dimensioned dynamic between environmental cleaning and infection control. For instance, even though clinicians recognize the significance of cleaning procedures, there is a clear need for official coordination among facility management teams to establish uniformity in cleaning procedures and infection prevention. As noted by the observations of (May et al., 2012), technological mechanisms that monitor and provide quantifiable data for the standards of cleaning can facilitate coordination and advance infection control practices at large. By fostering a culture where cleanliness is supported and given priority as the precursor to patient safety, hospitals can further minimize HAIs rates and maximize patient outcome (Figure 9.8).

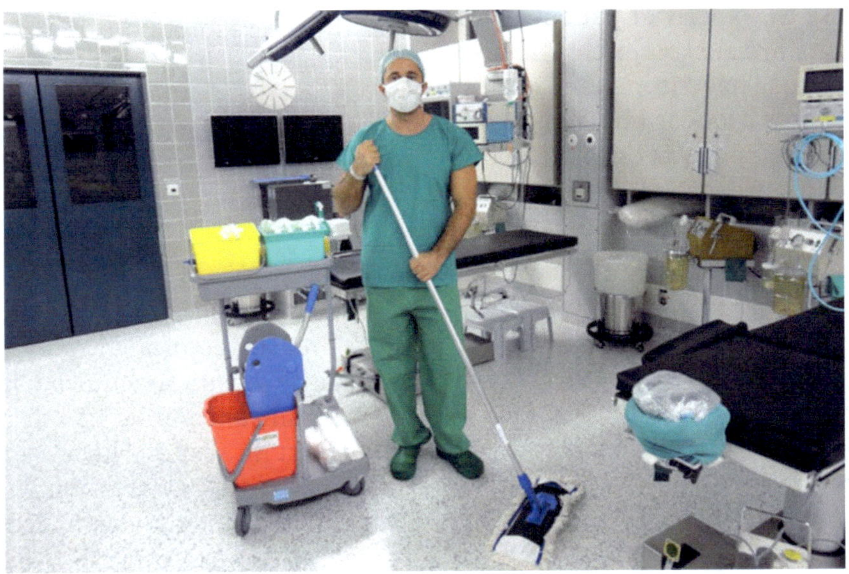

Figure 9.8. Cleanliness and hygiene in hospitals.

Source: https://miro.medium.com/v2/resize:fit:780/1*4qsj6eFGPxxjJDFDhDMcrA.jpeg.

Test Your Knowledge

1. What patient-related factors increase the risk of acquiring hospital-acquired infections?
2. How do healthcare-related factors, , such as invasive procedures, contribute to the development of HAIs?

9.3. Impact of Hospital-Acquired Infections (HAIs) on Patient Outcomes

Learning Outcome

1. Describe rising morbidity and mortality rates;
2. Know recovery time and duration of hospital stays for hospital-acquired infections (HAIs);
3. Call attention to the cost implications for health systems.

The role of hospital-acquired infections (HAIs) on patient outcomes is significant and multifaceted, exerting a substantial impact on both the health and the economic interests of health systems. HAIs lead to increased morbidity and mortality among patients, particularly when high-risk groups like the elderly or patients with comorbid conditions are susceptible. HAIs also carry an economic cost beyond patient health, with higher expenses for longer hospitalization periods, which account for a total estimated 90% of all HAI-related costs (Giraldi et al., 2019). Thus, the need for effective infection control interventions is paramount to avoid these adverse repercussions. Understanding of the delicate connection between HAIs and patient health is essential to formulate significant interventions that can enhance patient safety and overall care quality. Beyond health outcomes, hospital-acquired infections impose considerable economic costs on healthcare systems. The cost of HAIs is brought about by increased hospital stay time, additional treatment, and lost productivity due to increased recovery times. As explained in the context of the National Health Service (NHS), these infections impart high economic burdens not just on healthcare organizations but also to individuals and society at large (Mullings et al., 2019). For the patient, the economic implications are supplemented by potential out-of-pocket expenditures for other medical procedures. Furthermore, the psychological implications of carrying an HAI can yield decreased quality of life and increased anxiety over hospitalization. Thus, the economic implications of HAIs necessitate keen awareness of their effects on patient outcomes as well as a demand for effective infection control measures. Measurement of the HAI-related results highlights the urgent need for additional research and improvement in infection control practices. Research, , such as the Evaluation of Cost of Nosocomial Infection study (ECONI), aims to provide valuable information on the incidence of HAIs, costs, and broader effects on patient health (Mullings et al., 2019). Through the observation of patients who contract HAIs and comparing them to patients with no infections, scientists can better determine risk factors and refine prevention. This serves to inform policy and practice that is targeted at patient protection and enhancing recovery pathways. Lastly, the resolution of the impact of HAIs on the outcomes of patients by quality research and good infection control can significantly improve the quality of care provided in the health care facilities.

9.3.1. Increased Morbidity and Mortality Rates

The prevalence of high rates of morbidity and mortality hospital-acquired infections (HAIs) is a significant public health as well as health care system issue. These types of infections that occur in patients while they are in the care of the hospital or shortly after they are discharged are caused by various reasons that can include surgical procedures, medical equipment, and even the hospital environment. The treatment complications arising from these infections usually lead to extended periods of hospitalization, increased healthcare expenses, and, most significantly, enhanced possibilities of severe health complications. The necessity of effective infection control programs emerges as HAIs continue to raise concerns, requiring multifaceted approaches to guarantee patient safety and quality treatment programs. Aforementioned is of utmost importance in the prevention of HAIs is knowledge of their epidemiology and associated health hazards, particularly among susceptible patient populations. There is research to suggest that some of these infections, including Methicillin-resistant *Staphylococcus aureus (*MRSA) and Clostridium difficile, play a significant role in higher rates of morbidity, with patterns of resistance and spread in healthcare settings being alarming. Enhanced diagnostic testing and innovative use of point-of-care testing have the potential to bring enormous economic savings in addition to improved patient outcomes through early intervention. The initiatives by organizations , such as the Technology Strategy Board and the Department of Health emphasize the importance of goal-oriented research and investment towards the design of beneficial diagnostic instruments, eventually aiming to mitigate the effect of HAIs on patient health and healthcare resources (Szczepura & Osipenko , 2009). Moreover, there is new evidence suggesting a connection between respiratory infections and increased cardiovascular events, indicating the wider reach of HAIs on the overall outcomes of health. There has been evidence put forward wherein infections due to opportunistic pathogens , such as *Streptococcus pneumoniae* and influenza viruses, have been found to lead to acute cardiovascular events, with higher myocardial infarction and stroke rates among infected patients. This correlation highlights the imperative for enhanced vaccination rates and aggressive infectious disease control within clinical practice. Through facing the double threat of infection and its consequent cardiovascular ramifications, medical practitioners can better design prevention strategies that not just reduce HAIs but also enhance the overall health landscape of patients and demonstrate that controlling infection is critical to reducing morbidity and mortality due to these infections (Hayward et al., 2018).

9.3.2. Length of Hospital Stay and Recovery Time

Hospitalization and recovery durations are crucial factors managed by hospital-acquired infections (HAIs) that play a decisive role in patient outcomes and healthcare costs. HAIs-infected patients might have extended hospitalization duration since they can receive prolonged treatments, observation, and, in certain cases, surgical intervention. For instance, in CDI, strict antibiotic policies have been linked to improved outcomes, reducing the overall incidence of such infections, and possibly shortening the length of stay in hospitals. However, the existing evidence shows that whereas mortality rates may decrease following severe infection, secondary outcomes like stay do not change, which implies that there is an intelligent relationship between infection control measures and patient recovery periods (Helps et al., 2017). Thus, prevention of HAIs through implementation of effective infection control practices is necessary for ensuring maximum recovery of patients and efficient utilization of resources within healthcare facilities. Recovery times from hospital-acquired infections can likewise be very diverse from patient to patient, based on comorbidities, severity of infection, as well as timing of commencement of treatment. With community acquired pneumonia (CAP), time to first antibiotic treatment has been proven to directly relate with the recovery of the patient. A study indicated that patients waited for extended durations, averaging 7 hours and 48 minutes, before receiving their initial dose of antibiotics, which can prolong recovery and make hospital stays complicated (Callus et al., 2012). Effective infection control measures, , such as prompt diagnosis and treatment, play a significant role in mitigating the adverse effects of HAIs on recovery time. By streamlining processes and applying standardized management practices, healthcare facilities are able to reduce hospital stay and enhance patient outcomes. In the end, addressing the issue of reducing hospital stay duration and recovery times must entail an integrated approach of infection control practices. This entails not only the implementation of guidelines for HAIs but also continuous training and education of healthcare workers. The use of stringent infection control practices can help in providing a safer environment for patients and decrease the risk of HAIs and related complications. The connection between patient outcomes, infection control, and antibiotic stewardship underscores the necessity of healthcare institutions making an investment in evidence-based interventions that advance both patient safety and organizational effectiveness. These activities not only increase recovery rates and lengths of stay, but also contribute to enhancing the utilization of resources in healthcare systems, and emphasize the coordination between quality care and proper infection management (Figure 9.9).

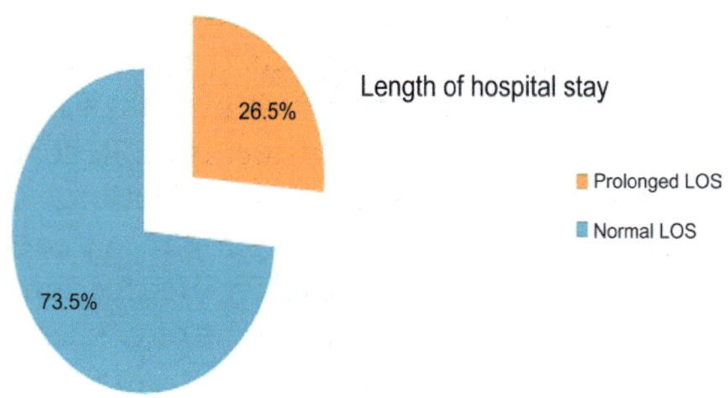

Figure 9.9. Length of hospital stay.

Source: https://www.medrxiv.org/content/medrxiv/early/2023/12/09/2023.12.07.23299680/F1.large.jpg.

9.3.3. Financial Implications for Healthcare Systems

The economic impact of hospital-acquired infections (HAIs) is a significant burden on healthcare systems, impacting a large number of operational and clinical outcomes. Direct costs of HAIs include prolonged hospitalization, additional laboratory work, and treatment requirement as a result of infection control. Moreover, the infections might encourage long-term complicated issues, requiring extended patient care. Health centers typically bear the cost of higher rates of readmission as well as penalty charges from payers like Medicare, which now entail financial penalties against high-HAIs rate hospitals. With increasing importance being placed on patient safety outcomes, it is evident that hospitals have to spend a lot of resources on infection control efforts in order to avert such economic losses as well as adhere to healthcare regulations. Additionally, HAIs bear consequences beyond immediate clinical costs to extend to implications for healthcare financing and policy. As an illustration, the total cost of HAIs in the United States has been put at billions of dollars each year. The economic burden is compounded further by the high morbidity and mortality rates caused by infections, not just overburdening hospital facilities, but also undermining public confidence in healthcare systems. Efforts at improving infection control, ranging from increased sanitation practices to application of new technologies, are investments that are necessitated. However, these systems entail the upfront cost of financial investments that can be stressful for budgets in the short run. Because of this reason, hospitals must weigh the costs in the short run against savings in the long run, since preventive infection control practices can greatly offset the long-run economic cost of HAIs and enhance patient outcomes overall. The fiscal condition of health-care systems with HAIs is also worsened by antibiotic resistance. The misuse of antibiotics has led to the creation of resistant bacterial strains, which disrupt treatment protocols and double healthcare costs. In HAIs, infections caused by resistant organisms are more likely to require more expensive and longer-duration treatments. This can lead to extended stays in the hospital, higher intensive care use, and increased rates of negative health outcomes. As the problem of antibiotic resistance grows more widespread, healthcare systems need to place top priority on financing research, training staff, and implementing effective antibiotic stewardship programs to fight this vital challenge. Epidemiological disease burden due to hospital-acquired infections and resistant infections is not only going to save lives but will also reduce the economic burden on healthcare systems in the long run, by restraining the spending on lengthened hospital stays and complex treatment regimens (D'Alessandro et al., 2016; Lillestolen et al., 2018).

Test Your Knowledge

1. In what ways do hospital-acquired infections add to morbidity and mortality rates among patients?
2. How does HAIs affect patient recovery time and hospital stay?
3. What are the direct and indirect financial costs of HAIs to the healthcare system?

9.4. Infection Control Strategies

Learning Outcome

1. Discuss hand hygiene practices;
2. Describe the use of personal protective equipment (PPE);
3. Learn about sterilization and disinfection procedures.

Implementation of good infection control practices is critical towards containing Hospital-Acquired Infections (HAIs) within healthcare centers. Among such measures, building a culture of safety is core. According to the European Federation of Nurses Associations (EFN), the healthcare services must establish an environment where mistakes may be reported and learned from without fear of any repercussions, thereby enabling ongoing improvement to patient safety as well as infection control (Burke et al., 2008). This approach also inclines healthcare professionals to report events without fear of victimization, a condition necessary in identifying where correction can be executed. Furthermore, by employing the optimal practices garnered from research and exchanges, infection control can be organized and optimized in preventing HAIs. Another strong component of infection control measures is the implementation of Antimicrobial Stewardship Programs (ASPs). As highlighted by recent studies, such interventions do have a great impact among children's populations through reducing inappropriate use of antibiotics and the subsequent risks (Barbieri et al., 2020). From what the evidence indicates, when hospitals incorporate ASPs, not only do they save on unnecessary antibiotic use but also combat the development of antimicrobial resistance—a developing issue in hospitals. Through the implementation of a systematic antibiotic prescribing system, hospitals can enhance treatment outcomes while limiting the deleterious effects of inappropriate use of antibiotics. ASPs thus constitute an integral part of good infection control that is in line with overall approaches to maximizing patient safety and quality of care. Furthermore, enhancing hand hygiene among healthcare workers becomes an imperative infection control measure. The Centers for Disease Control and Prevention (CDC) emphasizes hand cleanliness as one of the first measures against HAIs. Washing hands with soap and water or using alcohol-based hand rubs greatly reduces the transmission of microorganisms within healthcare facilities.

Educating and reminding employees to follow hand hygiene protocols can drastically lower infection rates. As various studies and reports have demonstrated, even minimal improvements in hand hygiene compliance are linked to dramatic decreases in HAIs, thereby making such a straightforward yet effective strategy more relevant. Consequently, integrating rigorous hand hygiene training with overall infection control measures improves the effectiveness of interventions designed to combat hospital-acquired infections, which drives better patient outcomes and safety (Figure 9.10).

Figure 9.10. Logo of the U.S. Centers for Disease Control and Prevention since 2024.

Source: https://upload.wikimedia.org/wikipedia/commons/thumb/7/71/CDC_logo_2024.svg/800px-CDC_logo_2024.svg.png.

9.4.1. Hand Hygiene Practices

Effective hand hygiene practices are key components in the path to preventing hospital-acquired infections (HAIs) and play a significant role in enhancing patient safety within healthcare facilities. Effective handwashing practices, in the opinion of the World Health Organization, reduce the transmission of pathogens and thus reduce HAIs incidence. Various methods , such as hand washing with soap and water, alcohol-based antiseptic rubs, and surgical hand scrubs, are recommended based on clinical situations. This multi-faceted approach allows for healthcare professionals to select appropriate hand hygiene practice in accordance with situations for maximizing infection control interventions. Most significantly, the integration of these practices into everyday care routines promotes a safety and accountability culture among healthcare professionals that is essential in mitigating risk related to HAIs and ultimately improving patient outcomes. The complexity of hand hygiene is compliance beyond, yet it is establishing a safe environment for the patient and the workforce. Healthcare environments are known to be significant reservoirs for cross-transmission of infection, and therefore the rigorous application of disinfectants is important. Literature demonstrates that high-reliability organizations implement systematic hand hygiene programs, which not only encompass direct hand washing but also emphasize disinfection of surfaces and instruments in a bid to limit the risk of infection even more. These practices address the evidence for the necessity of a multi-faceted infection control strategy of monitoring hand hygiene adherence and maintaining protocols updated with novel research on a continuous basis. From the literature, the use of "bundles" of more than one best evidence practice is a very efficient strategy in HAIs prevention and in establishing a culture of patient safety (Cammalleri et al., 2019). Moreover, ongoing education and training play a crucial role in ensuring the effectiveness of hand hygiene techniques within healthcare settings. Research indicates that health care professionals often misinterpret policies or lack the awareness of their contribution toward preventing infection (Burke et al., 2008). Programs of continuous professional development, including awareness and effective application of hand hygiene techniques, can help enhance rates of compliance. By developing an infection prevention culture, healthcare administrators improve patient safety and reduce the burden of HAIs, which has economic and clinical implications. Hence, the inclusion of hand hygiene education within the overall infection control strategy reinforces its pivotal role as drivers of organizational practice change to facilitate patient safety as a highest priority in health care (Figure 9.11).

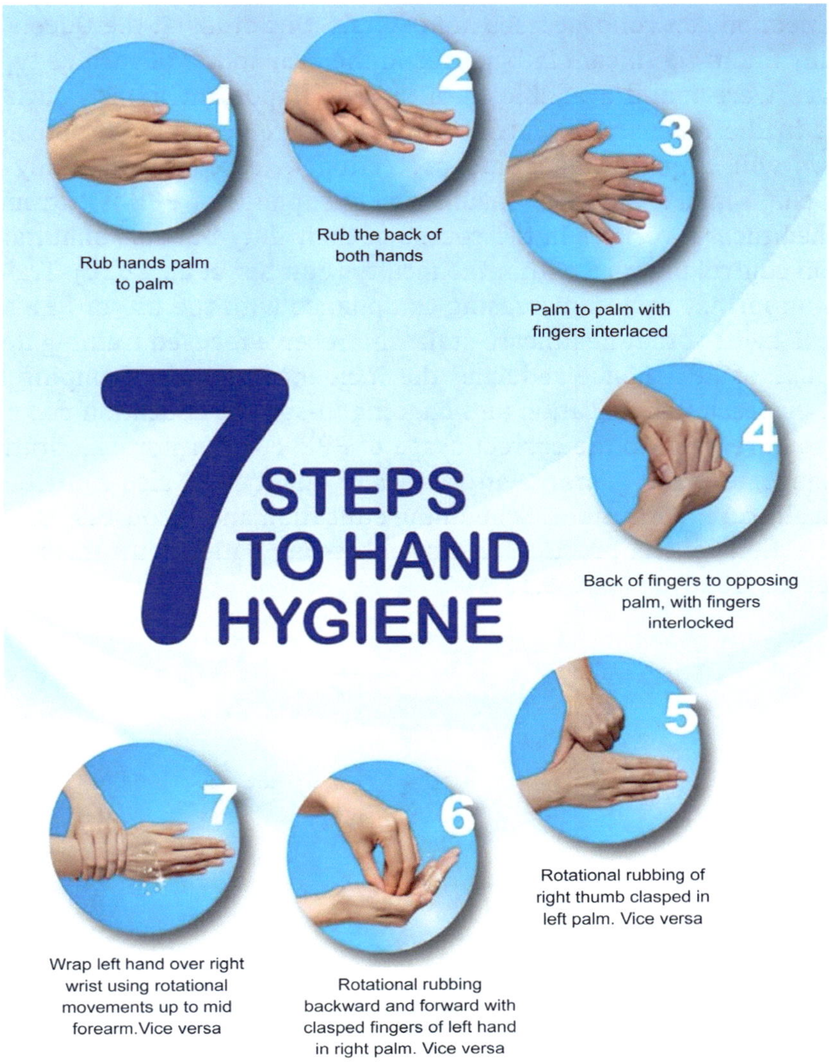
1
Rub hands palm to palm
2
Rub the back of both hands
3
Palm to palm with fingers interlaced
4
Back of fingers to opposing palm, with fingers interlocked
7 STEPS TO HAND HYGIENE
5
Rotational rubbing of right thumb clasped in left palm. Vice versa
6
Rotational rubbing backward and forward with clasped fingers of left hand in right palm. Vice versa
7
Wrap left hand over right wrist using rotational movements up to mid forearm.Vice versa

Figure 9.11. 7 steps of hand hygiene.

Source: https://i.pinimg.com/736x/ae/5f/b5/ae5fb5e5c395cfd84285e526e5e156b9.jpg.

9.4.2. Use of Personal Protective Equipment (PPE)

PPE usage is a life-sustaining intervention in the prevention of hospital-acquired infection (HAI), safeguarding health professionals during care provision for vulnerable groups. PPE is employed to offer a barrier against the transmission of pathogens between patients and health professionals, especially in high-risk environments. There are still ongoing issues, however, particularly with the adherence of health professionals to prescribed PPE protocols. Studies at St. Mary's Hospital

Lacor showed that few participants knew why PPE is used and even fewer adhered to proper techniques in donning and doffing the equipment. These findings justify plugging training gaps and awareness as key to improving compliance and, by extension, infection control practices in healthcare settings (Burke et al., 2008). Also important are the availability and accessibility of PPE for effective infection control processes in hospitals. One study at the Queen Elizabeth Central Hospital had already found significant imbalances in the availability of various types of PPE among wards. While gloves were found available in all wards, important items , such as goggles were not even available in the majority of wards. This imbalance comes with enormous risks, where healthcare workers will employ inadequate protection in case of potentially infectious cases. Enhancing supply chain management to ensure timely supplies of PPE is extremely important. It not only benefits healthcare workers in the course of their duty but also simultaneously improves the overall infection control practice within the facility (Comber et al., 2020). Training and ongoing education play an important role in increasing compliance with the use of PPE among healthcare workers. Evidence is evident that healthcare staff who receive focused training demonstrate better adherence to the use of PPE, hence reducing the incidence of HAIs. Pumping rigorous training programs through professional education and ongoing in-service education can significantly boost the knowledge base in relation to the correct usage of PPE. Furthermore, institutional support like monitoring by management and guaranteeing access to quality PPE also contributes to fostering a safety culture in healthcare institutions. Scheduling education and resources can assist hospitals in enhancing their infection control practices, hence enhancing patient outcomes and reducing HAIs' burden (Comber et al., 2020) (Figure 9.12).

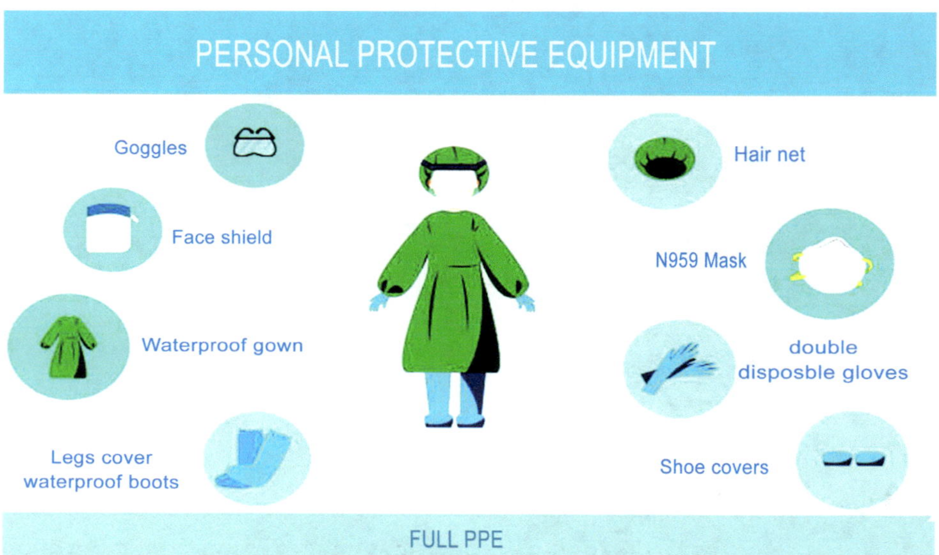

Figure 9.12. Personal protective equipment (PPE).

Source: https://www.netmeds.com/images/cms/wysiwyg/blog/2021/05/1620809350_PPE_big_2.jpg.

9.4.3. Sterilization and Disinfection Protocols

Good practice in sterilization and disinfection is an integral part of the fight against hospital-acquired infection (HAI), which remains a potential threat to healthcare facilities at all times. Infections not only affect patient outcomes but also place significant logistical and financial pressures on health systems. Good practice in sterilization and disinfection must be utilized to prevent the transmission of microorganisms, particularly in high-risk environments , such as operating theaters and intensive care units. Interventions , such as targeted hand hygiene, surface disinfection, and environmental cleaning have been proven to dramatically reduce infection rates. The inclusion of routine and rigorous sterilization measures enables a culture of safety within health care facilities, enabling the workers to combat HAIs effectively. According to hospital sanitation studies, maintaining such infection control practice focus is paramount to the protection of patient health and maximal outcomes for the delivery of medical care (Mohamed et al., 2023). In the exercise of surgical intervention, stringent sterilization and disinfection practices are especially important. Surgical wounds are especially sensitive to infection, and this can be caused by a variety of vectors , such as direct contact with the medical team or cross-infection between patients. To reduce these risks, procedures include thorough surgical scrubbing, operating theatre disinfection, and sterilization of all surgical instruments. Uses of newer techniques of sterilization , such as steam sterilization and ethylene oxide, for sensitive equipment are a demonstration of the need for specialization of technique to specific clinical uses.

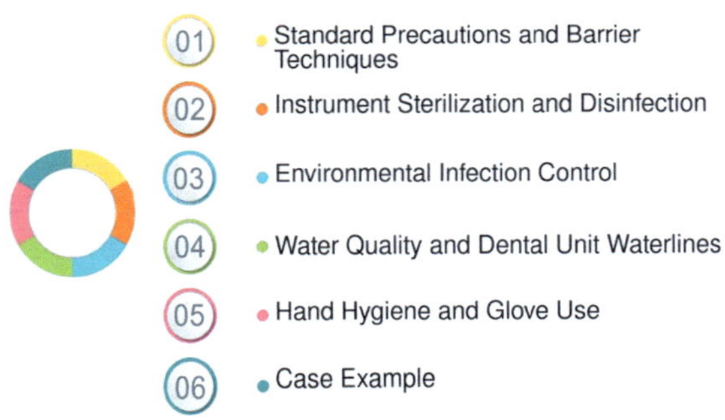
01
Standard Precautions and Barrier Techniques
02
Instrument Sterilization and Disinfection
03
Environmental Infection Control
04
Water Quality and Dental Unit Waterlines
05
Hand Hygiene and Glove Use
06
Case Example

Figure 9.13. Infection control and sterilization practices.

Source: https://fastercapital.co/i/Dental-quality-assurance-Ensuring-Dental-Excellence--Quality-Assurance-Strategies-for-Dental-Entrepreneurs--Infection-Control-and-Sterilization-Practices.webp.

Furthermore, training programs for surgical staff are inevitable, ensuring team members have the skills in the use and preparation of disinfectants as well as the carrying out of sterilization procedures. Overall, these steps create a strong platform for infection control, culminating eventually with reduced incidence of HAIs in surgical environments (Alam et al., 2024). Furthermore, the development of sterilization methods keeps evolving with new technologies that provide improved infection control solutions within healthcare settings. New developments , such as ultraviolet light sterilization and cold plasma technologies, are potential substitutes for traditional means, with the potential to provide more effective and faster means of pathogen destruction. These new solutions can supplement existing measures, strengthening the integrity of the sterilization process as a whole. As hospitals face the dual demons of antibiotic-resistant pathogens and repeated HAIs, the integration of new disinfection technologies into routine procedure becomes increasingly imperative. By developing an infrastructure in which conventional and advanced sterilization processes are prioritized, healthcare facilities can both enhance patient safety and improve health outcomes. Lastly, the strict adherence to sterilization and disinfection protocols is an essential pillar of effective infection control practices that is pivotal in the war against HAIs (Mohamed et al., 2023) (Figure 9.13).

Test Your Knowledge

1. Why is hand hygiene the most vital practice in hospital-acquired infection prevention?
2. In what way does proper use of personal protective equipment (PPE) reduce infection spreading in hospitals?

9.5. Role of Healthcare Professionals

Learning Outcome

1. Priority on education and training for infection control;
2. Identify a multidisciplinary infection prevention strategy;
3. Report and monitor HAIs.

Healthcare professionals' role against HAIs is imperative to ensuring patient safety and healthcare outcomes. The professionals are directly involved in combating infections using skills and training to assess, prevent, and treat HAIs effectively. Their responsibility extends beyond direct patient care; healthcare providers have a responsibility to embrace evidence-based practice, maintain rigorous infection control policies, and instill a culture of safety in healthcare settings. This involves continued education and training on how to remain up to date with the latest guidelines and practices in infection control, which is essential in minimizing the possibility of HAIs. Secondly, collective cooperation among healthcare workers is also imperative when formulating a broader infection control strategy. Effective communication and coordination among nurses, physicians, pharmacists, and infection control personnel are required to identify potential risks of infections and offer timely interventions. This employee participates in multidisciplinary rounds and committees to become familiar with infection cases and obtain information. The emphasis on a culture of safety, promoted by organizations like the European Federation of Nurses Associations (EFN), once again underscores the importance of immediate reporting of mistakes and exchange of best practices among health professionals (Burke et al., 2008). This effort not only enhances patient outcomes but also provides a firm basis for learning and quality enhancement. With the growing problem of antibiotic resistance, healthcare providers should be better equipped with information and tools to combat this issue more effectively. Antibiotic misuse has made it possible for resistant strains to thrive, rendering HAIs more difficult to treat and promoting morbidity and mortality (Lillestolen et al., 2018). Health workers must adopt good prescribing practices as well as enlighten patients on the management of antibiotics. They play a core role in encouraging research and funding to address the intricate issues of HAIs and antibiotic resistance. By facilitating an informed patient base and following antimicrobial stewardship measures, healthcare professionals can dramatically curb the incidence of HAIs and enhance overall patient safety.

9.5.1. Training and Education on Infection Control

Education and training in infection control play a necessary role in curbing the incidence of HAIs. Effective IPC practices are inherent features of health care delivery, which directly impact patient outcomes and organizational integrity. Continuous education of healthcare workers generates a culture of safety wherein caregivers are equipped with the required knowledge and competency to implement IPC principles and practices effectively. WHO guidance outlines that enhancing knowledge of IPC principles and practices not only reduces the incidence of HAI but also instills confidence in health systems. The edu-critical function is also illustrated through the simplicity with which a majority of HAIs can be avoided using thoroughly documented IPC guidelines, therefore placing strong importance on the necessity for frequent training programs in every healthcare facility, from nursing professionals to administrative experts within hospitals, hence successfully addressing the intricate patterns of patient care and safety (Higgins et al., 2017).

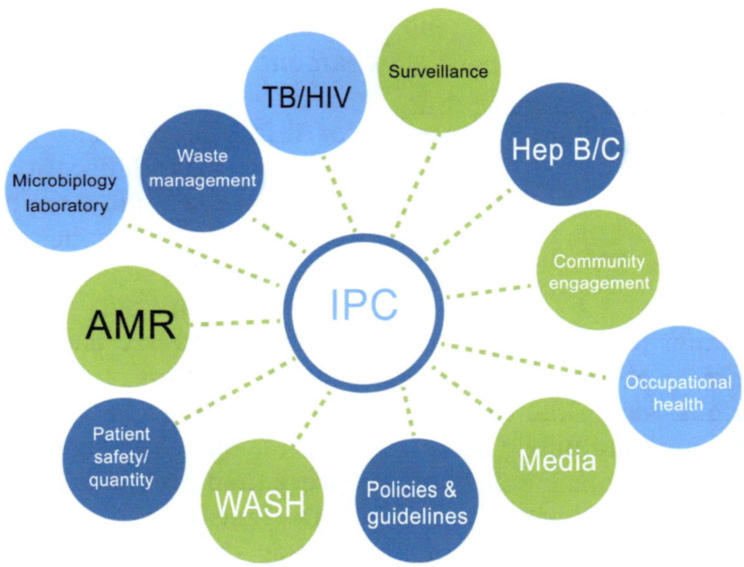

Figure 9.14. Infection prevention and control (IPC).

Source: https://d3f1iyfxxz8i1e.cloudfront.net/courses/course_image/b195c88b17a8.jpg.

Moreover, a successful training system requires a holistic approach integrating theory and practice. Simulation instruction and experiential training workshops are of utmost importance in instilling competence in infection control procedures among healthcare staff. These processes allow for instantaneous feedback and determination of areas requiring improvement, thus facilitating a culture of continuous learning. Training programs must also incorporate evaluations to assess the effectiveness of training interventions and keep healthcare staff up to date on evidence-based practice protocols. In addition, the engagement of healthcare professionals in ongoing professional development through continued education credits can help ensure high standards of practice. As revealed by the many studies, including those which the European Federation of Nurses Associations has placed in the limelight, the creation of a safety culture through extensive training can significantly contribute to reducing HAIs and overall enhancing patient safety (Burke et al., 2008). Moreover, the incorporation of IPC teaching into medical and nursing students' curriculum for healthcare education is crucial to the enhancement of infection control in the long term. By incorporating these principles into early training, future healthcare professionals are more likely to prioritize infection prevention in their work throughout their careers. This forward-thinking approach is central to building a workforce that is cognizant of HAIs' ramifications and the importance of sound IPC practices. An interprofessional educational approach, where various healthcare professions learn together, can also improve understanding and implementation of best practices. This kind of training also helps teams because it encourages team cohesion and a more cohesive patient safety strategy. It is, in the end, an investment in healthcare quality and safety, important in reducing the burden of HAIs in healthcare facilities (Higgins et al., 2017) (Figure 9.14).

9.5.2. Multidisciplinary Approach to Infection Prevention

Multidisciplinary infection prevention is vital in the quest to minimize HAIs. By bringing knowledge from various fields like nursing, epidemiology, microbiology, and public health, healthcare systems can establish a holistic approach that embodies the complexity of HAIs. Mixing together various professionals ensures that the complexity of infection control is addressed comprehensively, opening up the way for innovative interventions that cross through traditional silos. This intersubjective process not only facilitates enhanced communication within health care teams but also enhances compliance with best practice sustained by evidence-based research, which is critical to enhanced patient safety and outcomes. Moreover, as in research summarizing the culture of highly reliable organizations, the intermixing of various professional perspectives can facilitate gigantic leaps forward in learning about and avoiding risks associated with HAIs (Burke et al., 2008). Effective infection prevention activities also include the engagement of clinical personnel who can learn from the real-time implementations and adapt effective practices in their own facilities. Case reports of various healthcare organizations provide valuable information on what has been implemented to reduce HAIs, results of the interventions, and the valuable lessons learned in the process (Blumenthal et al., 2006). By analyzing these types of case studies, multidisciplinary teams can decide on reproducible and achievable best practices to apply in their settings. This evidence-based problem-solving allows for customization of infection control measures to meet institutional goals and patient demands. Moreover, building a learning culture among healthcare staff leads to continual improvement, hence enhancing the effectiveness of infection prevention activities. With the benefits of collaboration among healthcare providers, a multidisciplinary approach also emphasizes stakeholder engagement, including administrative support. Engagement by hospital administrators and policy-makers is vital for efficient resource allocation, interprofessional communication, and adoption of innovative infection control measures. Administrative professionals' engagement ensures infection prevention programs receive adequate funding and institutional backing for successful implementation. As noted in the discussions on patient safety culture, collaborative work between frontline healthcare workers and organizational leaders creates an environment that encourages transparency and accountability. In the long term, a multidisciplinary approach allows for a comprehensive platform against HAIs to improve the overall quality of infection prevention and control within healthcare institutions (Burke et al., 2008).

9.5.3. Reporting and Monitoring HAIs

Effective reporting and monitoring of HAIs are important for enhancing patient safety and healthcare practice. Improved timeliness of infection reporting, as well as related incident reporting, can be encouraged through a culture of transparency and honesty by healthcare organizations. This allows infections to be detected early and interventions to be directed. Under the European Federation of Nurses Associations (EFN), one needs to establish an open culture in which reporting errors immediately takes the central stage in guaranteeing patient safety maximization (Burke et al., 2008). Furthermore, dissemination of outcomes and best practices is critical in the maintenance of high standards in the different healthcare institutions. Since health facilities strive to achieve excellence, standards for regular monitoring and reporting can significantly reduce HAIs, thereby ensuring better patient outcomes and encouraging staff to trust reporting systems. The implementation of evidence-based guidelines is required to facilitate the proper monitoring of HAIs. Studies indicate that employing standardized practices can reduce infection rates significantly, particularly for procedures with higher risk levels, e.g., central line insertions. Specialized groups tasked with ensuring these processes are necessary for ensuring compliance with set procedures, as well as ongoing education of healthcare staff. Participation in cooperative networks also ensures the ability to track results and offer rich lessons learned between institutions. Through putting in place such interventions, hospitals are able to lay a solid groundwork for infection control practices in line with up-to-date research and clinical guidelines (Silow-Carroll & Edwards, 2011). In the long run, such methods not only improve patient care but also improve the integrity of healthcare systems overall. HAIs are not only tracked by data gathering but also through such information being used to drive change. Use of sophisticated data analysis software can facilitate real-time tracking of infection rates, enabling hospitals to respond quickly to outbreak developments. Further, the active participation of frontline staff in data collection and analysis can enhance ownership and responsibility for patient safety. Coordination between administrative entities and clinical teams is essential to transform data into policies that reduce HAIs. Emphasis on this aspect of infection control enhances the process of reporting because results are linked directly to improvement activities, resulting in a cycle of continuous improvement in patient care. Through experience and as evidenced by many studies, comprehensive reporting and monitoring of HAIs is significant in establishing a culture of patient safety and quality infection control practice (Figure 9.15).

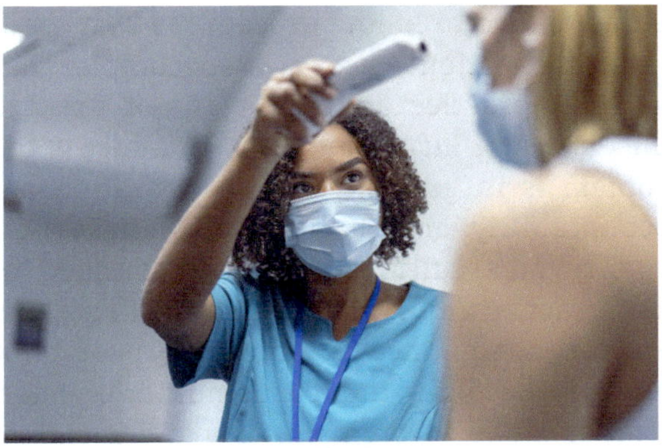

Figure 9.15. Monitoring of hospital-acquired infections (HAIs).

Source: https://www.coordinare.org.au/assets/Uploads/CTA/GettyImages-1319877948__FitWzE5MjAsMTA4MF0.jpg.

Test Your Knowledge

1. How is ongoing training and education among health professionals improving infection control processes in hospitals?
2. What is the significance of a multidisciplinary approach to hospital-acquired infection prevention and management?

9.6. Challenges in Infection Control

Learning Outcome

1. Identify antibiotic resistance and its meaning;
2. Deal with compliance with infection control procedures;
3. Prioritize healthcare facility resource constraints.

There are quite a number of challenges facing hospitals in infection control of hospital-acquired infections. One such challenge is compliance by healthcare providers with evidence-based prevention of infection protocols. There are policies, but the inconsistency weakens the effectiveness of the interventions. High staff turnover rates and poor training are the reasons behind failure to follow procedures that are in place, and patient cases are so complex that stringent practice adherence is not feasible, hence causing increased HAIs. To address this problem is to guarantee stern education and accountability of patient care teams on the urgency of a culture of safety grounded on clear practice and regular scrutiny of stringent practice compliance to infection protection measures. Secondly, the role of multidisciplinary teams cannot be overemphasized in the triumph over infection control problems. Organizations that support collaboration between various healthcare providers are better placed to identify, monitor, and act on the causes of HAIs. This is particularly relevant for interventions , such as central line-associated bloodstream infection prevention, which have been demonstrated to be significantly improved with specialist team monitoring as well as participation in collaboratives. Through integrated teams focused on infection prevention, hospitals can make the most of collaborative knowledge and expertise in performing and maintaining strict infection control measures. Increased communication between the teams also allows for timely action against developing infirmities to infection, leading to improved patient care and preventing the occurrence of HAIs as in high-reliability organizations (Silow-Carroll & Edwards, 2011). Besides, instilling a work culture for the reporting of mistakes in an honest way and passing on the best practices on a systematic scale is necessary to ensure infection control. It has been established through research that a safety culture can significantly reduce the incidence of HAIs since it ensures the work environment where mistakes become traceable and can be learned from. It demands efforts towards encouraging transparency and hands-on learning in policy reporting and infection control guidelines. European Federation of Nurses Associations reports that it demands a focus on safety to unite healthcare services for a shared purpose of patient care through continuous development from continuous research and recommendations (Burke et al., 2008). By embracing this culture of safety, healthcare institutions are not only positioning themselves to fend off the risk of HAIs but also establishing a setting in which there can be ongoing improvement in infection control procedures.

9.6.1. Antibiotic Resistance and Its Implications

Antibiotic resistance has developed into a globally recognized public health threat, particularly against the backdrop of hospital-acquired infections (HAIs). Antibiotic overuse and abuse have created resistant strains of bacteria that make infection control an issue in hospitals. With hospitals now theatres of war for several pathogens, the need for effective infection control measures has never been more important. For instance, erstwhile touted cure-alls , such as broad-spectrum antibiotics have unwittingly provided a platform for resistance, and education and awareness among healthcare personnel about prescribing habits are urgently required. Unless these knowledge gaps are addressed, the resistance cycle will continue to fuel itself, leading to morbidity and mortality in HAIs, especially among those high-risk patient populations. The implications of resistance to antibiotics extend beyond patient result to impact health care systems and society in general. Of greatest concern is the potential for increased health care costs in terms of increased hospitalization, testing, and need for more expensive, often cytotoxic, alternative therapy. The association between suboptimal initial antimicrobial therapy and poor patient outcomes warrants stringent practice of antibiotic stewardship. In the case of intra-abdominal infections (IAIs), one does not need to stress the importance of effective and timely source control as well as proper antimicrobial therapy. Untreated infections result in increased rates of resistance as well as death. The inclusion of strong antibiotic stewardship programs in healthcare facilities is thus necessary to assist in countering the effects as well as optimize the quality of patient care, ultimately redefining HAIs. Further, the global aspect of antibiotic resistance heightened the necessity of an organized campaign against this disaster. Efforts like AGORA attempt to optimize the proper use of antimicrobials in battle against challenging IAIs, engaging all forms of global stakeholders in this fight. Resistance to multiple drugs, particularly by Gram-negative bacteria, is a task uphill that none country alone can overcome and hence entails collaborative efforts. Increased anxiety about resistance by bacteria is also contributed to by flattening of the curve for the emergence of new antimicrobial products, and thus cooperation becomes the sine qua non. Through the establishment of a shared information culture and best practice, clinicians can enhance patient outcomes and ultimately regain antibiotic efficacy against HAIs, demonstrating loyalty to the care of the individual, alongside global health communities (Figure 9.16).

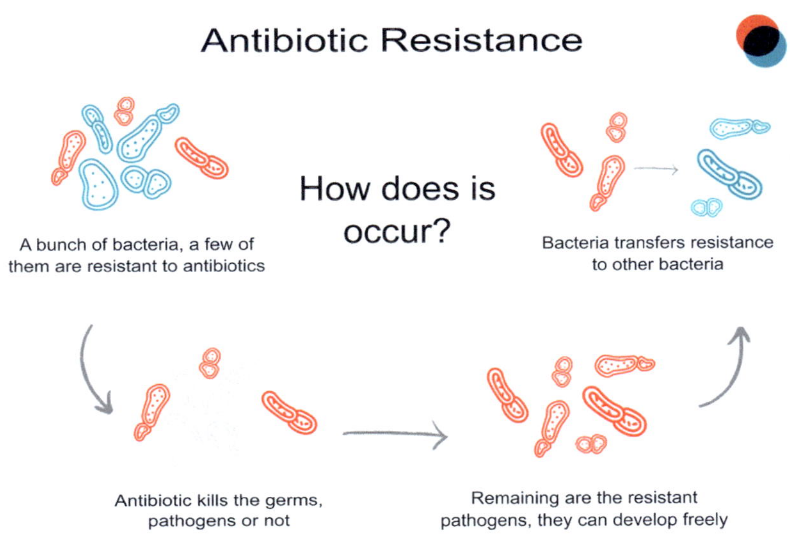

Figure 9.16. Antibiotic resistance.

Source: https://www.labtoo.com/hs-fs/hubfs/Antibiotic%20resistance%20680x482.png?width=680&height=482&name=Antibiotic%20resistance%20680x482.png.

9.6.2. Compliance with Infection Control Protocols

Compliance with infection control guidelines is crucial in the prevention of HAI, a significant problem in medical facilities. When health care providers are compliant with standard guidelines, they help create a safer environment for health care for patients by reducing the risk of infection related to invasive procedures, , such as central line placement. Best practices are highlighted by research to be applied, the very foundations of the guidelines. For instance, central line insertion teams have been advanced as being at the forefront of good infection control (Silow-Carroll & Edwards, 2011). This systematic strategy not only encourages compliance but also sets up a culture of responsibility for the healthcare staff by asserting that it is each provider's responsibility to be compliant with these processes. The organization's safety culture that prioritizes patient safety cannot be overstated in any discussion regarding compliance with infection control measures. Good safety culture facilitates open communication, under which staff members feel comfortable reporting a suspected infraction without fear of retaliation. An environment that does such is compliant with the recommendations set by the European Federation of Nurses Associations and thus facilitates a culture of error reporting and exchange of best practices (Burke et al., 2008).

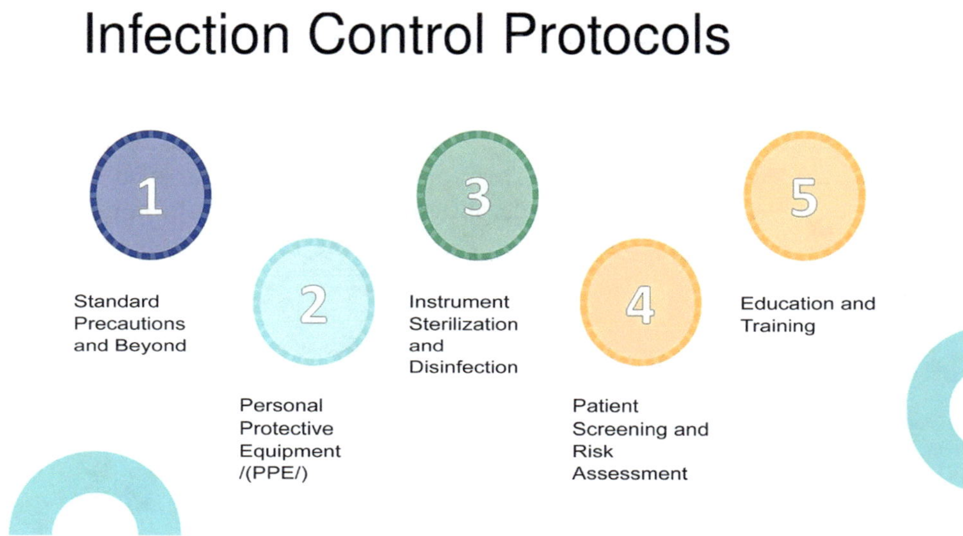
Infection Control Protocols
1
Standard Precautions and Beyond
2
Personal Protective Equipment /(PPE/)
3
Instrument Sterilization and Disinfection
4
Patient Screening and Risk Assessment
5
Education and Training

Figure 9.17. Infection control protocols.

Source: https://fastercapital.co/i/Dental-regulation-and-compliance-Navigating-Dental-Regulations--A-Guide-for-Entrepreneurs--Infection-Control-Protocols.webp.

By combining these aspects, hospitals are able to improve infection control procedures, not just to the level of guideline compliance but also active engagement in quality of safety improvement. Most importantly, the active involvement should be promoted because this builds a learning and development culture through which HAIs can be managed. Education and training are powerful drivers for having all the healthcare personnel conversant with infection control procedures. Ongoing education programs that equip employees with up-to-date evidence-based practices applied in infection prevention are important in monitoring compliance. These programs can include simulation training for appropriate technique, value of hand hygiene training sessions, and infection control guidelines refresher courses. The effectiveness of training programs is of highest importance as the learning obtained immediately impacts day-to-day practice and indirectly influences patient outcomes. Institutions are also required to offer assurance that conformity is monitored and measured consistently by audit and feedback mechanisms as not only does it deliver conformity, but it also offers a sneak peek at areas requiring improvement. This methodical training benefits the safety organizational culture, making hospitals better poised to handle HAIs (Figure 9.17).

9.6.3. Resource Limitations in Healthcare Facilities

The availability of resources within health facilities largely contributes to diluting the efforts of HAI control. Staff shortage is a widespread occurrence, and it contributes significantly to diluting the ability to put in place effective infection prevention policies. A study reveals that most health care facilities suffer from invariability in the reporting of infection control measures, an aspect that is further driven by understaffed manpower. From the evidence of national and local studies, hospitals are likely to undertake a reactive approach towards staffing indicators rather than a proactive one, which is a critical requirement for further enhancing infection prevention interventions (Ahmad et al., 2016). Aside from the fact that these constraints pose danger to patient safety, they also consolidate the pattern of poor reactions towards infections occurring in outbreaks, which again requires revisiting the operational capacity of healthcare systems. The organizational culture of healthcare also plays an important part in overcoming limitations in resources. Infection control is not merely a matter of following guidelines, but a safety culture in general that permits open communication and the timely reporting of mistakes. As the European Federation of Nurses Associations came to understand, this type of culture can equal better patient safety outcomes and HAIs (Burke et al., 2008). However, in the environment of scarce resources, engaging staff in open communication on safety becomes challenging. Such disengagement can halt the building and growth of cooperative partnerships upon which proactive infection control of HAIs leans heavily. The mutual dependence of the organizational culture and resource budgeting challenges the healthcare leaders to invest in the human and systemic factors promoting effective infection control. Lastly. Strategic resource alignment with infection control practice is crucial to healthcare outcome improvement. Failure to harmonize national regulations and local hospital practices is a prevalent phenomenon because there are insufficient resources. Periodic review of the regulatory guidelines indicates that guidelines to help prevent infection are in place, but hospitals' utilization of these indicators varies greatly owing to the insufficiency of resources (Ahmad et al., 2016). The sheer need for hospitals to create space to support routine reporting and implementation of operational protocols cannot be overestimated. Hospital infrastructure investment and resource planning are essential, since apart from encouraging standard compliance, they also support a welcoming environment for systematic prevention of HAIs. Thus, limitation in resources becomes a significant factor in the overall fight against HAIs in healthcare settings.

Test Your Knowledge

1. How does antibiotic resistance complicate the management and control of hospital-acquired infections?
2. What are some of the determinants of non-adherence with infection control measures among health workers?

SUMMARY

The conclusion drawn from the study of HAIs confirms the absolute need for thorough infection control measures in healthcare facilities. HAIs not only identify the susceptibility of the patients but also the inbuilt weaknesses of the prevailing healthcare protocols. For instance, HAIs and sepsis in intensive care units detail the dismal fate of inadequate infection control protocols; ICU-acquired sepsis patients exhibit extremely high mortality and hospital stay, reflecting the need for more effective monitoring and intervention strategies. According to SPIN-UTI project results, the connection between HAIs and preventable health burdens cannot be overemphasized, and therefore, the remedy has to be multidisciplinary in nature if there is to be improved patient outcomes in all hospitals. Lastly, systemic programs targeting strict adherence to hygiene practices, sterilization procedures, and environmental cleaning are of the utmost significance. The extensive HAIs report informs that healthcare facilities are reservoirs of cross-transmission and the implementation of proper cleaning and disinfection protocols should be embraced. In an awareness that there exist varied hand hygiene protocols with high infection risk reduction potential, healthcare facilities need to give priority to education on the essence of such guidelines among healthcare workers. As literature shows, adherence to established regulations, , such as those in place from Spaulding's classification, remains a pillar in the combat against HAIs. That aspect of providing a culture of accountability within hospitals will not only reduce infections but also improve overall provision of healthcare as a whole. Decreasing HAIs is thus an all-hands-on-deck effort that involves everyone in the healthcare sector, from administrators to clinicians, and even support workers.

As uncovered in the research, practice bundles involving more than one preventive strategy have been found effective for decreasing HAIs. It is essential, therefore, to develop an environment that promotes continuous education, awareness, and adherence to evidence-based practice. Emphasis on a research agenda for improving current preventive practice will be essential. The general outlook ensures that the healthcare systems engage not only in a battle of quantities of HAIs but also their causes for their diffusion, in order to finally offer safer patient care and improved health outcomes at institutions (Agodi et al., 2018; Cammalleri et al., 2019). Proper comprehension of HAIs is essential to a discussion of the primary prevention methods and their implementation in healthcare settings.

Primary findings emphasized in more recent works verify evidence-based infection control measures as an imperative. For instance, having specialized teams perform procedures, , such as central line insertions, is found to significantly reduce infection-related events. These specialty teams play an important role in enforcing best practices and a safety culture within healthcare facilities. Moreover, collaborative efforts by healthcare centers may lead to learning from each other and benchmarking against infection rates and thereby enhancing the practices performed for the prevention of HAIs. Observations and evaluation of infection rates need to be carried out from time to time so that these interventions can be readjusted and enhanced on a continuous basis, ultimately leading to improved patient outcomes through effective infection control practices (Silow-Carroll & Edwards, 2011). In addition, the widespread application of antibiotics has also been a prominent contributor to curing as well as complicating the issues surrounding HAIs. Penicillin was a medical miracle, but the ensuing abuse of broad-spectrum antibiotics has been a prime source of concern regarding antibiotic resistance. Misuse of these powerful drugs without sufficient knowledge of their biochemical mechanisms has permitted the entrance door for resistant bacterial strains to proliferate, and infection control in hospitals has become very challenging. The tragic reality is that resistance to antibiotics results in thousands of fatalities annually in the United States alone, and even in Third World countries, it's worse. To overcome the challenges, rigorous research and funding to identify the unique genetic cause of resistance and mechanisms behind it must be conducted to enable healthcare to combat HAIs effectively (Lillestolen et al., 2018). In conclusion, an infection control plan for healthcare facilities should be put in place to reduce the rate of HAIs.

This entails the use of evidence-based practice, specialized monitoring units, as well as constant monitoring of rates of infection, which supplements the strong basis for effective infection control. While so, the threat of antibiotic resistance serves as a reminder to clinicians of the small margin in antimicrobial treatment and the need to find new lines of treatment. While the war continues against infection due to antibiotic resistance, healthcare centers are forced to place greater importance on prevention and research initiatives in order to protect patients. The ever-changing aspect of HAIs and the resistance pattern requires that there should always be measures that bring clinical practice in line with innovative research to provide improved care and safety for hospitals in the future.

KEY TERMS FROM THIS CHAPTER

Alcohol-based disinfection
Antibiotic stewardship programs
Comorbid vulnerabilities
Educational interventions
Gastrointestinal infections
Health complications
Healthcare environment
Healthcare organizations
Healthcare resources
Healthcare systems
Hospital-acquired infections
Hygienic environments
Antibiotic resistance
Community acquired pneumonia
Complicated-infection patients
Evidence-based intervention
Hand hygiene techniques
Health institutions
Healthcare facilities
Healthcare professionals
Healthcare settings,
Hospital environments
Hospitalization rate
Infection control measure

CRITICAL THINKING QUESTIONS

1. **Which of the following is NOT a hospital-acquired infection (HAI)?**
   a. Catheter-associated urinary tract infection (CAUTI)
   b. Central line-associated bloodstream infection (CLABSI)
   c. Community-acquired pneumonia
   d. Surgical site infection (SSI)
2. **What is one of the major risk factors for ventilator-associated pneumonia (VAP) in hospital inpatients?**
   a. Ambulation within 24 hours
   b. Endotracheal intubation
   c. Oxygen nasal cannula use
   d. Low body temperature
3. **Which of the following best describes the effect of HAIs on patient outcomes?**
   a. Shorter hospital stay
   b. Lower healthcare expenses
   c. Improved patient satisfaction
   d. Enhanced morbidity and mortality
4. **Which one of the following is an ordinary infection control measure used to reduce HAIs?**
   a. Adherence to hand hygiene
   b. General use of broad-spectrum antibiotics
   c. Isolation of hospital patients
   d. Permanently limiting family visitation
5. **What is a usual obstacle to effective infection control in health-care centers?**
   a. Excessive availability of personal protective equipment (PPE)
   b. Reporting too many infection rates
   c. Infection control practice low staff adherence
   d. No electronic health records

Short Answer Questions

1. What are the most common hospital-acquired infection (HAI) types, and from which hospital departments are they most typically seen?
2. What are the essential risk factors and causes that contribute to the development of HAIs in hospital patients?
3. How do invasive devices , such as catheters and ventilators contribute to infection in hospitals?

4. How do hospital-acquired infections impact patient outcomes , such as length of stay, morbidity, mortality, and cost of care?
5. What are the essential elements of effective infection control practices in hospitals?
6. How does compliance in hand hygiene among healthcare providers impact HAIs, and what can be done to increase adherence?
7. What is the role of antimicrobial stewardship in preventing and controlling HAIs with the increasing prevalence of multidrug-resistant organisms (MDROs)?
8. What are the most critical challenges for healthcare facilities in implementing and sustaining effective infection control programs?

Answer to Critical Thinking Questions

1. (c); 2. (b); 3. (d); 4. (a); 5. (c)

REFERENCES

1. Agodi, A., Barchitta, M., Auxilia, F., Brusaferro, S., D'Errico, M. M., Montagna, M. T., Pasquarella, C., Tardivo, S., Arrigoni, C., Fabiani, L., Laurenti, P., Mattaliano, A. R., Orsi, G. B., Squeri, R., Torregrossa, M. V., Mura, I., & Collaborators (2018). Epidemiology of intensive care unit-acquired sepsis in Italy: results of the SPIN-UTI network. *Annali di igiene : medicina preventiva e di comunita*, *30*(5 Supple 2), 15–21. https://doi.org/10.7416/ai.2018.2247(accessed on 13th June 2025).
2. Ahmad, R., Birgand, G., Castro-Sánchez, E., Holmes, A., et al. (2016). Capacity of English NHS hospitals to monitor quality in infection prevention and control using a new European framework: A multilevel qualitative analysis. https://core.ac.uk/download/323057614.pdf (accessed on 13th June 2025).
3. Alam, M., & Singh, M. (2024). A clinical review on importance of sanitizing the operating room. https://core.ac.uk/download/613230116.pdf (accessed on 13th June 2025).
4. Ali, Y. (2018). Decreasing CAUTI rates by educating staff on reinforcing the CAUTI bundle. https://core.ac.uk/download/217228547.pdf (accessed on 13th June 2025).
5. Allardice, G. M., Coubrough, S., Noone, A., Reilly, J., et al. (2008). Results from the Scottish national HAI prevalence survey. https://core.ac.uk/download/9023284.pdf (accessed on 13th June 2025).
6. Apio, J. A., Kansime, F., Odora, J., Okello, T. R., & Pecorella, I. (2017). Barriers and factors affecting personal protective equipment usage in St. Mary's Hospital Lacor in Northern Uganda. https://core.ac.uk/download/188828828.pdf (accessed on 13th June 2025).
7. Barbieri, E., Daverio, M., Donà, D., Giaquinto, C., et al. (2020). Implementation and impact of pediatric antimicrobial stewardship programs: A systematic scoping review. https://core.ac.uk/download/286270886.pdf (accessed on 13th June 2025).
8. Berdini, S., De Luca, A., Di Ninno, F., Ferretti, M., et al. (2016). Healthcare associated infections: Educational intervention by "adult learning" in an Italian teaching hospital. https://core.ac.uk/download/84928307.pdf (accessed on 13th June 2025).
9. Bernard, D. (2014). Public transportation: Perceptions of filth contributing to poor health. https://core.ac.uk/download/56326277.pdf (accessed on 13th June 2025).
10. Blumenthal, D., & McCarthy, D. (2006). Committed to safety: Ten case studies on reducing harm to patients. https://core.ac.uk/download/71350251.pdf (accessed on 13th June 2025).
11. Bocicor, M. I., Molnar, A. J., & Taslitchi, C. (2016). Preventing hospital acquired infections through a workflow-based cyber-physical system. https://arxiv.org/abs/1702.08010 (accessed on 13th June 2025).
12. Burke, J., Smith, L.N., Sveinsdóttir, H. and Willman, A. (2008) Patient safety in Europe: medication errors and hospital-acquired infections. Workgroup of European Nurse Researchers. (accessed on 13th June 2025).
13. Cairns, S., Gibbons, C., King, H., Llano, M., et al. (2018). Results from the third Scottish National Prevalence Survey: Is a population health approach now needed to prevent healthcare-associated infections? https://core.ac.uk/download/293863931.pdf (accessed on 13th June 2025).

14. Callus, R., Mamo, J., Micallef, J., Montefort, S., et al. (2012). Hospital management of community-acquired pneumonia in Malta. https://core.ac.uk/download/46602322.pdf (accessed on 13th June 2025).

15. Cammalleri, V., Protano, C., Romano Spica, V., Valeriani, F., et al. (2019). Hospital environment as a reservoir for cross transmission: Cleaning and disinfection procedures. https://core.ac.uk/download/296244490.pdf (accessed on 13th June 2025).

16. Ceccarelli, G., Di Gregorio, V., Falcone, M., Farcomeni, A., et al. (2015). The spread of multi drug resistant infections is leading to an increase in the empirical antibiotic treatment failure in cirrhosis: A prospective survey. https://core.ac.uk/download/54521158.pdf (accessed on 13th June 2025).

17. Comber, A., Madziatera, D., Mkandawire, S. D., Msofi, C., et al. (2020). Availability, accessibility and proper use of personal protective equipment in wards at Queen Elizabeth Central Hospital (QECH) Blantyre, Malawi: An observational study. https://core.ac.uk/download/388986613.pdf (accessed on 13th June 2025).

18. D'Alessandro, D., Napoli, C., & Nusca, A. (2016). Are liquids an efficient vehicle of healthcare associated infections? A review of reported cases in Italy (2000–2014). https://core.ac.uk/download/84928144.pdf (accessed on 13th June 2025).

19. S. Silow-Carroll, and J. N. Edwards, Eliminating Central Line Infections and Spreading Success at High-Performing Hospitals, The Commonwealth Fund, December 2011.(accessed on 13th June 2025).

20. Epstein, S. E., Westropp, J. L., & Wong, C. (2015). Antimicrobial susceptibility patterns in urinary tract infections in dogs (2010–2013). https://core.ac.uk/download/323068134.pdf (accessed on 13th June 2025).

21. Gabbard, S. E. (2016). Post Foley removal guideline process and outcome evaluation. https://core.ac.uk/download/232575773.pdf (accessed on 13th June 2025).

22. Giraldi, G., Iachini, M., Montesano, M., Orsi, G., et al. (2019). Excess length of hospital stays due to healthcare acquired infections: Methodologies evaluation. https://core.ac.uk/download/227029126.pdf (accessed on 13th June 2025).

23. Hauck, K., & Zhao, X. (2025). A structural equation model of adverse events and length of stay in hospitals. https://core.ac.uk/download/pdf/6340780.pdf (accessed on 13th June 2025).

24. Hayward, A. C., Warren-Gash, C., Whitaker, H., Huijskens, E., Hung, I., McMenamin, J., Ren, X., et al. (2018). Laboratory-confirmed respiratory infections as triggers for acute myocardial infarction and stroke: A self-controlled case series analysis of national linked datasets from Scotland. https://core.ac.uk/download/153570271.pdf (accessed on 13th June 2025).

25. Helps, A., Irvine, S. C., Jones, B. L., Ritchie, L., et al. (2017). Restrictive antibiotic stewardship associated with reduced hospital mortality in gram-negative infection. https://core.ac.uk/download/46558800.pdf (accessed on 13th June 2025).

26. Higgins, A., Jamal, A., Lipitz-Snyderman, A., Pinto, A., Vicca, A. F., Howie, A. J., Yinnon, A. M., et al. (2017). Core components for effective infection prevention and control programmed: New WHO evidence-based recommendations. https://core.ac.uk/download/293884656.pdf (accessed on 13th June 2025).

27. Kilale, A., Prüss-Üstün, A., Reda, A. A., Doebbeling, B., Gumodoka, B., Denise, C., Kessler, C.

S., et al. (2013). Estimated risk of HIV acquisition and practice for preventing occupational exposure: A study of healthcare workers at Tumbi and Dodoma Hospitals, Tanzania. https://core.ac.uk/download/pdf/18410863.pdf (accessed on 13th June 2025).

28. Lillestolen, D. (2018). Infections not fought: Antibiotic resistance in underserved communities. https://core.ac.uk/download/158970352.pdf (accessed on 13th June 2025).

29. Listiowati, E., Rosa, E. M., & Sari, N. (2019). The infection control risk assessment and strategies to reduce HAIs at hospital in Yogyakarta, Indonesia. https://core.ac.uk/download/333842324.pdf (accessed on 13th June 2025).

30. May, D., & Pitt, M. (2012). Environmental cleaning in the NHS since the NHS Plan: A policy and evidence-based context. https://core.ac.uk/download/157852848.pdf (accessed on 13th June 2025).

31. McCarthy, D., & Klein, S. (2011). Keeping the commitment: A progress report on four early leaders in patient safety improvement. https://core.ac.uk/download/71358579.pdf (accessed on 13th June 2025).

32. Mohamed, K., Moussa, M., & Ali, A. (2023). Hospital hygiene challenges: An overview of issues and solutions. https://core.ac.uk/download/618379289.pdf (accessed on 13th June 2025).

33. Mullings, A., McFarland, A., Leanord, A., Ross, E., Mason, H., Reilly, J., Ritchie, L., et al. (2019). How do we evaluate the cost of nosocomial infection? The ECONI protocol: An incidence study with nested case-control evaluating cost and quality of life. https://core.ac.uk/download/293866892.pdf (accessed on 13th June 2025).

34. Szczepura, Ala and Osipenko, Leeza (2009) Point of care tests for hospital-acquired infections (HAIs) : economic analysis report. Coventry: Warwick Medical School. (Unpublished)(accessed on 13th June 2025).

35. Sartelli, M., Weber, D. G., Ruppé, E., Bassetti, M., Wright, B. J., Ansaloni, L., et al. (2016). Antimicrobials: A global alliance for optimizing their rational use in intra-abdominal infections (AGORA). *World Journal of Emergency Surgery, 11*, 33. https://doi.org/10.1186/s13017-016-0089-y (accessed on 13th June 2025).

MICROBIOLOGICAL DIAGNOSIS OF INFECTIOUS DISEASES

10

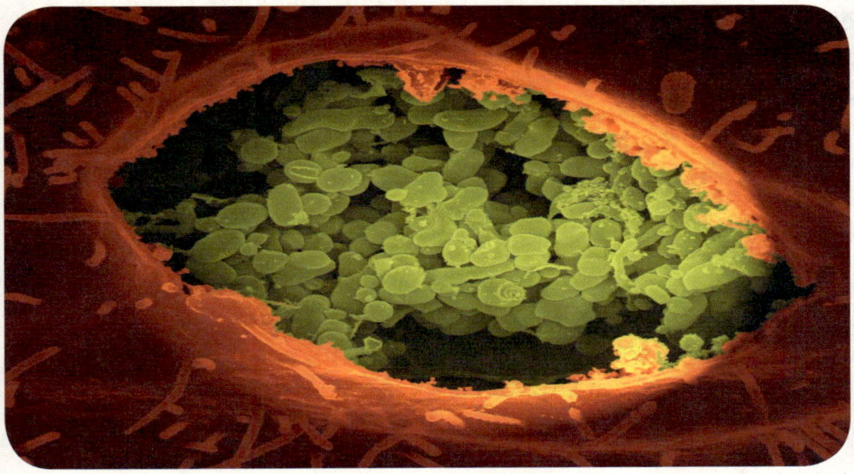

LEARNING OBJECTIVES

After studying this chapter, you will be able to:

1. Define blood cultures;
2. Describe urine cultures, a diagnostic test of utmost significance;
3. Understand cerebrospinal fluid (CSF) cultures;
4. Discuss the function sputum cultures play in the microbiological diagnosis of infectious disease;
5. Highlight the function of serological tests in the microbiological diagnosis of infectious disease.

Introduction

Diagnosis of infectious diseases in microbiology plays a central role in patient management and treatment efficacy. Accurate identification of the pathogens responsible using various diagnostic tests can significantly enhance outcomes, particularly in severe cases requiring urgent treatment. The advances in laboratory testing have given clinicians a three-dimensional arsenal of blood, urine, cerebrospinal fluid (CSF), and sputum cultures, as well as serological tests. Each of these tests has certain strengths and limitations, thus making it a necessity to possess a comprehensive understanding of their functions in establishing infection diagnosis. A positive application of these microbiologic tools leads to timely therapy, and that is imperative in light of rising antibiotic resistance and potential for life-threatening complications from untreated infection. Of the diagnostic approaches employed by clinical microbiology, culture techniques are a cornerstone of recovery and identification of infecting agents. These techniques are particularly helpful in the analysis of samples from various body fluids , such as blood and sputum, which could offer information about the causal infectious agent. For instance, the use of sputum culture is crucial when diagnosing respiratory infections, while the blood cultures are crucial in identifying systemic infections. Recent developments in antigens detection have been encouraging, especially in resource-limited countries where traditional culture techniques would not be so convenient. Studies have also shown antigen detection has the ability to outmatch conventional culture under some circumstances, especially in children who have had prior antimicrobial therapy (Lankinen et al., 2003).

This indicates a shift toward integrating various diagnostic tools that can produce timely and accurate results for a variety of clinical scenarios. Serological tests have proven to be a valuable complement to culture and antigen detection methods, especially in cases where it might be challenging to identify the pathogen directly. They can identify antibodies or antigens to some infectious pathogens and are commonly employed for the diagnosis of infections , such as viral infections, where culture may not be possible. Their application is even more evident where diagnosis is necessary urgently to prevent further transmission, e.g., in the diagnosis of TB. In the high-burden setting, specialty techniques like the Microscopic Observation Drug Susceptibility Assay have been shown to be more sensitive than traditional techniques, which lends urgency to the development of novel diagnostic approaches that are both cost-effective and efficient (Dang, 2012). In summary, an interplay approach using several microbiological diagnostic mechanisms must be employed in order to optimize infectious disease detection and control.

Definition of Microbiological Diagnosis

Microbiological diagnosis is a cornerstone of infectious disease identification and treatment that employs a number of laboratory techniques to detect the pathogens. The process is a series of techniques capable of isolating and detecting microorganisms, including bacteria, viruses, fungi, and parasites. Employing clinical samples , such as blood, urine, cerebrospinal fluid (CSF), and sputum, microbiological diagnosis assists clinicians in the diagnosis or rule-out of specific infections. A significant aspect of a diagnostic approach like this is that it relies on both culture-based and non-culture-based methods, which are distinct from one another in sensitivity and specificity. For instance, culture methods have been the historical gold standard, while advances in molecular technology , such as the polymerase chain reaction (PCR) enhance pathogen identification even in situations where the bacterial burden is poor. The validity of microbiological diagnosis can be appreciated in its application in several clinical settings, including tuberculosis (TB) and pneumonia diagnosis. In TB, the advent of new culture techniques, like the Microscopic Observation Drug Susceptibility Assay (MODS), has proven to be more sensitive compared to the conventional smear microscopy, detecting additional cases that otherwise go undetected. This is of prime significance in resource-limited environments where the TB burden continues to remain high and effective diagnosis plays a pivotal role in its control and treatment. Apart from this, advancements in antigen detection methods have also been encouraging in the detection of pathogens like pneumococci, which are generally difficult to culture through conventional culturing methods. Furthermore, the employment of a number of diagnostic tools raises overall diagnostic accuracy to get an accurate view of the infectious disease scenario among a given patient population (Dang, 2012). The appreciation of the significance of standardization of microbiological diagnostic methods is essential in ensuring accuracy and enabling comparability between studies. Development of protocols, for instance, the World Health Organization's proposed pneumococcal disease ones, emphasizes the necessity for standardized approaches in making clinical diagnosis results more consistent. These are not just included in the clinical diagnosis but also epidemiological research and vaccine trials, where proper identification of pathogens is essential in order to assess public health programs. Moreover, ongoing research and development in molecular techniques and immunoassays continue to push the boundaries of microbiological diagnosis, with increasingly sensitive and discriminating tests. As the science evolves, a commitment to rigorous validation of new methods continues to be crucial to maintaining the integrity of microbiological diagnosis, eventually leading to better patient outcomes in the fight against infectious disease (Lankinen, 2003) (Figure 10.1).

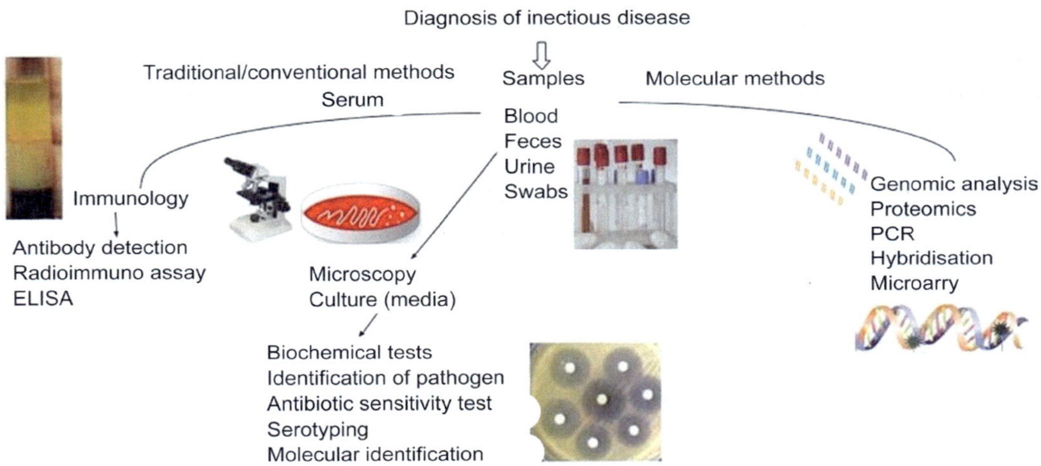

Figure 10.1. Sample processing for the diagnosis of infectious disease using conventional and molecular methods.

Source: https://www.researchgate.net/profile/Muazzam-Sheriff-Maqbul/publication/350878009/figure/fig1/AS:1012773744025604@1618475485473/Sample-processing-for-the-diagnosis-of-infectious-disease-using-conventional-and.jpg.

Importance in Clinical Settings

In clinical practice, the significance of microbiological diagnosis cannot be overemphasized, particularly in the identification and control of infectious diseases. Precise and early diagnosis of pathogens by blood, urine, and other body fluid cultures has a significant impact on the outcome of patient treatment. For instance, blood cultures allow for the identification of systemic infections , such as septicemia, and this can assist healthcare providers to implement pertinent antimicrobial interventions in a timely fashion. Moreover, sensitive methods , such as serological tests and enzyme immunoassays are capable of identifying the occurrence of specific antibodies or antigens, thus further delineating clinical data regarding the patient's condition. Implementation of these diagnostic techniques is essential in guiding treatment, optimizing the use of antibiotics, and avoiding the generation of antimicrobial resistance, thereby promoting public health and patient survival. The significance of employing appropriate diagnostic protocols is also manifested in managing diseases like tuberculosis (TB), whereby traditional methods of diagnosis prove to be insufficient. As an example, use of the Microscopic Observation Drug Susceptibility Assay (MODS) has shown increased sensitivity compared to conventional smear microscopy, particularly in low-resource settings where timely diagnosis is imperative for effective treatment. Comparative evaluation of MODS and other technologies, like the Mycobacteria Growth Indicator Tube (MGIT), shows their effectiveness in accurate diagnosis of TB and multidrug-resistant TB. These advances underscore the importance of the adoption of new diagnostic techniques and technologies that enable more detection of infections. Therefore, healthcare providers are in a position to provide timely and specific interventions, leading to better patient outcomes and reduced broader transmission of infectious pathogens within populations, according to recent research (Dang, 2012). Furthermore, serological tests have an important function in the clinic in that they are capable of detecting those pathogens less readily grown. Antigen detection, for instance, has been successful in the diagnosis of some infections, , such as pneumococcal infection, where standard culture may be of reduced value, especially after past antimicrobial treatment, as mentioned with respiratory infections. The enhanced sensitivity of antigen detection, coupled with enrichment techniques, can lead to more accurate diagnosis in challenging situations. This feature is particularly useful in epidemiological surveys, where detection of incidence patterns is crucial to public health activities. Thus, the inclusion of many microbiological diagnostic tools in healthcare facilities not only enhances infectious disease diagnosis accuracy but also plays a role in informing healthcare policies that are geared to improving patient care and limiting the spread of infections (Lankinen, 2003).

Overview of Diagnostic Methods

Various diagnostic techniques are necessary in the case of microbiological diagnosis in order to detect infectious diseases. These methods are grouped into three broad categories: culture-based methods, molecular tests, and serological tests. The gold standard for identifying pathogens in clinical specimens, e.g., blood, urine, cerebrospinal fluid (CSF), and sputum, is through culture methods. For instance, in the diagnosis of tuberculosis, emerging liquid culture technologies , such as Microscopic Observation Drug Susceptibility Assay (MODS) offer higher sensitivity compared to traditional smear microscopy and therefore improve detection rates within resource-limited settings (Dang, 2012). But culture methods generally have long incubation times and are influenced by sample manipulation and bacterial titer, leading to treatment delays, hence the need for adjunct diagnostic modalities. Molecular tests like polymerase chain reaction (PCR) have become invaluable tools in the quick detection of pathogens. These methods offer speed and sensitivity advantages over traditional culture, with the ability to detect specific genetic material from microbes in patient samples. Furthermore, PCR is employed in diagnosing infections with difficult-to-culture causative organisms, e.g., some viruses and fastidious bacteria. Among various applications, antigen detection tests have been shown to hold much promise, particularly in out-patient contexts, since they can significantly hasten diagnosis where rapid clinical decisions are called for. For instance, one study on pneumococcal infections illustrates the way in which antigen detection may prove superior to conventional culture methods, especially when prior antibiotic treatment renders bacteria less amenable to growth (Lankinen, 2003). By utilizing molecular techniques, the clinician can react rapidly to infectious illness and therefore improve patient outcomes. Serological tests are the foundation of another critical part of diagnostic protocols with the emphasis being on the immune response to infection. In numerous cases, these tests quantify antibodies or antigens in serum as indirect evidence of infection. The utility of serological tests is their ability not only to assist in the diagnosis of ongoing infections but also to establish prior exposure. Particularly, enzyme-linked immunosorbent assays (ELISA) have also gained popularity for being sensitive and capable of analyzing several samples simultaneously. However, serological results interpretation is usually closely associated with the timing of sampling and the established epidemiological framework of the disease. Consequently, serological tests may sometimes give false positives or negatives and must be carefully confirmed with clinical findings and other modalities of diagnosis. Overall, the combination of various methods of diagnosis enhances microbiological diagnosis accuracy and dependability for various infectious diseases.

10.1. Blood Cultures

Learning Outcome

1. Understand the purpose and significance of blood cultures;
2. Discuss common pathogens isolated in blood cultures;
3. Interpret blood culture results.

Blood cultures are extremely significant in the microbiological diagnosis of infectious diseases, particularly when sepsis or bacteremia is suspected. This is a laboratory test in which blood samples are obtained and incubated to detect the presence of pathogenic microorganisms in the blood. The early detection of these pathogens has a profound impact on patient management since timely initiation of relevant antimicrobial therapy can dramatically alter patient outcomes. The sensitivity of blood culture is most important since delays in detection are associated with increased morbidity and mortality, especially in critically ill patients. Furthermore, the interpretative difficulty of blood culture results necessitates a good understanding of local infection epidemiology and clinical condition of the individual patient, and thus involves the necessity to correlate microbiological findings with clinical experience for effective therapy. In Streptococcus pneumoniae diagnosis, new methods , such as antigen detection may enhance sensitivity of blood culture. Research has indicated that antigen detection, with a coupled enrichment process, may be better than traditional culture techniques in the identification of pneumococcal pathogens from clinical samples. This is especially applicable in populations , such as children who have been exposed to antimicrobials previously, where traditional culture techniques can be false negatives. Development of targeted assays, , such as enzyme immunoassays for pneumococcal capsular antigens, is a diagnostic method breakthrough that provides options that could enhance outcomes in situations where advanced lab facilities are not available. Therefore, the constant upgrading of diagnostic approaches is critical against infections, highlighting the importance of collaboration between researchers and clinicians to standardize and improve these techniques for wider use. Blood cultures are not without issues either; they require strict attention in the areas of sample collection, storage, and processing. Blood cultures' clinical value is compromised if samples become contaminated during sampling or handled inappropriately prior to testing. Effective methods to minimize these risks include maintaining aseptic technique strictly while collecting blood and the use of adequate blood volume for optimal positive culture yield. Additionally, the rise of antibiotic-resistant organisms poses further challenges in the therapy of infections found on blood cultures and requires a focus on antibiotic stewardship. Because sepsis remains one of the leading causes of morbidity and mortality in intensive care settings, it is essential for clinicians to be properly informed regarding how blood culture results affect therapy advice while being mindful of not adding to the development of antimicrobial resistance (Chan et al., 2017) (Figure 10.2).

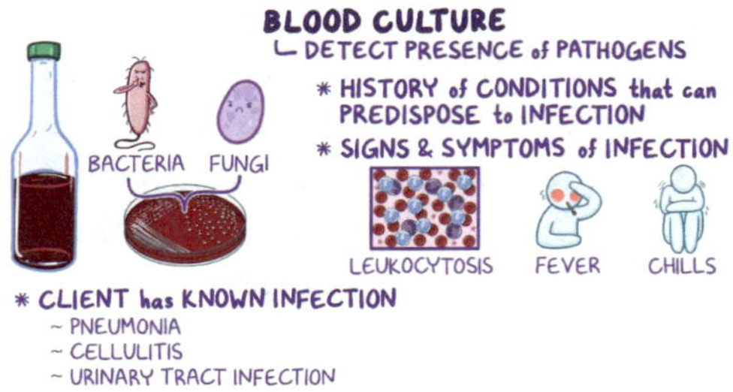

Figure 10.2. Blood culture.

Source: https://www.osmosis.org/_next/image?url=https%3A%2F%2Fd16qt3wv6xm098.cloudfront.net%2FGKnPOKI5TYCcBlYP5KdR3ORVQh2NSHNt%2F_.jpg&w=3840&q=75.

10.1.1. Purpose and Significance of Blood Cultures

The role of blood cultures is primarily in their ability to provide an accurate indication of the presence of microbial infection in the bloodstream, termed bacteremia or fungemia. These tests have a significant role in the diagnosis, monitoring, and control of infectious diseases, including sepsis, which might develop severe systemic complications if untreated. By allowing clinicians to remove and identify the etiologic pathogens of an infection, blood cultures enable the implementation of focused antimicrobial treatment, enhancing the potential for favorable outcome. Such diagnostic precision is particularly urgent in life-threatening cases in which timely action is paramount, illustrating the extreme importance of blood cultures as a core cornerstone within infectious disease management and microbiologic diagnosis. The value of blood cultures extends far beyond mere identification; they provide vital information about the etiologic infecting organisms and their antibiotic susceptibility. Knowing this information is essential to the development of successful therapeutic regimens and the management of antibiotic resistance, a worldwide growing problem. Early diagnosis by blood culture can significantly reduce septic disease morbidity and mortality by allowing clinicians to administer the best therapy early in the course of the illness. In addition, technologies , such as molecular diagnostics are enhancing the speed and viability of getting diagnostic results, and this further underscores the ongoing relevance of blood cultures in practice today and their impact on antimicrobial stewardship programs for the avoidance of resistance. In addition to their clinical use, blood cultures play an important role in monitoring the epidemiology of causative organisms as well as informing public health efforts.

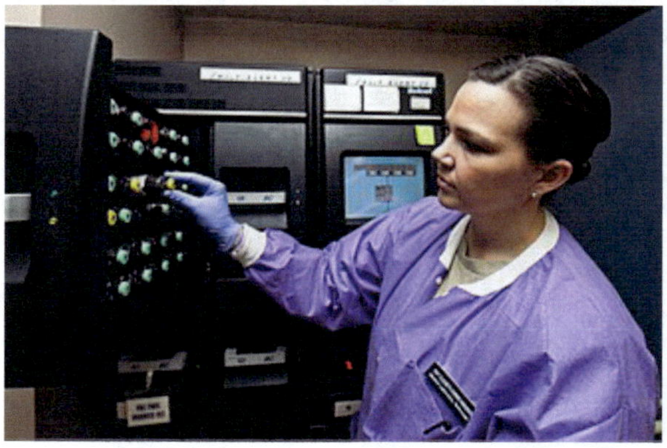

Figure 10.3. A laboratory worker unloads blood culture bottles from a BACT/Alert machine, an automated system used to incubate blood cultures and detect microbial growth.

Source: https://upload.wikimedia.org/wikipedia/commons/thumb/f/ff/National_Lab_Week_130410-F-TT327-090.jpg/330px-National_Lab_Week_130410-F-TT327-090.jpg.

Data collected from such cultures can give evidence of the trends in the prevalence of pathogens and resistance patterns among specific groups, thereby facilitating the implementation of targeted prevention programs. Such epidemiological data have widespread uses, particularly in veterinary medicine, where details of infectious disease dynamics in animal populations are essential for disease control programs. For instance, studies on enteric swine diseases have heightened concern for the necessity of robust diagnostic tests like blood culture to assess and manage health concerns in a befitting way, validating their increased impact on human as well as animal health interventions (Blackburn et al., 2006; Jacobson et al., 2003) (Figure 10.3).

10.1.2. Common Pathogens Detected in Blood Cultures

Blood cultures are a fundamental diagnostic method for the identification of pathogens causing bloodstream infections, which may be described as sepsis and other critical illness. One of the most common pathogens isolated, *Staphylococcus aureus,* methicillin-resistant *Staphylococcus aureus* (MRSA), is a primary clinical concern due to its increasing prevalence and drug resistance to standard antibiotic therapy. Identification of such pathogens in blood cultures is significant since it determines proper antibiotic treatment and infection control measures.

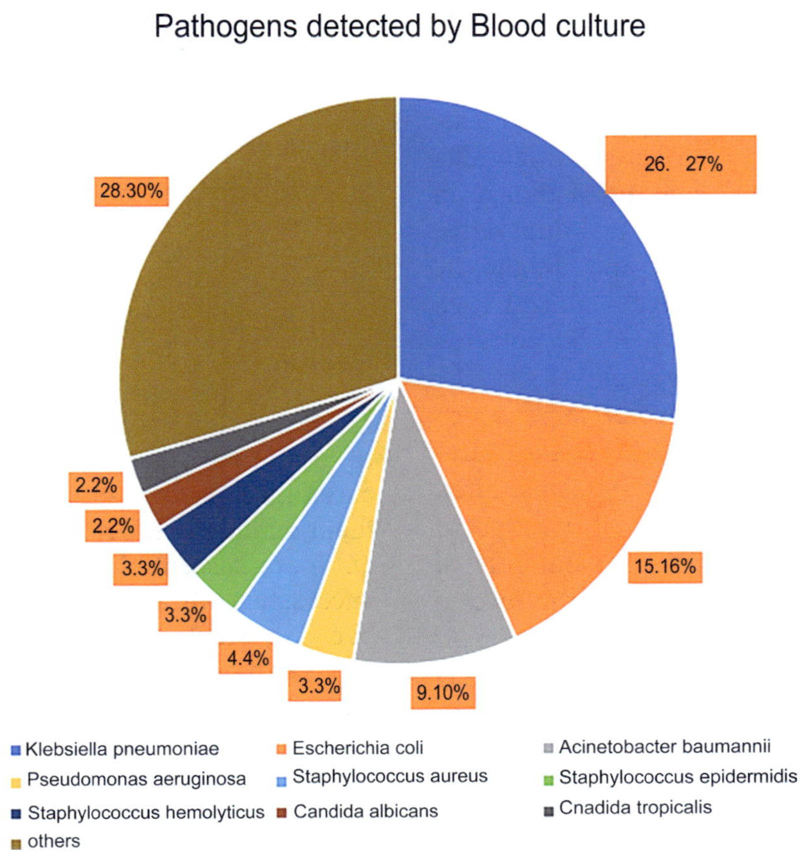

Figure 10.4. Pathogens detected by blood culture.

Source: https://www.researchgate.net/publication/368418187/figure/fig2/AS:11431281254264552@1719101784756/Pathogens-detected-by-blood-culture.tif.

In addition, the detection of *Escherichia coli,* long known to be involved in urinary tract infections but more recently employed for sepsis diagnosis, shows the importance of extensive microbiological examination. Understanding the dominance of such microorganisms in blood culture is important for the purpose of gaining positive outcomes in treating deadly infections. Another highly visible pathogen that one can generally identify in blood cultures is Streptococcus pneumoniae. This organism produces a range of diseases, , such as pneumonia and meningitis, and identification in bloodstream infections is associated with extensive morbidity and mortality. While blood culture remains the present gold standard for identification, advances in technology for antigen detection methods, i.e., enzyme immunoassay for pneumococcal polysaccharides, have shown promising gains in sensitivity, particularly in patients who have received prior antibiotic exposure. These diagnostic advances simply show the ongoing need for more advanced methodologies in microbiological diagnosis, particularly for those persistent infectious disease trends. With the continuing change in the infectious disease scenario, it is imperative to have robust surveillance and diagnostic capability in order to effectively control such pathogens (Lankinen, 2003). Blood cultures tend to reveal enteric bacteria , such as *Klebsiella* spp. and *Enterobacter* spp., which are significant etiologic agents of healthcare-associated infections. These organisms, often multidrug resistant across a wide range of antibiotic classes, highlight the vital role of effective antibiotic stewardship in the face of mounting resistance rates. The best management centers on the necessity of accurate and timely identification of these organisms in order to guide appropriate therapeutic interventions. Also, the utilization of blood culture data is not only for the treatment of individual patients but also extends to influencing the broader public health interventions toward containing the spread of multidrug-resistant organisms in healthcare settings. Continuous evaluation of blood culture systems, as well as incorporation of new diagnostic tests, is fundamental to minimizing the impact these organisms have on patient outcomes and healthcare systems (Chan et al., 2017) (Figure 10.4).

10.1.3. Interpretation of Blood Culture Results

Blood culture result interpretation is the cornerstone of infectious disease diagnosis, particularly sepsis-causing ones. Blood cultures are designed to detect pathogens in the blood and, through their result, inform clinicians how best to craft proper antimicrobial therapy. The result of blood cultures varies with the time of sampling, volume of blood drawn, and method adopted in culturing. Immediate reporting of these results is justified, particularly in sepsis, since early identification of the causative agent may prove useful to patient outcome. Studies have indicated that awareness of the spectrum of pathogens can inform effective management practices and maximize the selection of particular antibiotics and thereby reduce morbidity and mortality associated with infectious disease (Lankinen, 2003). A rational approach to interpreting the findings of blood culture, therefore, guarantees that clinicians effectively manage potential infections. Upon acquiring blood culture results, it is important to assess both negative and positive findings carefully. A positive blood culture also requires identification of the recovered organism and its antibiotic susceptibility, which can be critical for successful clinical management. Contaminating bacteria, which are usually seen with skin flora, can lead to misinterpretations and unwarranted panic unless correlated with proper clinical findings. Apart from this, negative blood cultures can be useful at times; they report the absence of detectable microorganisms by culture but can cause one to seek alternative potential foci of infection. Novel technologies of diagnostic testing, , such as the utilization of molecular techniques, are capable of improving sensitivity and specificity for the detection of pathogens and consequently overall diagnostic yield in complex cases of interpretation of blood cultures (Lankinen, 2003). This two-step process emphasizes the complexity and significance of correct interpretation of results in overall diagnosis. Finally, familiarity with the epidemiological context in where blood cultures are to be interpreted is essential. The differential list of possible pathogens may be extremely heterogeneous based on geography, patient population, and local epidemiologic trends, as has been explained through several studies of community-acquired sepsis (Asia et al., 2017). For instance, clinicians must consider endemic infections in specific populations , such as Dengue viruses or Leptospira spp that are not present elsewhere. The diagnostic approach would have to be adjusted according to these variations. Additionally, ongoing efforts in the education of clinicians about updated guidelines and protocols of blood culture interpretation can lead to better diagnostic performance and treatment outcomes. Continuities of feedback from laboratory to clinical results are also of great significance in the refinement of diagnostic processes, ultimately providing improvement in treatment of infectious diseases through evidence-based decision-making (Figure 10.5).

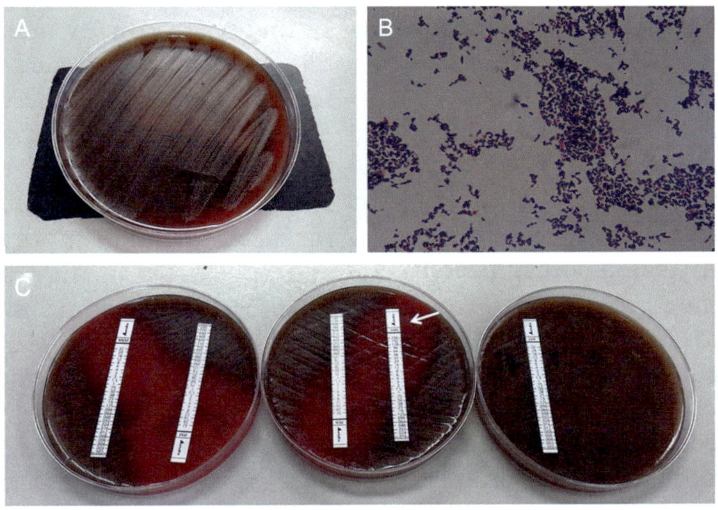

Figure 10.5. Blood culture results. (A) Growth of colonies of *Abiotrophia defectiva* in the blood agar; (B) Gram stain reveals Gram-positive pleomorphic coccobacilli, arranged in chains (original magnification, 1,000X); and (C) Antimicrobial susceptibility testing demonstrated susceptibility to vancomycin, imipenem, and meropenem, but was resistant to penicillin and levofloxacin.

Source: https://www.researchgate.net/publication/359192467/figure/fig2/AS:11431281187924415@1694450724459/Blood-culture-results-A-Growth-of-colonies-of-Abiotrophia-defectiva-in-the-blood-agar.tif.

Test Your Knowledge

1. What is the main reason for performing blood cultures in clinical practice?
2. What are the typical common pathogens to be detected by blood cultures, and how is this variable for each patient group?

10.2. Urine Cultures

Learning Outcome

1. Identify the indications for isolation of urine cultures;
2. Describe common urinary pathogens and their importance;
3. Describe urine sample collection and processing methods.

Urine cultures are a critical diagnostic step in the assessment of urinary tract infections (UTIs), which are among the most prevalent infectious diseases across the globe. The process is to collect a sample of urine that is subsequently tested microbiologically to identify and quantify microbial organisms present. Previously, urine culture has successfully isolated pathogens , such as *Escherichia coli,* which accounts for the majority of UTIs, as well as other bacteria , such as Klebsiella pneumoniae and Proteus mirabilis. Not only does analysis detect the existence of infection, but it also provides details regarding the antibiotic resistance of isolated pathogens to guide effective therapy. The ability to identify these microorganisms accurately is crucial, especially in complex UTI or recurrent infection patients, since infection left untreated may lead to serious complications, including pyelonephritis and renal failure, highlighting the value of urine culture in practice. In addition to bacterial culture, urine analysis is currently also utilized for detecting a variety of biomarkers associated with specific infections. For instance, the identification of microbial antigens or nucleic acid amplification tests can complement the diagnostic quality of traditional urine cultures in some cases, , such as when routine cultures are able to yield negative results. This is especially significant considering that heterogeneity of pathogens involved in UTIs, along with bacterial pathogens, can include viral and fungal organisms, but are less common. Besides, as illustrated in a study of fever of unknown origin (FUO), the prevalence of UTIs as an infection cause supports the inclusion of thorough urinary analysis as a step in differential diagnosis. This multi-dimensional consideration emphasizes the importance of urine cultures in untangling the cause of infectious diseases and guiding targeted therapeutic interventions (Thangamathi, 2006). Technical advancements have also improved the effectiveness of urine cultures, particularly with the introduction of automated systems that facilitate rapid sample processing and analysis. With these advancements, the time to obtain culture results has been significantly reduced, which is a critical factor in the clinical setting where timely interventions are crucial. The use of enriched media, as explained in the recent research, enhances the identification of demanding microbes that may be in limited quantities but are causative of severe clinical symptoms (Lankinen, 2003). With sustained research and the improvement of sensitivity and specificity in diagnostic tests, there can be improved outcomes in the cure of UTIs and other infection diagnoses using urine testing. It is essential for healthcare professionals to regularly update their knowledge and procedures on urine cultures so that they can produce optimal patient results in the microbiological diagnosis of infectious disorders (Figure 10.6).

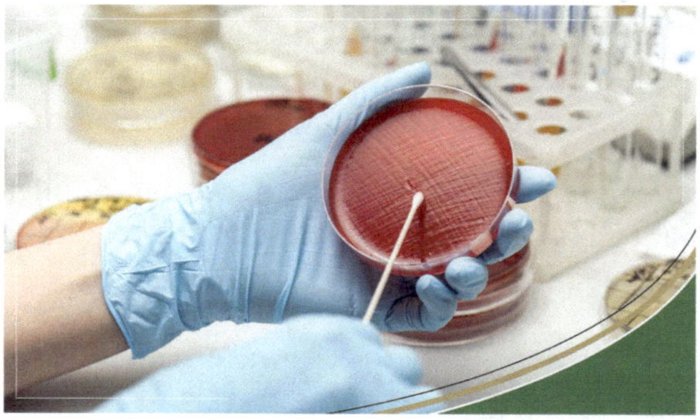

Figure 10.6. Urine culture test.

Source: https://www.sweetcures.co.uk/cdn/shop/articles/Urine-Culture-Test-Finding-the-Cause-of-UTI_2b3b778e-2fb8-46a7-9def-c08cf785d2ab.jpg?v=1633102104.

10.2.1. Indications for Performing Urine Cultures

Performs urine cultures as a critical area of microbiological diagnostics, especially in the evaluation of urinary tract infections (UTIs). Urine cultures are basically ordered whenever a patient presents with symptomatology typical of infection, , such as dysuria, frequency or urgency, or flank pain. The presence of these symptoms requires thorough investigation to identify the causative pathogenic organisms responsible for the infection. In clinical practice, early diagnosis by urine cultures is particularly important in directing the appropriate antibiotic therapy and preventing complications of untreated infections. Moreover, the sensitivity and specificity of urine cultures make them a worthy diagnostic tool for UTI diagnosis, thus ensuring that the patient is treated with targeted therapy addressing the etiologic microorganism. Furthermore, urine cultures are particularly beneficial in specific patient populations , such as the elderly, pregnant women, and patients with intrinsic diseases, placing them at risk of complicated infections.

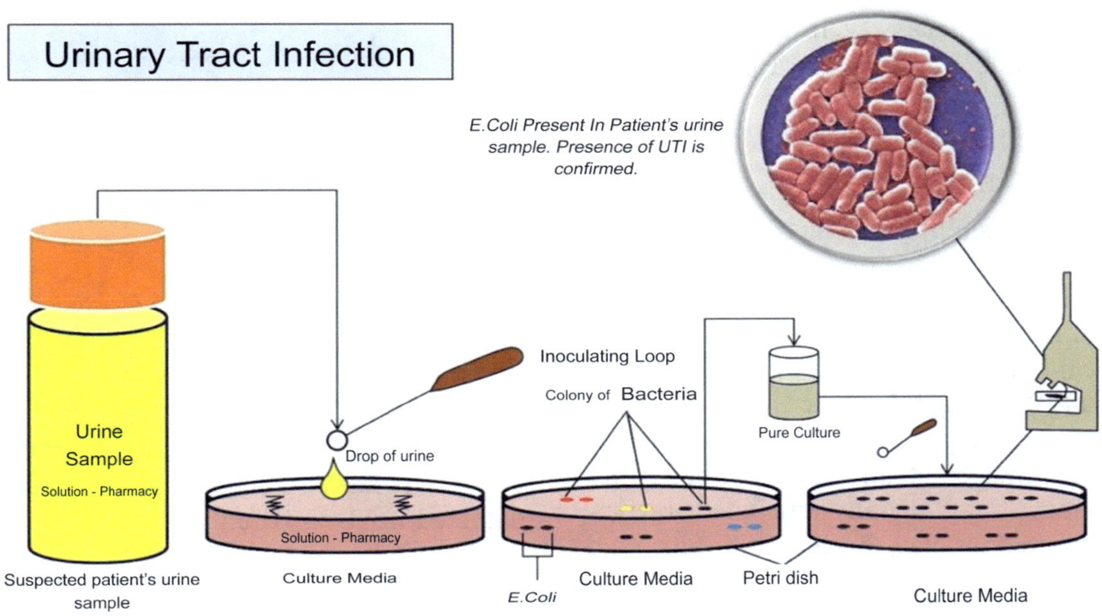

Figure 10.7. Urinary tract infections (UTIs).

Source: https://bookmerilab.com/tests/wp-content/uploads/2022/04/maxresdefault-1024x576.jpg.

In such patients, the risk of asymptomatic bacteriuria must be carefully evaluated because inadequately treated infection will cause severe morbidity. In pregnant women, for instance, bacteriuria can potentially lead to pyelonephritis, which affects both the mother and the baby. Additionally, the use of urine cultures for patients with recurrent UTIs is critical to identifying current infections or complications, , such as anatomical problems or antibiotic resistance, to enable more targeted prophylaxis or treatment strategies. Ultimately, these considerations highlight the importance of urine cultures beyond their usefulness as a diagnostic tool, with implications for patient management that are more critical. Other than the usual diagnostic indications, urine cultures can also be very useful in guiding empirical antibiotic treatment, especially with the increasing pattern of resistance. With the increasing resistance, urine cultures can provide useful data to guide treatment. For instance, in most cases, classical culture techniques can identify pathogens in a significant percentage, but long-term infections would need advanced diagnostic methods, , such as mNGS, to achieve the highest detection rate and offer more focused therapies in complex cases. Classical culture techniques fall short at times, particularly when the pathogens are hard to identify in the case of mixed or atypical infections (Chen et al., 2022). Therefore, urine cultures not only allow for accurate diagnosis but also inform paradigms of treatment in multifarious and complex clinical scenarios, making them a necessity in microbiological diagnosis of infections (Figure 10.7).

10.2.2. Common Urinary Pathogens and Their Implications

For the sake of comprehending common urinary pathogens and implications, it is important to determine the most prevalent pathogens responsible for UTIs. Of the pathogens, *Escherichia coli* is the most prevalent cause, accounting for some 80% of infections. This organism is highly suited to infection of the gastrointestinal tract and is introduced into the urinary tract usually via the urethra. Klebsiella pneumoniae, Proteus mirabilis, and the Enterococcus are other common pathogens and each are particularly difficult to treat and diagnose. The implications of such pathogens are worse than simple UTIs; recurrent UTIs, for instance, lead to complications like pyelonephritis and renal scarring. Moreover, the emergence of antibiotic-resistant types of such pathogens poses significant public health issues, necessitating efficient microbiological diagnostic methods for the timely and effective treatment. The traditional diagnosis of UTIs includes urine culture, which identifies these common pathogens. However, advances in serological tests and molecular techniques have progressed the field, allowing for quicker and more accurate diagnosis. Rapid antigen detection assays, for example, have been developed to allow for quicker diagnosis of certain pathogens. These types of diagnosis not only allow for appropriate antimicrobial therapy but also help with the overall epidemiologic management of these diseases. The importance of early microbiological diagnosis is particularly realized in vulnerable groups, including the elderly and immunocompromised patients, who can suffer serious consequences from otherwise treatable infections.

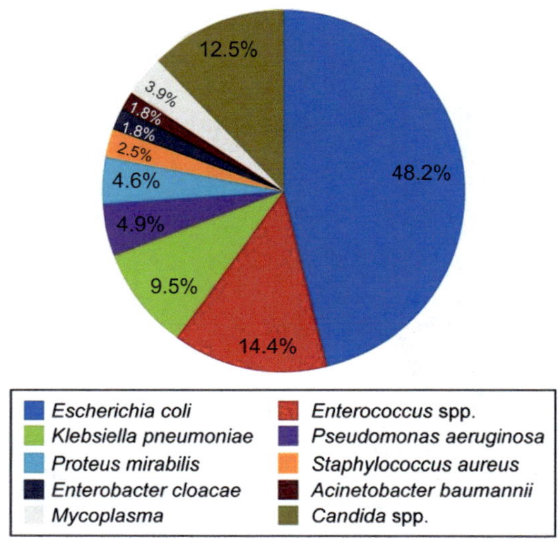

Figure 10.8. The most common pathogens detected in cUTI patients.

Source: https://www.researchgate.net/publication/320942080/figure/fig1/AS:11431281256676657@1719560982853/Most-common-pathogens-detected-in-cUTI-patients.jpg.

Thus, an unambiguous understanding of the common urinary pathogens is necessary for effective disease management and population-based surveillance. In addition to typing the pathogens, it is crucial to understand their resistance patterns due to the growing burden of antimicrobial resistance. Resistance most commonly follows overuse and abuse of antibiotics, leading to the development by organisms like *E. coli* of mechanisms that render standard therapies ineffective. The increasing frequency of multidrug-resistant urinary pathogens complicates treatment, and prescribers are compelled to reconsider prescribing patterns. Clinical guidelines emphasize the importance of tailoring antibiotic therapy based on culture reports and sensitivity patterns. Further, integrating microbiological diagnosis with novel treatment methods, , such as targeted antimicrobial therapy, has the ability to decrease patient outcomes compromised by resistant bacteria. Thus, accurate knowledge of common urinary pathogens and their implications not only facilitates immediate clinical interventions but also acts as a guide for future infection control and prevention (Lankinen, 2003) (Ali et al., 2015) (Figure 10.8).

10.2.3. Techniques for Collecting and Processing Urine Samples

Urine sampling collection is an essential process in the microbiological diagnosis of infectious diseases, particularly UTIs. The accuracy of diagnostic outcomes highly relies on the sampling collection methods employed. Another key technique of urination collection is the clean catch midstream method, which minimizes the contamination with the external genital area and thus maximizes the test validity.

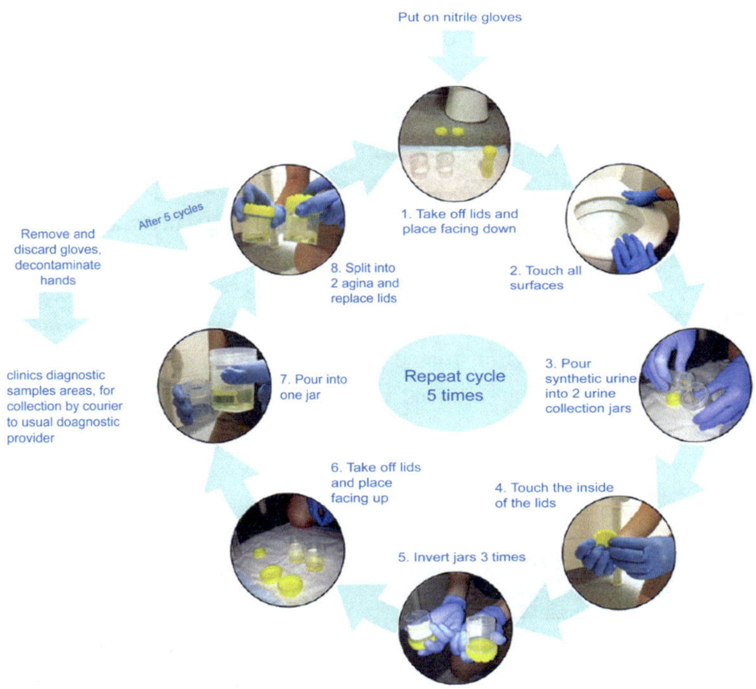

Figure 10.9. The method for the simulation of the collection of urine specimens using a urine surrogate solution.

Source: https://www.researchgate.net/profile/Patiyan-Andersson-2/publication/267742581/figure/fig1/AS:295741949005841@1447521783730/The-method-for-simulation-of-collection-of-urine-specimens-using-a-urine-surrogate.png.

The test involves having the patient start urinating, stopping the stream, and then collecting urine midstream in a clean container. In some circumstances, , such as collecting from infants and toddlers or patients who cannot collect midstream specimens, catheterization is utilized. Each method of collection has particular merits and pitfalls, ultimately impacting the microbial profile gained and, therefore, the subsequent clinical decision on treatment and management. Upon collection of urine specimens, prompt and effective processing is then very important for a valid microbiological diagnosis. The work of the microbiology laboratory is involved at this level, where specimens are filtered, centrifuged, and plated on selective media to identify possible pathogens. In using traditional culture techniques, laboratories can detect the presence of urinary pathogens , such as *Escherichia coli,* a typical causative organism of UTIs. Rapid tests like urine dipsticks for leukocyte esterase and nitrites can also provide initial hints for urinary tract infection, as cultures confirm the results. Using standard protocols allows reproducibility of results, making clinicians more confident in infectious disease diagnosis by association with urine samples and thereby efficiently and effectively guiding patient treatment plans, as highlighted by expert recommendations on test procedures (Baron et al., 2013). Storage and transport of urine samples are other issues that can affect microbial viability and analytical outcomes. For the preservation of urine samples, It is crucial that the samples are kept at the correct temperatures, typically between 2 to 8 degrees Celsius, to prevent overgrowth or degradation of the bacterial population. Delaying the processing may lead to increased false-negative rates or errors in reading microbial counts due to bacterial multiplication or death. Based on microbiological best practices, the sample is to be analyzed within two hours of collection; however, where this is not feasible, appropriate precautions, including the use of preservatives, need to be taken to maintain sample integrity. These practices are in place to ensure the accuracy of microbiological analysis, which enables improved clinical decision-making regarding infectious disease control according to urine testing (Morabe, 2022) (Figure 10.9).

Test Your Knowledge

1. What are the principal clinical indications for the collection of a urine culture?
2. What pathogens are most commonly found in urine cultures and what do they signify clinically?
3. What are the optimal methods for the collection of urine samples to minimize contamination?

10.3. Cerebrospinal Fluid (CSF) Cultures

Learning Outcome

1. Understand the role of CSF cultures in diagnosing central nervous system infections;
2. List the common pathogens that cause infection with CSF;
3. Summarize how to collect and analyze CSF.

CSF culture examination is a significant part of microbiological diagnosis of infectious illness, particularly CNS infection. CSF cultures play a vital role in the diagnosis of pathogens that cause diseases , such as meningitis and encephalitis, whose prognosis is based on their early diagnosis. In clinical practice, sterile CSF samples have to be collected by lumbar puncture. The samples may then be treated using various culture techniques to isolate bacteria, viruses, and fungi. Early CSF sample processing significantly enhances the possibility of successful pathogen identification, and prompt initiation of appropriate therapeutic interventions is crucial to the outcome of patients. Familiarity with the specific microbiological processes and culture conditions that various pathogens require is very significant in establishing an effective protocol of CSF culture in clinical labs. The pathogenesis of infection , such as viral encephalitis, can be elucidated through thorough examination of CSF cultures. One pediatric patient study approximated the prevalence of enterovirus 71 as the primary etiologic factor for viral encephalitis, followed by herpes simplex virus and measles (Beig et al., 2010). Employing various isolating techniques, like viral growth in some cell lines and serology for IgM antibodies, researchers can augment diagnostic efficiency significantly.

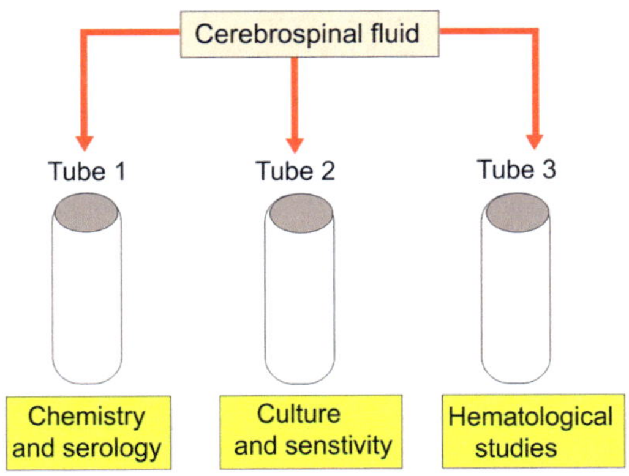

Figure 10.10. Cerebrospinal fluid.

Source: https://labpedia.net/wp-content/uploads/2020/01/CSF-tubes-collection.jpg.

As the study indicated, the prevalence of generalized convulsions and altered sensorium in patients matches positive CSF culture findings. The understanding of clinical presentations as well as laboratory findings, therefore, increases with knowledge of both, emphasizing the role of CSF cultures in the effective management of cases. Moreover, CSF cultures are highly significant in detecting less common but clinically significant pathogens, especially fungi. Cryptococcus neoformans is a fungal pathogen that can cause severe CNS infection, hence the need for both accurate identification and treatment (Calandra et al., 2010). The emergence of new antifungal agents has been necessitated by the inefficacy of existing drugs in controlling some of the fungal pathogens. CSF culture plays a crucial role in the identification of such an organism, thereby availing customized therapeutic interventions, thereby improving the outcomes of the patient. The incorporation of new diagnostic techniques, including the development of new antifungal peptides that specifically target elements of the fungal cell, is a testament to the ongoing growth of the microbiology department. This innovation plays a pivotal role in expanding our understanding and intervention with infectious diseases linked to CSF abnormalities (Figure 10.10).

10.3.1. Role of Cerebrospinal Fluid (CSF) Cultures in Diagnosing Central Nervous System Infections

In diagnosing infections of the central nervous system, cerebrospinal fluid cultures are priceless. The cultures form an important clue to diagnosis in the detection of causative pathogens of different types of infections, including meningitis and encephalitis. In studying CSF obtained by lumbar puncture, clinicians can determine microbial agents, as the fluid is an environment that reflects the status of the central nervous system. Early CSF culture diagnosis is crucial since early treatment with appropriate antibiotic therapy significantly improves patient outcomes. Also, the specificity of CSF cultures facilitates discrimination between bacterial, viral, and fungal infections, which is useful in the planning of the proper treatment regimen. This accuracy is most vital, since ill treatment has the potential to cause severe patient deterioration or allow antibiotic resistance to occur, making further clinical management difficult (Chan et al., 2017). Though CSF cultures are very informative, their utility is not unrestrained. False negatives can occur from a number of causes, including prior antibiotic administration, contamination with fastidious organisms, or inadequacies in sampling technique. Thus, clinicians are forced to make their diagnosis based on a combination of clinical aids, including imaging and clinical symptom assessment, with CSF examination. Diagnosis is reinforced even more when culture is augmented by PCR techniques, which detect pathogens' nucleic acids in cases where conventional culture fails. Such an integrated management ensures that central nervous system infections are accurately diagnosed and treated to minimize the risk of long-term neurological complications in patients.

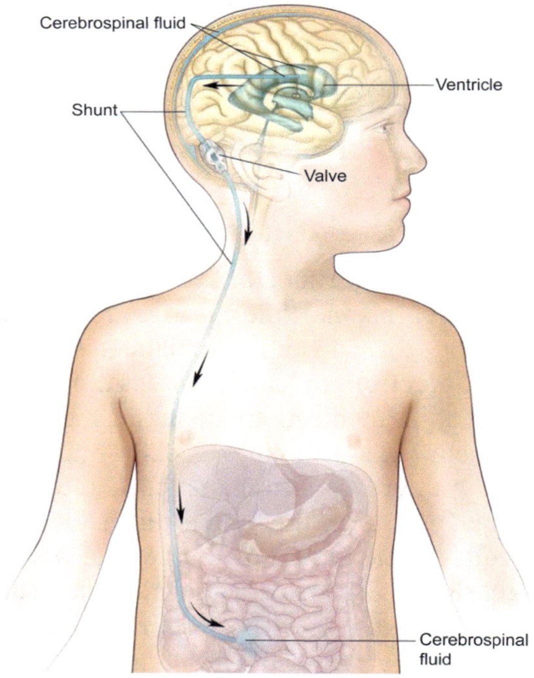

Figure 10.11. Cerebrospinal fluid has an important function of protecting the central nervous system.

Source: https://storage.googleapis.com/prod-diagcorp/images/ckeditor/FZ3VknqPLDQpKYPIdDmrhTpzdhHe2rfO1awuZBhdyDUNOKBf9PpSmVMsdooc4EKg4xEQXd9k9KWHRoHk_1612430552.jpg.

Additionally, awareness of the etiology of febrile illnesses, as articulated in the principle of fever of unknown origin (FUO), underscores the need for thorough investigations, including CSF cultures, for optimal patient care (Thangamathi, 2006). The role of CSF cultures is not only diagnosis; they are central to informing public health response to new infectious disease emergence. Through the detection of resistant strains or pathogens of public health concern, health authorities can implement measures needed to control outbreaks. Also, bulk data derived from CSF cultures are source material for epidemiologic studies tracking the prevalence and incidence of central nervous system infection, which highlights the importance of surveillance in public health policy. As the emerging trend is antibiotic resistance, data from CSF cultures can even be utilized in antimicrobial stewardship programs to optimize the use of drugs and avoid the development of resistant microorganisms. Thus, CSF cultures not only contribute to diagnostic accuracy but also have a considerable effect on treatment decisions and public health policy (Chan et al., 2017) (Figure 10.11).

10.3.2. Common Pathogens Associated with Cerebrospinal Fluid (CSF) Infections

Infections of the CSF and central nervous system (CNS) are usually due to a variety of pathogens that differ in virulence factor and presentation. Acute bacterial meningitis is most commonly caused by *Neisseria meningitidis*, *Streptococcus pneumoniae*, and *Haemophilus influenzae*. Meningococcal disease, most commonly occurring in young adults, can have severe complications in the forms of sepsis and morbidity if not promptly treated. Pneumococcal disease is still a leading morbidity and mortality illness despite vaccine availability, particularly in the immunocompromised or elderly, where *S. pneumoniae* is capable of causing meningitis, pneumonia, and bacteremia. Lastly, H. influenzae type b was a frequent cause of infection in children before the widespread implementation of effective conjugate vaccines but remains problematic in unimmunized populations. Apart from bacterial pathogens, viral agents are also frequently implicated in CSF infections. Viruses , such as herpes simplex virus (HSV), especially types 1 and 2, are known to be the etiologic agents of viral meningitis and sporadic encephalitis, which can be debilitating for the nervous system if not promptly treated. Enteroviruses and cytomegalovirus are some of the other viruses that significantly contribute to the overall incidence of viral meningitis, especially in immunocompromised hosts. Enteroviruses, for instance, are responsible for the most common viral meningitis in children and appear as epidemics in summer seasons. Detection of these viruses would mostly be by using PCR technology for greater sensitivity and specificity since older technologies like viral cultures fall behind and cannot keep pace with the enormous numbers of strains available. Serological tests also have an important role in viral and bacterial etiological differentiation and allow for more individualized therapeutic approach in the patient's treatment. Fungal and also parasitic agents have been reported to raise significant issues in specific populations, particularly in immunocompromised individuals. *Cryptococcus neoformans* is a frequent agent of CNS infection in AIDS patients and leads to cryptococcal meningitis, for instance. Diagnosis in most cases involves the identification of the organism in CSF by India ink prep or cryptococcal antigen, which reflects on the need for increased awareness of opportunistic infection in high-risk groups. Similarly, the protozoan *Toxoplasma gondii* can lead to cerebral toxoplasmosis in immunocompromised hosts, further complicating CSF infection. With the heterogeneous collection of pathogens, solid microbiological diagnosis with cautious CSF analysis, combined with appropriate serologic tests, is still essential in effective treatment results (Lankinen, 2003; Chan et al., 2017). Being informed about the common pathogens causing CSF infection not only helps in correct diagnosis but also in public health interventions to lower rates of infection among high-risk groups (Figure 10.12).

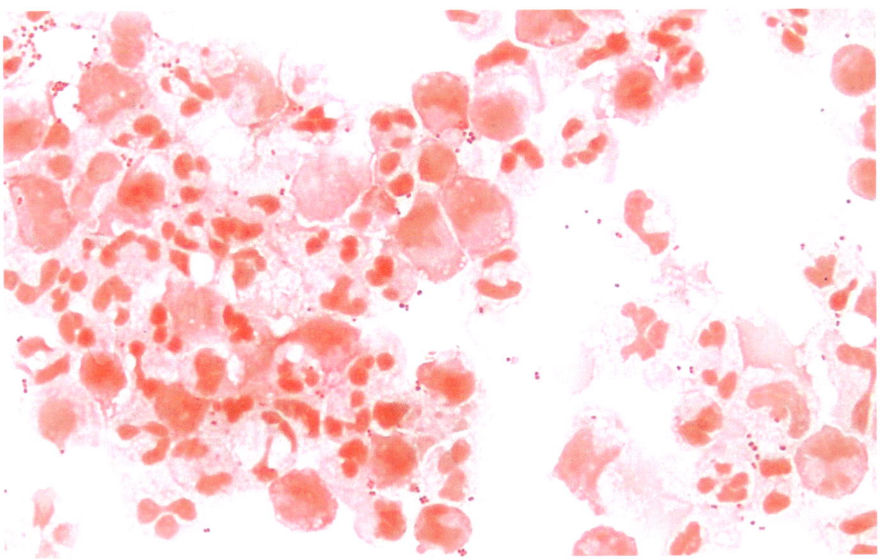

Figure 10.12. *Neisseria meningitidis* in cerebrospinal fluid (CSF) seen by Gram stain at 1000× magnification.

Source: https://upload.wikimedia.org/wikipedia/commons/thumb/e/e6/Neisseria_meningitidis_CSF_Gram_1000.jpg/1024px-Neisseria_meningitidis_CSF_Gram_1000.jpg.

10.3.3. Procedures for Cerebrospinal Fluid (CSF) Collection and Analysis

Collection and analysis of CSF is a critical procedure in microbiological diagnosis of infectious diseases, particularly central nervous system infections. The examination is typically conducted by lumbar puncture, whereby the needle is very slowly introduced into the subarachnoid space in order to aspirate the fluid for analysis. The procedure should be conducted under asepsis to prevent contamination and infection in the patient. Once obtained, CSF is examined with various tests, including cytological examination, biochemistry, and microbiology, to identify potential pathogens and markers of inflammation. Careful handling and transportation of CSF samples are essential, as delays or unsuitable conditions are destructive to sample integrity, eventually undermining diagnostic validity. As a result, adhering to set protocols and guidelines is of utmost importance for effective CSF sample collection followed by examination. After being collected, CSF is analyzed for a series of diagnostic markers that could reflect infections , such as meningitis or encephalitis. Important microscopy techniques, including Gram staining, as well as culture techniques are used to identify whether there is bacteria, fungus, or virus. Polymerase Chain Reaction (PCR) tests have also become an essential tool for quick and proper identification of particular pathogens, particularly in cases where standard cultures take more time to give results. In addition, biochemical tests like glucose and protein estimation provide more evidence regarding the inflammatory status of the meninges. In some contexts, serological examination can complement CSF analysis, especially for immune conditions (Bani et al., 2020). Interpretation of such results hinges on the expertise of the practitioner because correlations between parameters in CSF and clinical presentation symptoms are key to accurate diagnosis. Clinical application of CSF analysis extends beyond its diagnostic utility; treatment planning and patient prognosis assessment are also fundamental parts of it. As an example, a CSF pattern in keeping with bacterial meningitis would usually mandate immediate broad-spectrum antibiotic coverage, while viral infection may sometimes allow more cautious treatment. Furthermore, CSF nuances' understanding aids in differentiating among competing central nervous system infection etiologies, thereby rendering inappropriate therapeutic maneuvers less probable. There have also been the latest studies that have indicated the efficiency of the combination of traditional methods and new diagnostics, i.e., the utilization of urine Xpert and urine-lipoarabinomannan (LAM) tests, to aid the detection of simultaneously occurring systemic infections (Barr et al., 2017). Thus, the labor-intensive procedure of collection and analysis of CSF is the essential part in the entire microbiological assessment of infectious disease.

Test Your Knowledge

1. What is the value of cerebrospinal fluid (CSF) cultures in the diagnosis of central nervous system infections?
2. Which pathogens are most frequently isolated in CSF cultures, and how do they vary with patient age and clinical presentation?
3. What are the proper procedures for safe and effective collection of cerebrospinal fluid for culture analysis?

10.4. Sputum Cultures

Learning Outcome

1. Form an understanding of the role of sputum cultures in respiratory infections;
2. Mention regarding pathogen identification in sputum samples;
3. Summarize factors influencing sputum culture results.

Sputum cultures are a critical diagnostic tool in microbiological diagnosis of respiratory infections, and they provide useful information concerning causative pathogens of pneumonia and other lung diseases. Sputum analysis and collection can provide information on the causative agent's identity, enabling individualized therapy. This type of diagnosis is particularly effective in determining the presence of bacteria , such as Streptococcus pneumoniae, which is associated with community-acquired pneumonia. It has been revealed in the recent research that certain antigen detection methods could be more sensitive than the standard culture practices, especially in patients with past exposure to antibiotics, and incorporation of enrichment steps must be planned as a step towards better diagnostic outcome. The above advancements reflect the requirements to employ effective methodologies subject to patient history and regional prevalence, thus leading to improved clinical outcome for patients with respiratory infection (Lankinen, 2003). Furthermore, application in a clinical environment of sputum cultures promotes overall epidemiological understanding of infectious disease. For example, research into various pathogens, including pneumococci and atypical bacteria, demonstrates the importance of conducting sputum tests in an effort to track spread among such organisms in a population. In Southeast Asia, where severe respiratory infection and sepsis are due to a wide range of pathogens, recognition of particular microbiological patterns will guide health interventions and antibiotic stewardship programs. With the problem of precise diagnosis of pneumonia in resource-constrained environments, standard uniform practices are critical in interpreting sputum culture. Such practices are not only augmenting diagnostic accuracy but also preparedness against public health threats of emerging pathogens, thereby strengthening healthcare systems (Asia et al., 2017). Precision in sputum cultures also relies on technical factors involved in sample collection, processing, and interpretation. Sample acquisition as high-quality samples is crucial because contamination with oral flora will most likely generate false results, hence diagnosis of infection being cumbersome.

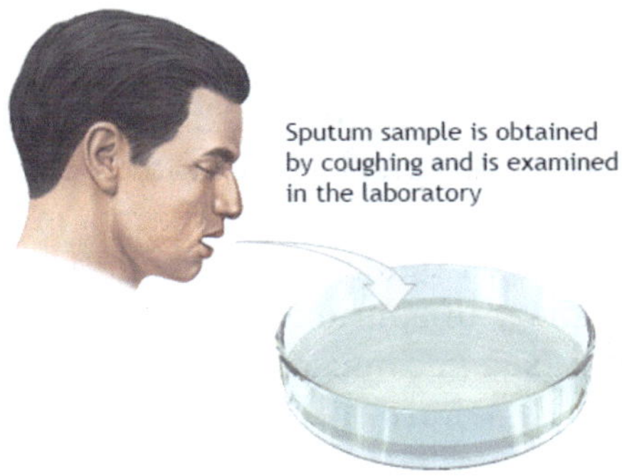

Figure 10.13. Sputum culture illustration.

Source: https://ssl.adam.com/graphics/images/en/9945.jpg.

Therefore, compliance with standardized procedures is very important in an effort to obtain viable results. More sensitive diagnostic tests, such as enzyme immunoassays for the detection of specific antigens, are also becoming adjunct tools to culturing methods, increasing sensitivity and specificity. This complementarity between traditional and newer methods enables treatment plan decision making for health practitioners as it minimizes the risk of misdiagnosis. With advancing diagnostic techniques, the continuous upgrading of sputum culture techniques is required in order for successful management of respiratory infections and total quality patient care (Lankinen, 2003) (Figure 10.13).

10.4.1. Importance of Sputum Cultures in Respiratory Infections

Sputum cultures play a critical role in microbiological diagnosis of respiratory infections, particularly in making decisions on causative agents of infections like pneumonia, chronic bronchitis, and tuberculosis. Sputum sampling and culture allow direct inspection of the bacterial pathogens in the respiratory tract. Isolation and identification of specific microorganisms allow clinicians to adjust antibiotic treatment, a necessity in light of rising trends towards antibiotic resistance. The sensitivity of sputum culture in detecting pathogens, especially with polymicrobial infections or atypical pneumonia, cannot be overstressed. According to research, methods , such as antigen detection are able to enhance the sensitivity of sputum culture, making them justifiably used in clinical settings in many cases, particularly where routine microbiological resources are limited (Lankinen, 2003). Moreover, the utilization of sputum cultures extends to the diagnostic arena; they find use in epidemiological research and public health surveillance as well. Pathogenic organism identification from sputum may be used to demonstrate evidence of trends in respiratory infection within a population to guide the use of specific vaccination and prevention measures. Interestingly, studies have found that the study of sputum is significant for determining the incidence of Streptococcus pneumoniae, a leading cause of community-acquired pneumonia (Lankinen, 2003). With advancement in molecular techniques, the rapidity and efficiency of sputum cultures are on the rise with the potential to make an early diagnosis and initiate early intervention. Therefore, data gathered using sputum cultures not only influence patient treatment but also contribute to public health interventions aimed at controlling respiratory infections. In addition to influencing therapeutic decisions and public health interventions, sputum cultures influence clinical outcomes among patients. Early diagnosis of the etiologic organisms enables clinicians to treat with the most effective antimicrobial agents, possibly reducing complications and hospitalization from respiratory infections. There is mounting evidence to support the opinion that delays in appropriate antibiotic therapy will expand morbidity and mortality rates, particularly in high-risk patients. Sputum cultures also provide for appropriate isolation techniques for infectious patients, an important factor in the avoidance of transmission of highly infectious pathogens, , such as those causing tuberculosis. They are hence a pillar of the entire care of respiratory infections, underlining their intrinsic worth in the overall practice of microbiological diagnosis of infectious diseases (Figure 10.14).

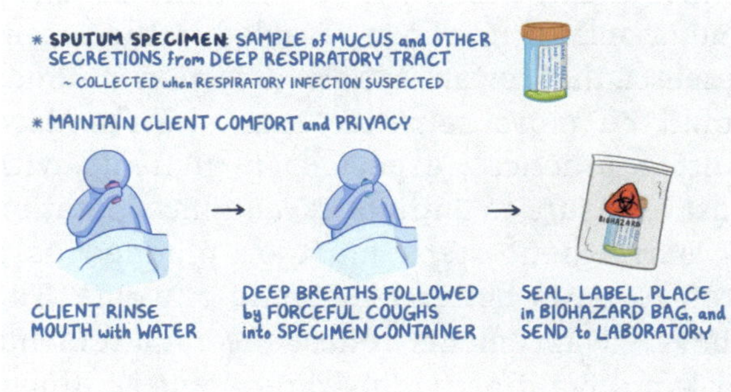

Figure 10.14. Sputum cultures for respiratory infections.

Source: https://www.osmosis.org/_next/image?url=https%3A%2F%2Fd16qt3wv6xm098.cloudfront.net%2F9PtTvA5oRN_0ChsyNEtD3JFwSNmD2EqC%2F_.jpg&w=3840&q=75.

10.4.2. Identification of Pathogens in Sputum Samples

The identification of pathogens from sputum samples is important in the diagnosis of respiratory infections, , such as pneumonia, which remains an emerging health issue worldwide. Traditional methods, , such as culture techniques, have been the mainstays of microbial diagnosis. However, these are frequently wanting since they are not sensitive and specific enough, especially with fastidious organisms or polymicrobial infections. In addition, the correct determination of pathogens has a direct impact on treatment planning, highlighting the importance of having reliable diagnostic tools. Developments in molecular diagnostics are meeting these needs well and allowing clinicians to identify a wider variety of pathogens with greater accuracy. With the addition of new techniques, the process of diagnosis is evolving and therefore it is important that clinicians are aware of the newer techniques that further enhance patient care by way of early and correct identification of microorganisms. Molecular techniques, , such as polymerase chain reaction (PCR), have revolutionized the identification of pathogens from sputum samples. These methods allow for the rapid amplification and detection of specific microbial RNA or DNA to detect a wide range of pathogens, including viruses, bacteria, and fungi. The advantage of these technologies is particularly evident in situations where traditional culture methods are ambiguous because they can detect pathogens with low numbers or those that have unique growth requirements.

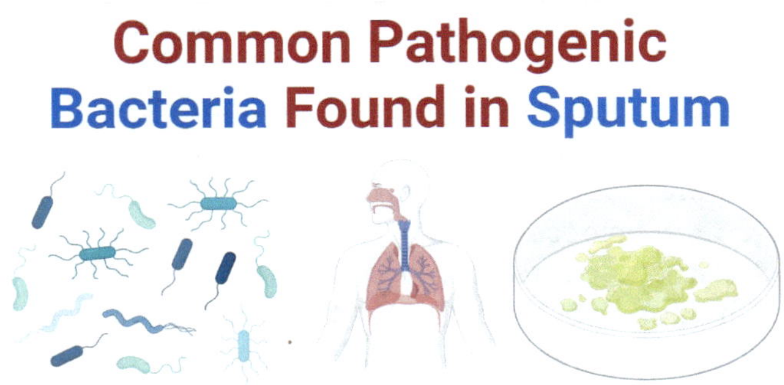

Figure 10.15. Common pathogenic bacteria found in sputum.

Source: https://microbenotes.com/wp-content/uploads/2022/05/Common-Pathogenic-Bacteria-Found-in-Sputum.jpeg.

Furthermore, the utilization of multiplex PCR assays makes it possible to identify multiple pathogens simultaneously, significantly increasing the speed of diagnosis. These developments not just enhance the sensitivity of pathogen detection but also facilitate the earlier initiation of effective antibiotic treatment, which is fundamental towards improved patient outcomes in the case of serious respiratory infections, as seen with the latest study showing the clinical utility of molecular diagnostics in treating pneumonia (Cillóniz et al., 2019). Incorporating technology , such as microarray analysis into sputum diagnosis also enhances the identification process. The Virochip, in turn, is one huge screening platform for various viral pathogens and thus an example of advances. One particular example of detection of human parainfluenzavirus 4 by endotracheal aspirate showed the strength of microarray technology in unveiling pathogens that potentially might not be discovered using normal diagnostic procedures. Infamously, this case not only illustrated the presence of a previously underemphasized pathogen but also showed the far-reaching practice implications—supporting early treatment of patients with life-threatening disease (Blackburn et al., 2006). As our understanding of the lung microbiome evolves, it is increasingly apparent that the microbiological flora is heterogeneous, making it imperative that complicated diagnostic instrumentation be capable of unraveling the web of respiratory infections. This advancement in diagnostic techniques therefore promises a bright future in the effective control of infectious diseases (Figure 10.15).

10.4.3. Factors Affecting Sputum Culture Results

The validity of sputum culture findings is based on a variety of crucial factors, including the quality of the specimen submitted for analysis. Proper collection techniques for the sample are of critical concern; e.g., over-salivation contamination will hide the presence of the pathogens and lead to false-negative results. In addition, the time of collection, ideally early morning when the patient's secretions are most concentrated, can enhance the possibility of recovery of infectious agents. Socioeconomic status and patient groups also enter into this; certain groups will have higher prevalences of specific infections, which will affect which organisms are cultured and identified. Furthermore, chronic medical disease, e.g., immunosuppressive disease, will influence how many and what types of pathogens are present, making diagnosis and treatment regimens more challenging (Thangamathi, 2006). Maximizing sputum culture yields thus needs to be diligent with strict collection protocol. Another important determinant of sputum culture outcomes is sample transportation and processing. Once the sample has been collected, it ought to be transported and processed in such a manner that maintains the viability of the organisms within the sample. Delays in transportation may allow overgrowth of saprophytic flora and compromise the viability of non-desired organisms, particularly in the case of fastidious pathogens. In addition, temperature variations and environmental conditions involved in shipping can affect microbial integrity. Proper culture media and techniques should be employed to isolate and identify pathogens appropriately, as some pathogens require special growth conditions or may take longer to develop. New technologies , such as the GeneXpert assays documented in other microbiological studies indicate that rapid diagnostic tools can enhance the sensitivity of the detection of pathogens in sputum cultures, therefore enhancing patient outcomes (Morabe, 2022). Sputum culture interpretation is also influenced by the reality that antibiotic therapy was administered prior to specimen sampling. Patients who have been treated with antibiotics may have results that are biased due to such treatment being well known to suppress the growth of specific pathogens, thus making them underrepresented in culture results. This underscores the importance of obtaining a good history of the patient regarding past treatments in order to put culture results into their rightful context. Laboratory conditions, including the laboratory staff's proficiency and the methods employed, also contribute towards making sputum culture results reliable. Quality control procedures must be implemented and adhered to routinely because these ensure proper identification and susceptibility testing of the recovered organisms. Generally, the multifactorial variables affecting sputum culture results require an integrative approach in the clinical and laboratory practice to ensure proper diagnosis and treatment of infectious diseases (Thangamathi, 2006).

Test Your Knowledge

1. What is the clinical importance of sputum cultures in respiratory infection diagnosis?
2. What are the most common diseases found by sputum culture, and how does their result affect treatment?

10.5. Serological Tests

Learning Outcome

1. Understand methods of serological testing;
2. Describe infections diagnosed by serological tests;
3. Emphasize the limitations and strengths of serological tests.

Serological tests play a very significant role in the microbiological diagnosis of infectious diseases as they are used to identify specific antibodies or antigens in body fluids, predominantly serum. These tests utilize the immune response's capability of producing antibodies against infectious agents and, therefore, can detect a broad spectrum of infectious agents without the need to culture. A few advantages of serological tests include quick results and the potential to detect hidden infections that could be hard to detect through conventional culture. For instance, serological analysis has been found to be more sensitive in identifying pneumococcal infection, particularly if patients have undergone treatment with antimicrobial agents. The development of enzyme immunoassays against pneumococcal capsular polysaccharide antigens is an illustration of advances in serological methods that have developed a sensitive tool capable of generating useful epidemiological data (Lankinen, 2003). In addition to diagnosing specific pathogens like Streptococcus pneumoniae, serology plays a crucial role in understanding broader infection patterns, particularly in epidemiology. For example, a Southeast Asian study aimed to identify causative pathogens of community-acquired sepsis and significantly implicated the role of various serological markers in treatment and management planning. Particularly interesting, dengue viruses and leptospirosis were prevalent, mimicking the diverse microbial landscape in many areas. By including serological assays in diagnosis, clinicians can guide appropriate antimicrobial therapies, thereby improving clinical outcomes and potentially minimizing mortality from fulminant infections (Lankinen, 2003). This exemplifies the significance of serological assays as a diagnostic and public health intervention. Even though their benefits, serological tests are far from being limitation-free. In certain situations, the results can be masked by cross-reactivity among similar pathogens or similar serotypes and thus give false-positive or false-negative results. Furthermore, the timing of the test is also critical since the concentration of the antibodies is dramatically different based on the stage of infection. As techniques advance, there has to be a consensus on universal procedures for serological testing to enhance the accuracy of results from different labs. Ongoing research and cross-checking must be done in an attempt to maximize serological assays as well as ascertain optimal criteria for a positive outcome, particularly for regions beset by multiple endemic infections. Overcoming all these challenges will make serological tests a major component of microbiological diagnosis of infectious diseases and hence enhance global health programs (Lankinen, 2003) (Figure 10.16).

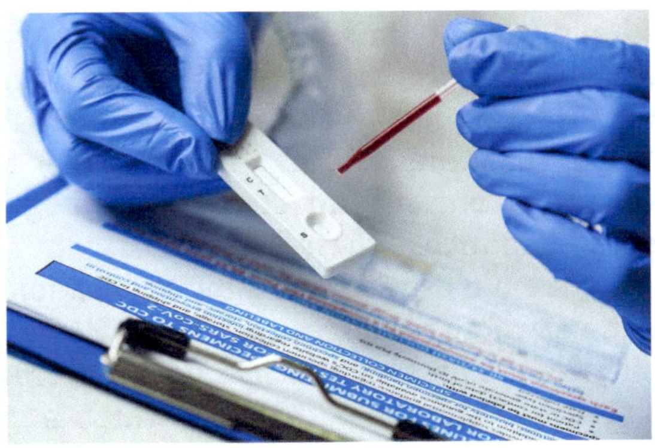

Figure 10.16. Performing a serological test.

Source: https://www.news-medical.net/images/news/ImageForNews_705943_16462272081747550.jpg.

10.5.1. Overview of Serological Testing Methods

Serological testing methods are extremely crucial in the microbiological diagnosis of infectious diseases since they identify the antibody or antigen in various biological samples. These methods are particularly valuable for illnesses where traditional culture techniques might take a long time or be less effective. Serological tests, for instance, can provide immediate diagnostic results for syphilis, HIV, and certain viral infections so that early clinical intervention can be undertaken. The ELISA and western blotting techniques are popular because they are highly sensitive and specific and can accurately identify pathogens. The ability to quantify the immune response to infection is not only of use for diagnosis but also for the design of vaccine strategy and for epidemiological investigations, validating the utility of serology testing to public health practice. The accuracy of serology tests depends largely on their antigen selection, the timing of when the sample is taken, and the underlying characteristics of the tests employed. For instance, the sensitivity of antigen detection methods under various conditions has been assessed, and findings indicated that such methods are, at times, more sensitive than traditional culture, particularly for individuals who have previously received antimicrobial therapy (Lankinen, 2003). Additionally, the presence of enrichment steps in serological assays enhances their sensitivity, hence making them more adaptable for application in situations where resources are limited. However, challenges are present, , such as potential cross-reactivity of similar pathogens, which might complicate its interpretation. Thus, it is essential to keep such resistance of the tests against such parameters in order to use them effectively in diagnosing infectious diseases clinically. Moreover, serological testing methodology can be utilized as an additional tool to support other diagnostic methods by offering a broad platform to control infectious diseases. For example, the combination of serum results with clinical data and other laboratory results, , such as polymerase chain reaction (PCR) testing, can provide a better explanation of the patient's condition. This multi-approach methodology is also necessary in the case of illness like tuberculosis because standard instruments may not be sensitive enough because of sensitivity fluctuations (Dang, 2012). Furthermore, the serological test technology keeps on progressing to ensure newer rapid and point-of-care test forms are being designed, thus enhancing access and efficiency within clinics. Such developments confirm the ongoing applicability of serological techniques in the microbiological diagnostic setting, particularly creating opportunities for enhanced healthcare.

10.5.2. Types of Infections Diagnosed Through Serological Tests

Serological tests constitute a fundamental tool of application in the diagnosis of numerous infections, allowing the identification of pathogens through the demonstration of characteristic antibodies or antigens in the serum of the patient. They have specific application in the diagnosis of viral diseases, , such as hepatitis B and C, where demonstration of viral antigens or anti-HBV and anti-HCV antibodies confirms active infection or exposure. Similarly, serological examinations are crucial to the diagnosis of infections like human immunodeficiency virus (HIV) infection, where early detection and treatment can be made possible. Serological methods are also useful to diagnose autoimmune conditions that may mimic infectious diseases and hence their utility in microbiological diagnostics is critical and varied. With the option for generating quick results, serological tests are a preferred option for acute clinical cases where prompt intervention is of great significance to ensure successful recovery for the patient. Apart from viral pathogens, serology is required for diagnosing bacterial infections, particularly where culture-based systems would be less sensitive or slow. For instance, such infections due to Streptococcus pneumoniae may be diagnosed by identifying specific pneumococcal antigens present in patient fluids , such as urine and nasopharyngeal secretions. It has been found that antigen detection is capable of outcompeting culture techniques in terms of sensitivity, especially among children who have previously been exposed to antibiotics (Lankinen, 2003). Furthermore, serological tests enable simpler diagnosis of illness , such as systemic lupus erythematosus, where the presence of autoantibodies can account for the causative infectious disease. In most cases, the incorporation of serological methods into the diagnostic procedure enables improved accuracy in the detection of bacterial infection, enabling improved treatment planning. Last but not least, serological tests are applicable to parasitic infestations, when usual methods of diagnosis prove inadequate. Malaria, *Leishmania*sis, and typhus fever are all diseases that can be diagnosed accurately with the help of serological testing, particularly in the application of rapid diagnostic tests. For instance, the identification of some antibodies in malaria diagnosis can prove exposure following the resolution of acute symptoms, which benefits epidemiologic investigation and public health initiatives to respond (Thangamathi, 2006). Likewise, use of serologic techniques for the identification of antibodies against leptospires in suspected leptospirosis underscores the utility of this diagnostic tool in endemic nations where the disease is an issue. With continued improvements in serological methods, the ability to detect a large number of infections is on the increase, covering loopholes other laboratory tests may have a tendency to leave.

10.5.3. Limitations and Advantages of Serological Tests

In microbiological diagnosis, serological tests are an important tool in the detection of infectious disease antibodies and antigens. One of the primary advantages of such tests is that they can provide relatively quick results, making it possible for early diagnosis and treatment initiation. For example, where suspected tuberculosis (TB) is a concern, serological tests could be employed to determine individuals who are asymptomatic yet are in the process of seroconverting, making it possible to intervene early to reduce disease transmission. Besides, serological testing is particularly valuable in poor-resource settings where blood culture testing can be less sensitive and specific, adding value to patient care in the highly prevalent areas. As per definition in Dang et al. (2012), simplicity of access to blood tests and affordability further strengthen their place in broadening the diagnosis of infectious diseases. Serological tests do have limitations that demotivate their utilization, however. One major drawback is the potential for false-negative or false-positive tests, which have a great effect on clinical judgment. For instance, serological detection of antibodies will lag behind infection and lead to missed diagnoses with acute illness. Cross-reaction among pathogens also gives false results and further confuses the clinical scenario. In candidemia, a rapidly rising bloodstream pathogen, serological assays may be non-reproducible due to the extensive prevalence of non-albican Candida species that are occasionally indistinguishable from one another through routine tests, as noted in Ali et al. (2015). Such limitations necessitate supplementing serological testing with other microbiological methods to verify outcomes and ensure diagnoses. In summary, while serological testing is extremely useful in the prompt and efficient diagnosis of infectious diseases, its limitations must be addressed meticulously. The validity of such tests is, in reality, paramount, particularly with conditions that must be treated urgently through therapeutic means, , such as TB and candidemia. With advances in medical science, there must be a rationale to integrate new methods and approaches that make serological testing more valid. Better assays with increased sensitivity and application of newer methods, i.e., multiplex serology, will rectify some of the current shortcomings. At the same time, recognition of the need for an integrated diagnostic system making use of both serological tests and culture techniques will ultimately improve clinical control of infectious disease and patient management in different medical environments.

Test Your Knowledge

1. What are the usual techniques used in serological testing for the diagnosis of infections?
2. Which types of infections are most commonly diagnosed or monitored routinely using serological testing?

SUMMARY

Microbiologic diagnosis of infectious diseases, particularly by blood, urine, cerebrospinal fluid (CSF), sputum cultures, and serologic tests, is the backbone of modern medicine. Improvements in the diagnostic techniques, , such as enzyme immunoassay and antigen detection tests, have significantly improved the sensitivity and specificity of identification of various pathogens and thus allowed effective and timely treatments to be offered to the patients. For instance, the development of improved pneumococcal antigen methods has registered promising results, which demonstrate antigen detection to be more sensitive than traditional culture methods, especially in cases where prior antimicrobial treatment has been employed, as demonstrated by findings of (Lankinen, 2003). These technologies demonstrate the potential for rapid pathogen detection and thus an improved response to infectious disease. Further, one should note the existing limitations in microbiological diagnosis. For example, despite monumental improvement in procedures like the Microscopic Observation Drug Susceptibility Assay (MODS) and LED fluorescence microscopy for tuberculosis diagnosis, problems with low sensitivity in detecting drug-resistant strains continue to be very prevalent, as evidenced in the analyzed studies (Dang, 2012). These limitations underscore the necessity for ongoing research and development in both the technology used and the training of manpower in diagnostic processes. Ensuring a very high level of diagnostic precision is critical for efficient management of public health conditions, implying that a combined effort by clinicians, researchers, and public health professionals is necessary to address the present challenges. Bottom line, the pursuit towards the optimization of microbiological diagnosis of infectious disease persists. Emphasizing the necessity of establishing international standards and protocols will facilitate better comparison of diagnostic results across different settings and ensure consistent quality of care. Integration of traditional and new diagnostic methods, backed by robust epidemiological support, will be a critical factor in guiding clinical decisions and optimizing patient outcomes. Given the changing landscape for the diagnosis of infectious diseases, it is necessary to remain committed to developing the available instrumentation and methodologies, as through experience drawn from the incorporation of innovations like have been made in pneumococcal diagnosis and tuberculosis examinations.

Microbiological diagnosis of infections by various biological samples like blood, urine, cerebrospinal fluid (CSF), and sputum forms a significant part of clinical practice. All these samples provide useful information about the etiology of infections and the causative agent responsible. For example, blood culture is crucial for the detection of infections like bacteremia and septicemia, while urine culture is crucial in the diagnosis of urinary tract infections. Sputum cultures are particularly crucial for respiratory infections like tuberculosis and pneumonia, wherein pathogens like *Mycobacterium tuberculosis* can be identified. The sensitivity of such diagnostic tests has a great bearing on patient care, determining the treatment course and outcome and thus highlighting the importance of accurate microbiological methods in clinical microbiology. Serological tests complement culture methods by detecting specific antibodies or antigens within the patient's serum and providing an added dimension to diagnostic capability. They are extremely helpful in cases where standard cultures may be too prolonged or not feasible. For instance, when it comes to opportunistic infections of the immunocompromised host, serological tests can quickly establish the presence of infections like those caused by Candida species or Aspergillus species, where time, most times, is of the essence in the initiation of treatment. The use of serological diagnosis facilitates the improved control of infectious diseases, particularly among cases of fungal infection. This early detection serves to significantly reduce morbidity and mortality rates among vulnerable groups (Akilamani, 2019).

The introduction of newer and more innovative techniques, , such as molecular techniques and quick diagnostic tests, has also revolutionized the microbiological approach to the diagnosis of infectious diseases. These technologies allow for faster and more accurate identification, particularly for difficult-to-culture pathogens or in cases where rapid treatment is indicated. For example, there has been recent evidence to show the utility of new diagnostic tools like the Microscopic Observation Drug Susceptibility Assay (MODS) in the diagnosis of tuberculosis, being more sensitive than traditional approaches (Dang, 2012). Similarly, the increased specificity and sensitivity of newer serological tests for the diagnosis of fungal infections can significantly enhance patient management. Taken together, these methods identify the increasing role of combined diagnostic methods towards the effective management of infectious diseases, ultimately connecting laboratory results and clinical application.

KEY TERMS FROM THIS CHAPTER

- Antifungal peptides
- Blood culture interpretation
- Bloodstream infections
- Causative organism
- Central nervous system
- Clinical scenarios
- CSF culture examination
- Enzyme immunoassays
- Healthcare-associated infections
- Lumbar puncture
- Microbiologic tools
- Biological samples
- Blood cultures
- Body fluids
- Causative organisms
- Cerebrospinal fluid
- Community-acquired pneumonia
- Culture-based methods
- Enzyme-linked immunosorbent assays
- Immunoassays
- Lung microbiome
- Microbiological diagnosis

CRITICAL THINKING QUESTIONS

1. **Which of the following is the MOST important factor in having a successful blood culture result?**
   a. Timing of the blood draw
   b. Amount of blood drawn
   c. Type of culture bottle
   d. Patient's diet before sample collection
2. **Which of the following causes a midstream urine culture is MOST characteristic of a urinary tract infection (UTI)?**
   a. $<10^3$ CFU/mL of mixed flora
   b. Epithelial cells
   c. $>10^5$ CFU/mL of a single bacterial species
   d. Negative leukocyte esterase test
3. **In cerebrospinal fluid (CSF) cultures, which of the following results is MOST suggestive of bacterial meningitis?**
   a. High glucose, low protein, lymphocytic pleocytosis
   b. Low glucose, high protein, neutrophilic pleocytosis
   c. Normal glucose and protein, eosinophilic pleocytosis
   d. High glucose, low protein, monocytic pleocytosis
4. **A sputum specimen properly obtained for culture should contain:**
   a. Predominantly squamous epithelial cells
   b. No leukocytes
   c. Predominantly alveolar macrophages and neutrophils
   d. Clear appearance with minimal mucus
5. **Serology is MOST useful in the diagnosis of infections when:**
   a. The pathogen can easily be cultured on routine media
   b. Treatment with antibiotics is not urgently needed
   c. The infection is limited and not systemic
   d. The organism cannot be cultured or grows slowly

Short Answer Questions

1. At what time and in what manner should a blood culture be taken from a patient with suspected septicemia, and why is timing so important?
2. How does one distinguish between a contaminated urine specimen and an actual urinary tract infection (UTI) based on colony count and organisms recovered?
3. When doing a lumbar puncture to diagnose meningitis, what are the key microbiological tests performed on the CSF, and what does each test detect?

4. Why is coagulase-negative staphylococci isolated from a single blood culture bottle important, and what would be the meaning of the result?
5. What is the most common cause of community-acquired UTIs, and how is it typically identified in urine culture?
6. How do IgM and IgG antibodies differ in diagnostic usefulness for acute vs. remote infections in serology?
7. Why is it imperative to process and incubate CSF specimens at the time of collection, and which organisms are most sensitive to delay in processing?

Answer to Critical Thinking Questions

1. (b); 2. (c); 3. (b); 4. (c); 5. (d)

REFERENCES

1. Beig, F. K., Malik, A., Rizvi, M., Acharya, D., & Khare, S. (2010). Etiology and clinico-epidemiological profile of acute viral encephalitis in children of western Uttar Pradesh, India. *International journal of infectious diseases : IJID : official publication of the International Society for Infectious Diseases, 14*(2), e141–e146. https://doi.org/10.1016/j.ijid.2009.03.035 (accessed on 13th June 2025).

2. Akilamani, M. (2019). A study on the pattern of fungal infections and clinical profile in immunocompromised patients with special reference to characterization and molecular study of *Candida* species in a tertiary care hospital. https://core.ac.uk/download/235670744.pdf (accessed on 13th June 2025).

3. Ali, F., Awan, S., Khanum, I., Mahmood, R., et al. (2015). Clinical characteristics and risk factors of candidemia in tertiary care hospital. https://core.ac.uk/download/132194744.pdf (accessed on 13th June 2025).

4. Bani, F., Battegay, M., Gingo, W., Hella, J., et al. (2020). Ultrasound in managing extrapulmonary tuberculosis: A randomized controlled two-center study. https://core.ac.uk/download/335373586.pdf (accessed on 13th June 2025).

5. Baron, E. J., Bourbeau, P., Carroll, K. C., Chapin, K., et al. (2013). A guide to utilization of the microbiology laboratory for diagnosis of infectious diseases: 2013 recommendations by the Infectious Diseases Society of America (IDSA) and the American Society for Microbiology (ASM). https://core.ac.uk/download/345206010.pdf (accessed on 13th June 2025).

6. Barr, D. A., Burton, R., Kerkhoff, A. D., Lawn, S. D., et al. (2017). Disseminated tuberculosis among hospitalized HIV patients in South Africa: A common condition that can be rapidly diagnosed using urine-based assays. https://core.ac.uk/download/96628002.pdf (accessed on 13th June 2025).

7. Blackburn, B. G., Chiu, C. Y., DeRisi, J. L., Eckburg, P. B., et al. (2006). Microarray detection of human parainfluenza virus 4 infections associated with respiratory failure in an immunocompetent adult. https://core.ac.uk/download/323072700.pdf (accessed on 13th June 2025).

8. Calandra, T., Mikulska, M., Poulain, D., Sanguinetti, M., Viscoli, C., & Third European Conference on Infections in Leukemia Group. (2010). The use of mannan antigen and anti-mannan antibodies in the diagnosis of invasive candidiasis: Recommendations from the Third European Conference on Infections in Leukemia. https://core.ac.uk/download/pdf/8646118.pdf (accessed on 13th June 2025).

9. Carvalho, A. C. C., Matin, N., Mello, F. C. D. Q., Pontali, E., et al. (2017). The cursed duet today: Tuberculosis and HIV-coinfection. https://core.ac.uk/download/158171520.pdf (accessed on 13th June 2025).

10. Chan, L., Ibrahim, N. A., Mat Nor, M. B., Tai, S. T., et al. (2017). Guide to antimicrobial therapy 2017. https://core.ac.uk/download/300453506.pdf (accessed on 13th June 2025).

11. Chen, J., Chen, Y., He, Q., Jalan, R., et al. (2022). Rapid pathogen detection for infected ascites in cirrhosis using metagenome next-generation sequencing: A case series. https://core.ac.uk/download/480394280.pdf (accessed on 13th June 2025).

12. Cillóniz, C., Lee, N., Torres Martí, A., Van der Eerden, M., et al. (2019). Laboratory diagnosis of pneumonia in the molecular age. https://core.ac.uk/download/237483570.pdf (accessed on 13th June 2025).

13. Dang, Thi Minh Ha (2012). *Diagnosis of tuberculosis in a high burden resource limited setting.* PhD thesis The Open University.

14. Diederen, B. M. W. (2007). New approaches to the laboratory diagnosis of Legionnaires' disease. https://core.ac.uk/download/pdf/15452626.pdf (accessed on 13th June 2025).

15. Edelstein, P. H., Jørgensen, C. S., & Wolf, L. A. (2020). Performance of the ImmuView and BinaxNOW assays for the detection of urine and cerebrospinal fluid *Streptococcus pneumoniae* and *Legionella pneumophila* serogroup 1 antigen in patients with Legionnaires' disease or pneumococcal pneumonia and meningitis. https://core.ac.uk/download/328720978.pdf (accessed on 13th June 2025).

16. Jacobson, M. (2003). *Enteric Diseases in Pigs from Weaning to Slaughter*. https://core.ac.uk/download/11694636.pdf (accessed on 13th June 2025).

17. Lankinen, K. S. (2003). *Catching the Pneumococcus: Studies Focusing on Carriage, Epidemiology and Microbiological Methods.* http://urn.fi/urn:isbn:9514270630(accessed on 13th June 2025).

18. Morabe, N. G. (2022). *Validation of GeneXpert Machine Using Extrapulmonary Samples at National Tuberculosis Referral Laboratory in Lesotho*. https://core.ac.uk/download/616422470.pdf (accessed on 13th June 2025).

19. Thangamathi, G. (2006). *Etiological Profile of Infectious Fever–Bacterial and Parasitical*. https://core.ac.uk/download/235655444.pdf (accessed on 13th June 2025).

20. Zhang, W., Zhang, X., & Zhao, Y. (2024). Application of metagenomic next-generation sequencing in the diagnosis of infectious diseases. https://core.ac.uk/download/635409553.pdf (accessed on 13th June 2025).

INDEX

Q

R

S

T

U

V

W

Z